THOMSON DELMAR LEARNING'S
NURSING REVIEW SERIES

Pediatric
Nursing

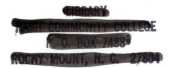

THOMSON DELMAR LEARNING'S NURSING REVIEW SERIES

Pediatric Nursing

Content taken from:
NCLEX-RN® Review

By:
Alice M. Stein EdD, RN
Retired
Senior Associate Dean for Student and Business Affairs
Drexel University
College of Nursing and Health Professions
Philadelphia, Pennsylvania

THOMSON
DELMAR LEARNING ™   Australia   Canada   Mexico   Singapore   Spain   United Kingdom   United States

THOMSON

★

^{TM}

DELMAR LEARNING

Nursing Review Series: Pediatric Nursing

by Alice M. Stein

Vice President, Health Care Business Unit:
William Brottmiller

Director of Learning Solutions:
Matthew Kane

Acquisitions Editor:
Tamara Caruso

Product Manager:
Patricia Gaworecki

Editorial Assistant:
Jenn Waters

Marketing Director:
Jennifer McAvey

Marketing Channel Manager:
Michele McTighe

Marketing Coordinator:
Danielle Pacella

Technology Director:
Laurie Davis

Technology Project Manager:
Mary Colleen Liburdi
Patricia Allen

Production Director:
Carolyn Miller

Production Manager:
Barbara Bullock

Art Director:
Robert Plante
Jack Pendleton

Content Project Manager:
Dave Buddle
Stacey Lamodi
Jessica McNavich

Production Coordinator:
Mary Ellen Cox

Library of Congress Cataloging-in-Publication Data
ISBN 10:1-4018-1177-9
ISBN 13:978-1-4018-1177-8

Notice to the Reader

Contents

Contributors

Margaret Ahearn-Spera, RN, C, MSN
Director, Medical Patient Care Services
Danbury Hospital
Danbury, Connecticut
Assistant Clinical Professor
Yale University School of Nursing
New Haven, Connecticut

Mary Mescher Benbenek, RN, MS, CPNP, CFNP
Teaching Specialist
School of Nursing
University of Minnesota
Twin Cities, Minnesota

Cynthia Blank-Reid, RN, MSN, CEN
Trauma Clinical Nurse Specialist
Temple University Hospital
Philadelphia, Pennsylvania
Clinical Adjunct Associate Professor
Drexel University College of Nursing and
    Health Professions
Philadelphia, Pennsylvania

Elizabeth Blunt, PhD (c), MSN
Assistant Professor and Director,
    Graduate Nursing Programs
Drexel University College of Nursing and
    Health Professions
Philadelphia, Pennsylvania

Margaret Brenner, RN, MSN
Senior Consultant, Pinnacle Healthcare
    Group, Inc.
Paoli, Pennsylvania

Margaret Brogan, RN, BSN
Registered Nurse/Expert
Children's Memorial Hospital
Chicago, Illinois

Mary Lynn Burnett, RN, PhD
Assistant Professor of Nursing
Wichita State University
Wichita, Kansas

Corine K. Carlson, RN, MS
Assistant Professor
Department of Nursing
Luther College
Decorah, Iowa

Nancy Clarkson, MEd, RN, BC
Professor and Chairperson
Department of Nursing
Finger Lakes Community College
Canandaigua, New York

Nancy Clarkson, RN, C, MEd
Associate Professor of Nursing
Finger Lakes Community College
Canandaigua, New York

Gretchen Reising Cornell, RN, PhD, CNE
Professor of Nursing
Utah Valley State College
Orem, Utah

Vera V. Cull, RN, DSN
Former Assistant Professor of Nursing
University of Alabama
Birmingham, Alabama

Deborah L. Dalrymple, RN, MSN, CRNI
Associate Professor of Nursing
Montgomery County Community College
Blue Bell, Pennsylvania

Laura DeHelian, RN, PhD, APRN, BC
Former Assistant Professor of Nursing
Cleveland State University
Cleveland, Ohio

Della J. Derscheid, RN, MS, CNS
Assistant Professor
Department of Nursing
Mayo Clinic
Mayo Clinic College of Nursing
Rochester, Minnesota

Judy Donlen, RN, DNSc
Executive Director, Southern New Jersey
Perinatal Cooperative
Pennsauken, New Jersey

Judith L. Draper, APRN, BC
Assistant Professor
Drexel University College of Nursing and
    Health Professions
Philadelphia, Pennsylvania

Theresa M. Fay-Hillier, MSN, RN, CS
Adjunct Faculty
Drexel University College of Nursing and
    Health Professions
Philadelphia, Pennsylvania

Marcia R. Gardner, MA, RN, CPNP, CPN
Assistant Professor
Drexel University College of Nursing and
    Health Professions
Philadelphia, Pennsylvania

Ann Garey, MSN, APRN, BC, FNP
Carle Foundation Hospital
Urbana, Illinois

Jeanne Gelman, RN, MA, MSN
Professor Emeritus, Psychiatric-Mental
    Health Nursing
Widener University
Chester, Pennsylvania

Theresa M. Giglio, RD, MS
Instructor, LaSalle University
Philadelphia, Pennsylvania

Beth Good, RN, MSN, BSN
Teaching Specialist
University of Minnesota
Minneapolis, Minnesota

Samantha Grover, RN, BSN, CNS
Psychiatric Mental Health Clinical
    Specialist
MeritCare Health System
Moorhead, Minnesota

Judith M. Hall, RNC, MSN, IBCLC, LCCE
Lactation Consultant and Childbirth
    Educator
Mary Washington Hospital
Fredericksburg, Virginia

**Judith M. Hall, RNC, MSN, IBCLC,
LCCE, FACCE**
Mary Washington Hospital
Fredericksburg, Virginia

**Jeanne M. Harkness, RN, BA, MSN,
BSN, AOCN**
Clinical Practice Specialist
Jane Brattain Breast Center
Park Nicollet Clinic
St. Louis Park, Minnesota

Marilyn Herbert-Ashton, RN, C, MS
Director, Wellness Center
F. F. Thompson Health Systems, Inc.
Adjunct Professor of Nursing
Finger Lakes Community College
Canandaigua, New York

Marilyn Herbert-Ashton, MS, RN, BC
Virginia Western Community College
Roanoke, VA

Holly Hillman, RN, MSN
Assistant Professor
Montgomery County Community College
Blue Bell, Pennsylvania

Lorraine C. Igo, RN, MSN, EdD
Assistant Professor
Drexel University College of Nursing and
    Health Professions
Philadelphia, Pennsylvania

Linda Irle, RN, MSN, APN, CNP
Coordinator, Maternal-Child Nursing
University of Illinois
Urbana, Illinois
Family Nurse Practitioner, Acute Care,
Carle Clinic,
Champaign, Illinois

Amy Jacobson, RN, BA
Staff Nurse
United Hospital
St. Paul, Minnesota

Nancy H. Jacobson, MSN, APRN-BC, CS
Staff Development Coordinator
Rydal Park
Rydal, Pennsylvania

Nancy H. Jacobson, RN, CS, MSN
Senior Manager
The Whitman Group
Huntington Valley, Pennsylvania

Nadine James, RN, PhD
Assistant Professor of Nursing
University of Southern Mississippi
Hattiesburg, Mississippi

Lisa Jensen, CS, MS, APRN
Salt Lake City VA Healthcare System
Salt Lake City, Utah

Ellen Joswiak, RN, MA
Assistant Professor of Nursing
Staff Nurse
Mayo Medical Center
Rochester, Minnesota

Charlotte D. Kain, RN, C, EdD
Professor Nursing, Health Care of Women
Montgomery County Community College
Blue Bell, Pennsylvania

Roseann Tirotta Kaplan, MSN, RN, CS
Adjunct Faculty
Drexel University College of Nursing and
    Health Professions
Philadelphia, Pennsylvania

**Betsy Ann Skrha Kennedy, RN, MS,
CS, LCCE**
Nursing Instructor
Rochester Community and Technical
    College
Rochester, Minnesota

**Robin M. Lally, PhD, RN, BA, AOCN,
CNS**
Teaching Specialist; Office 6-155
School of Nursing
University of Minnesota
Twin Cities, Minnesota

Penny Leake, RN, PhD
Luther College
Decorah, Iowa

Barbara Mandleco, RN, PhD
Associate Professor & Undergraduate
    Program Coordinator
College of Nursing
Brigham Young University
Provo, Utah

Mary Lou Manning, RN, PhD, CPNP
Director, Infection Control and
    Occupational Health
The Children's Hospital of Philadelphia
Adjunct Assistant Professor
University of Pennsylvania School of
    Nursing
Philadelphia, Pennsylvania

Gerry Matsumura, RN, PhD, MSN, BSN
Former Associate Professor of Nursing
Brigham Young University
Provo, Utah

Alberta McCaleb, RN, DSN
Associate Professor
Chair, Undergraduate Studies
University of Alabama School of Nursing
University of Alabama at Birmingham
Birmingham, Alabama

Judith C. Miller, RN, MSN
President, Nursing Tutorial and
    Consulting Services
Clifton, Virginia

Eileen Moran, RN, C, MSN
Clinical Educator
Abington Memorial Hospital
Abington, Pennsylvania

JoAnn Mulready-Shick, RN, MS
Dean, Nursing and Allied Health
Roxbury Community College
Boston, Massachusetts

Patricia Murdoch, RN, MS
Nurse Practitioner
University of Illinois, Chicago
Urbana, Illinois

Jayme S. Nelson, RN, MS, ARNP-C
Adult Nurse Practitioner
Assistant Professor of Nursing
Luther College
Decorah, Iowa

Janice Nuuhiwa, MSN, CPON, APN/CNS
Staff Development Specialist
Hematology/Oncology/Stem Cell
   Transplant Division
Children's Memorial Hospital
Chicago, Illinois

Kristen L. Osborn, MSN, CRNP
Pediatric Nurse Specialist
UAB School of Nursing
UAB Pediatric Hematology/Oncology
Birmingham, Alabama

Marie O'Toole, RN, EdD
Associate Professor, College of Nursing
Rutgers, The State University of New Jersey
Newark, New Jersey

Faye A. Pearlman, RN, MSN, MBA
Assistant Professor
Drexel University College of Nursing and
   Health Professions
Philadelphia, Pennsylvania

Karen D. Peterson, RN, MSN, BSN, PNP
Pediatric Nurse Practitioner
Division of Endocrinology
Children's Memorial Hospital
Chicago, Illinois

Kristin Sandau, RN, PhD
Bethel University's Department of
   Nursing
United's John Nasseff Heart Hospital
Minneapolis, Minnesota

Elizabeth Sawyer, RN, BSN, CCRN
Registered Nurse
United Hospital
St. Paul, Minnesota

Lisa A. Seldomridge, RN, PhD
Associate Professor of Nursing
Salisbury University
Salisbury, Maryland

Janice Selekman, RN, DNSc
Professor and Chair
Department of Nursing
University of Delaware
Newark, Delaware

Robert Shearer, CRNA, MSN
Assistant Professor
Drexel University College of Nursing and
   Health Professions
Philadelphia, Pennsylvania

Constance O. Kolva Taylor, RN, MSN
Kolva Consulting
Harrisburg, Pennsylvania

Magdeleine Vasso, MSN, RN
Assistant Professor
Drexel University College of Nursing and
   Health Professions
Philadelphia, Pennsylvania

Janice L. Vincent, RN, DSN
University of Alabama School of Nursing
University of Alabama at Birmingham
Birmingham, Alabama

Margaret Vogel, RN, MSN, BSN
Nursing Instructor
Rochester Community & Technical
   College
Rochester, Minnesota

Anne Robin Waldman, RN, C, MSN, AOCN
Clinical Nurse Specialist
Albert Einstein Medical Center
Philadelphia, Pennsylvania

Mary Shannon Ward, RN, MSN
Children's Memorial Hospital
Chicago, Illinois

Virginia R. Wilson, RN, MSN, CEN
Assistant Professor, Graduate Nursing
   Programs
Drexel University College of Nursing and
   Health Professions
Philadelphia, Pennsylvania

Preface

Congratulations on discovering the best new review series for the NCLEX-RN®! Thomson Delmar Learning's Nursing Review Series is designed to maximize your study in the core subject areas covered on the NCLEX-RN® examination. The series consists of 8 books:

Pharmacology

Medical-Surgical Nursing

Pediatric Nursing

Maternity and Women's Health Nursing

Gerontologic Nursing

Psychiatric Nursing

Legal and Ethical Nursing

Community Health Nursing

Each text has been developed expressly to meet your needs as you study and prepare for the all-important licensure examination. Taking this exam is a stressful event and constitutes a major career milestone. Passing the NCLEX is the key to your future ability to practice as a registered nurse.

Each text in the series is designed around the most current test plan for the NCLEX-RN® and provides a focused and complete content review in each subject area. Additionally, there are up to 400 review questions in each text: questions at the end of most every chapter and three 100 question review tests that support the chapter content. Each set of review questions is followed by answers and rationales for both the right and wrong answers. There is also a free PDA download of review questions available with the purchase of any of these review texts! It is this combination of content review and self assessment that provides a powerful learning experience for you as you prepare for you examination.

ORGANIZATION

Thomson Delmar Learning's unique Pharmacology review book provides you with an intensive review in this all important subject area. Drugs are grouped by classification and similarities to aid you in consolidating this pertinent but sometimes overwhelming information. Included in this text are:

- A section on herbal medicines, now being tested on the exam.
- Case studies that apply relevant drug content
- Prototypes for most drug classifications
- Mechanism of drug action
- Uses and adverse effects
- Nursing implications and discharge teaching
- Related drugs and their variance from the prototype

The review texts for Medical-Surgical Nursing, Pediatric Nursing, Maternity Nursing, Gerontological Nursing and Psychiatric Nursing follow a systematic approach that includes:

- The nursing process integrated with a body systems approach
- Introductory review of normal anatomy and physiology as well as basic theories and principles
- Review of pertinent disorders for each system including: general characteristics, pathophysiology/psychopathology
- Medical management
- Assessment data
- Nursing interventions and client education

Community Health Nursing and Legal and Ethical Nursing are unique review texts in the marketplace. They include aspects of community health nursing and legal/ethical subject matter that is covered on the NCLEX-RN® exam. Community Health topics covered are: case management, long-term care, home health care and hospice. Legal and ethical topics include: cultural diversity, leadership and management, ethical issues and legal issues for older adults.

FEATURES

All questions in each text in the series are compliant with the most current test plan from the National Council of State Boards of Nursing (NCSBN). All questions are followed by answers and rationales for both right and wrong choices. Included are many of the alternative format questions first introduced to the exam in 2003. An icon identifies these alternate types ⊙. The questions in each of these texts are written primarily at the application or analysis cognitive levels allowing you to further enhance critical thinking skills which are heavily weighted on the NCLEX.

In addition, with the purchase of any of these texts, a free PDA download is available to you. It provides you with up to an additional 225 questions with which you can practice your test taking skills.

Thomson Delmar Learning is committed to help you reach your fullest professional potential. Good luck on the NCLEX-RN® examination!

To access your free PDA download for Thomson Delmar Learning's Nursing Review Series visit the online companion resource at **www.delmarhealthcare.com** Click on Online Companions then select the Nursing discipline.

Reviewers

Judy Bourrand, RN, MSN
Ida V. Moffett School of Nursing
Samford University
Birmingham, Alabama

Mary Kathie Doyle, BS, CCRN,
Instructor
Maria College
Troy, New York

Mary Lashley, PhD, RN, CS
Associate Professor
Towson University
Towson, Maryland

Melissa Lickteig, EdD, RN
Instructor, School of Nursing
Georgia Southern University
Statesboro, Georgia

Darlene Mathis, MSN, RN APRN, BC,
NP-C, CRNP
Assistant Professor
Ida V. Moffett School of Nursing
Samford University
Birmingham, Alabama

Barbara McGraw, MSN, RN
Instructor
Central Community College
Grand Island, Nebraska

Carol Meadows, MNSc, RNP, APN
Eleanor Mann School of Nursing
University of Arkansas
Fayetteville, Arkansas

Maria Smith, DSN, RN, CCRN
Professor, School of Nursing
Middle Tennessee State University
Murfreesboro, Tennessee

Growth and Development

■ GENERAL PRINCIPLES

Definition of Terms

A. *Growth:* increase in size of a structure. Human growth is orderly and predictable, but not even; it follows a cyclical pattern.

B. *Development:* increased complexity in thought, behavior, skill, or function. Development includes growth and is a process that continues over time.

C. *Maturation:* physiologically determined pattern for growth and development.

D. *Cephalocaudal:* head-to-toe progression of growth and development.

E. *Proximodistal:* trunk-to-periphery (fingers and toes) progression of growth and development.

F. *Phylogeny:* development or evolution of a species or group; a pattern of development for a species.

G. *Ontogeny:* development of an individual within a species.

H. *Critical period:* specific time period during which certain environmental events or stimuli have greatest effect on a child's development.

I. *Developmental task:* skill or competency unique to a stage of development.

Rates of Development

Growth and development are not synonymous but are closely interrelated processes directed by both genetic and environmental factors. Although changes in growth and development are more obvious in some periods than others, they are important in all periods.

A. Infancy and adolescence: fast growth periods

B. Toddler through school-age: slow growth periods

C. Fetal period and infancy: the head and neurologic tissue grow faster than other tissues.

D. Toddler and preschool periods: the trunk grows more rapidly than other tissue.

E. The limbs grow most during school-age period.

F. The trunk grows faster than other tissue during adolescence.

Child Development Theorists

Sigmund Freud (Psychosexual Theory)

A. 0-6 months: oral passive (development of id; biologic pleasure principle)

B. 7-18 months: oral aggressive (teething); oral satisfaction of needs by mother decreases tension

C. 1½-3 years: anal (toilet training); projection of feelings onto others; elimination and retention as ways to control and inhibit

D. 3-6 years: phallic (love of opposite sex, parent-Oedipal complex); ego development; objective conscious reality

E. 6-12 years: latent; sexual drive repressed; socialization occurs; superego and morality development

Erik Erikson (Psychosocial Theory)

Core stages/psychosocial tasks or crises

A. Birth-1 year: trust vs mistrust

B. 1-3 years: autonomy vs shame and doubt

C. 3-6 years: initiative vs guilt

D. 6-12 years: industry vs inferiority

E. 12-18 years: identity vs role confusion

F. Young adult: intimacy vs isolation

G. Adult: generativity vs stagnation

H. Elderly: ego integrity vs despair

Jean Piaget (Cognitive Theory)

Development of thought

A. 0-2 years: sensorimotor (reflexes, repetition of acts)

B. 2-4 years: preoperational (preconceptual); no cause and effect reasoning; egocentrism; use of symbols; magical thinking

C. 4-7 years: intuitive/preoperational (beginning of causation)

D. 7-11 years: concrete operations

E. 11-15 years: formal operations (reality, abstract thought)

■ ASSESSMENT
Developmental Tasks

Developmental tasks are skills or competencies normally occurring at one stage and having an effect on the development of subsequent stages; fall into three categories

A. Physical tasks (e.g., learning to sit, crawl, walk; toileting)

B. Psychologic tasks (e.g., learning trust, self-esteem)

C. Cognitive tasks (e.g., acquiring concepts of time and space, abstract thought)

Measurement Tools

There are a number of different assessment tools for measuring the progress of growth and development.

A. Chronologic age: assessment of developmental tasks related to birth date

B. Mental age: assessment of cognitive development
  1. Measured by variety of standardized intelligence tests (IQ)
  2. Results from at least two separate testing sessions needed before determination of cognitive level is made
  3. Uses toys and language based on mental rather than chronologic age

C. *Denver Developmental Screening Test (DDST)*
  1. Generalized assessment tool; measures gross motor, fine motor, language, and personal-social development from newborn–6 years
  2. Does not measure intelligence

D. Growth parameters
  1. Bone age: X-ray of tarsals and carpals determines degree of ossification
  2. Growth charts: norms are expressed as percentile of height, weight, head circumference, and body mass index (BMI) for age; any child who crosses over multiple percentile lines or is above the 95th or below the 5th percentile needs further evaluation.

E. Correction for prematurity
  1. Subtract time premature from chronological age
  2. Use corrected age for developmental assessment until age 2

Developmental Stages

Infant (Birth through 12 months)

A. Physical tasks
  1. *Neonate (Birth to 1 month)*
    a. Weight: 6–8 lb (2750–3629 g); gains 5–7 oz (142–198 g) weekly for first 6 months
    b. Length: 20 inches (50 cm); grows 1 inch (2.5 cm) monthly for first 6 months
    c. Head growth
      1) head circumference 33–35.5 cm (13–14 inches)
      2) head circumference slightly larger than chest
      3) increases by ½ inch (1.25 cm) monthly for first 6 months
      4) brain growth related to myelinization of nerve fibers; increase in size of brain reflects this process, reaches ⅔ adult size at 1 year; 90% adult size at 2 years
      5) weak neck muscles result in poor head control
    d. Vital signs
      1) pulse: 110–160 and irregular; count for a full minute apically
      2) respirations: 32–60 and irregular; count for full minute; neonates are abdominal breathers and obligate nose breathers
      3) blood pressure: 75/49 mmHg

        4) poor development of sweating and shivering mechanisms; impaired temperature control
- **e.** Motor development
  - **1)** behavior is reflex controlled
  - **2)** flexed extremities
  - **3)** can lift head slightly off bed when prone
- **f.** Sensory development
  - **1)** hearing and touch well developed at birth
  - **2)** sight not fully developed until 6 years
    - **a)** differentiates light and dark at birth
    - **b)** rapidly develops clarity of vision within 1 foot
    - **c)** fixates on moving objects
    - **d)** strabismus due to lack of binocular vision

2. *1-4 months*
- **a.** Head growth: posterior fontanel closes
- **b.** Motor development
  - **1)** reflexes begin to fade (e.g., Moro, tonic neck)
  - **2)** gains head control; balances head in sitting position
  - **3)** rolls from back to side
  - **4)** begins voluntary hand-to-mouth activity
- **c.** Sensory development
  - **1)** begins to be able to coordinate stimuli from various sense organs
  - **2)** hearing: locates sounds by turning head and visually searching
  - **3)** vision
    - **a)** binocular vision developing; less strabismus
    - **b)** beginning hand-eye coordination
    - **c)** prefers human face
    - **d)** follows objects 180°
    - **e)** ability to accommodate is equal to adult

3. *5-6 months*
- **a.** Weight: birth weight doubles; gains 3-5 oz (84-140 g) weekly for next 6 months
- **b.** Length: gains ½ inch (1.25 cm) for next 6 months
- **c.** Eruption of teeth begins
  - **1)** lower incisors first
  - **2)** causes increased saliva and drooling
  - **3)** enzyme released with teething causes mild diarrhea, facial skin irritation
  - **4)** slight fever may be associated with teething, but not a high fever or seizures
- **d.** Motor development
  - **1)** intentional rolling over
  - **2)** supports weight on arms
  - **3)** creeping; pushes backward with hands
  - **4)** can grasp and let go voluntarily

              5) transfers toys from one hand to another
              6) sits with support
        e. Sensory development
              1) hearing: can localize sounds above and below ear
              2) vision: smiles at own mirror image and responds to facial expressions of others
              3) taste: sucking needs have decreased and cup weaning can begin; chewing, biting, and taste preferences begin to develop

4. *7–9 months*
        a. Teething continues
              1) 7 months: upper central incisors
              2) 9 months: upper lateral incisors
        b. Motor development
              1) sits unsupported; goes from prone to sitting upright
              2) crawls; may go backwards initially
              3) pulls self to standing position
              4) develops finger-thumb opposition (pincer grasp)
              5) preference for dominant hand evident
        c. Sensory development: vision
              1) can fixate on small objects
              2) beginning to develop depth perception

5. *10–12 months*
        a. Weight: birth weight tripled
        b. Length: 50% increase over birth length
        c. Head and chest circumference equal
        d. Teething
              1) lower lateral incisors erupt
              2) average of eight deciduous teeth
        e. Motor development
              1) creeps with abdomen off floor
              2) walks with help or cruises
              3) may attempt to stand alone
              4) can sit down from upright position
              5) weans from bottle to cup
        f. Sensory development: vision
              1) able to discriminate simple geometric forms
              2) able to follow rapidly moving objects
              3) visual acuity 20/50 or better
              4) binocularity well established; if not, amblyopia may develop

B. Psychosocial tasks
    1. *Neonatal period*
        a. Cries to express displeasure
        b. Smiles indiscriminately
        c. Receives gratification through sucking
        d. Makes throaty sounds

      2. *1-4 months*
- **a.** Crying becomes differentiated at 1 month
  - **1)** decreases during awake periods
  - **2)** ceases when parent in view
- **b.** Vocalization distinct from crying at 1 month
  - **1)** squeals to show pleasure at 3 months
  - **2)** coos, babbles, laughs; vocalizes when smiling
- **c.** Socialization
  - **1)** stares at parents' faces when talking at 1 month
  - **2)** smiles socially at 2 months
  - **3)** shows excitement when happy at 4 months
  - **4)** demands attention, enjoys social interaction with people at 4 months

      3. *5-6 months*
- **a.** Vocalization: begins to imitate sounds
- **b.** Socialization: recognizes parents, stranger anxiety begins to develop; comfort habits begin

      4. *7-9 months*
- **a.** Vocalization: verbalizes all vowels and most consonants
- **b.** Socialization
  - **1)** shows increased stranger anxiety and anxiety over separation from parent
  - **2)** exhibits aggressiveness by biting at times
  - **3)** understands the word "no"

      5. *10-12 months*
- **a.** Vocalization: imitates animal sounds, can say only 4-5 words but understands many more (ma, da)
- **b.** Socialization
  - **1)** begins to explore surroundings
  - **2)** plays games such as pat-a-cake, peek-a-boo
  - **3)** shows emotions such as jealousy, affection, anger, fear (especially in new situations)

C. Cognitive tasks

      1. *Neonatal period: reflexive behavior only*

      2. *1-4 months*
- **a.** Recognizes familiar faces
- **b.** Is interested in surroundings
- **c.** Discovers own body parts

      3. *5-6 months*
- **a.** Begins to imitate
- **b.** Can find partially hidden objects

      4. *7-9 months*
- **a.** Begins to understand object permanence; searches for dropped objects
- **b.** Reacts to adult anger; cries when scolded

      c. Imitates simple acts and noises

      d. Responds to simple commands

  5. *10–12 months*

      a. Recognizes objects by name

      b. Looks at and follows pictures in book

      c. Shows more goal-directed actions

D. Nutrition

  1. *Birth to 6 months*

      a. Breast milk is a complete and healthful diet; supplementation may include 0.25 mg fluoride, 400 IU vitamin D, and iron after 4 months.

      b. Commercial iron-fortified formula is acceptable alternative; supplementation may include 0.25 mg fluoride if water supply is not fluoridated.

      c. No solid foods before 5 months; too early exposure may lead to food allergies, and extrusion reflex will cause food to be pushed out of mouth.

      d. Juices may be introduced at 5–6 months, diluted 1:1 and preferably given by cup.

  2. *6–12 months*

      a. Breast milk or formula continues to be primary source of nutrition.

      b. Introduction of solid foods starts with cereal (usually rice cereal), which is continued until 18 months.

      c. Introduction of other food is arbitrary; most common sequence is fruits, vegetables, meats.

         1) introduce only one new food at a time.

         2) separate new foods by minimum of 3–4 days.

         3) decrease amount of formula to about 30 oz. as foods are added.

      d. Iron supplementation can be stopped.

      e. Finger foods such as cheese, meat, carrots can be started around 10 months.

      f. Chopped table food or junior food can be introduced by 12 months.

      g. Weaning from breast or bottle to cup should be gradual during second 6 months.

      h. Breastfeeding can continue beyond 12 months.

      i. No honey, nuts, egg whites until 12 months.

E. Safety

  1. *Birth to 4 months*

      a. Use car seat properly. Infants up to 9 kg (20 lb) and younger than 1 year should face rear.

      b. Ensure crib mattress fits snugly; do not use a pillow or comforters in the crib.

      c. Keep side rails of crib up.

      d. Position infant supine for sleep until infant is able to turn over. Prone position may increase risk for sudden infant death syndrome (SIDS).

      e. Do not leave infant unattended on bed, couch, table.

      f. Do not tie pacifier on string around infant's neck; remove bib before sleep.

      g. Remove small objects that infant could choke on.

      h. Check temperature of bath water and warmed formula or food.

      i. Use cool mist vaporizer.

  2. *5-7 months*

      a. Restrain in high chair or infant seat.

      b. Do not feed hard candy, nuts, food with pits.

      c. Inspect toys for small removable parts.

      d. Be sure paint on furniture does not contain lead.

      e. Keep phone number of poison control center readily available.

  3. *8-12 months*

      a. Keep crib away from other furniture and windows.

      b. Keep gates across stairways.

      c. Keep safety plugs in electrical outlets.

      d. Remove hanging electrical wires and tablecloths.

      e. Use child protective caps and cabinet locks.

      f. Place cleaning solutions and medications out of reach.

      g. Do not let child use fork to self-feed.

      h. Do not leave alone in bathtub.

F. Play (Solitary)

  1. *Birth to 4 months*

      a. Provide variety of brightly colored objects, different sizes and textures.

      b. Hang mobiles within 8–10 inches of infant's face.

      c. Expose to various environmental sounds; use rattles, musical toys.

  2. *5-7 months*

      a. Provide brightly colored toys to hold and squeeze.

      b. Allow infant to splash in bath.

      c. Provide crib mirror.

  3. *8-12 months*

      a. Provide toys with movable parts and noisemakers; stack toys, blocks; pots, pans, drums to bang on; walker and push-pull toys.

      b. Plays games: hide and seek, pat-a-cake.

G. Fears

  1. Separation from parents

      a. Searches for parents with eyes.

      b. Shows preference for parents.

      c. Develops stranger anxiety around 6 months.

  2. Pain

      a. Reacts with generalized body movement and loud crying.

      b. Can be distracted with talking, sucking opportunities.

Toddler (12 months to 3 years)

A. Physical tasks: this is a period of slow growth
1. Weight: gain of approximately 11 lb (5 kg) during this time; birth weight quadrupled by 2½ years
2. Height: grows 20.3 cm (8 inches); adult height about 2 times height at 2 years
3. Head circumference: 19½–20 inches (49–50 cm) by 2 years; anterior fontanel closes by 18 months
4. Pulse 110; respirations 26; blood pressure 99/64
5. Primary dentition (20 teeth) completed by 2½ years
6. Develops sphincter control necessary for bowel and bladder control
7. Mobility
    a. Walks alone by 18 months.
    b. Climbs stairs and furniture by 18 months.
    c. Runs fairly well by 2 years.
    d. Jumps from chair or step by 2½ years.
    e. Balances on one foot momentarily by 2½ years.
    f. Rides tricycle by 3 years.
B. Psychosocial tasks
1. Increases independence; better able to tolerate separation from primary caregiver.
2. Less likely to fear strangers.
3. Able to help with dressing/undressing at 18 months; dresses self at 24 months.
4. Has sustained attention span.
5. May have temper tantrums during this period; should decrease by 2½ years.
6. Vocabulary increases from about 10–20 words to over 900 words by 3 years.
7. Has beginning awareness of ownership (my, mine) at 18 months; shows proper use of pronouns (I, me, you) by 3 years.
8. Moves from hoarding and possessiveness at 18 months to sharing with peers by 3 years.
9. Toilet training usually completed by 3 years.
    a. Demonstrates readiness for toilet training between 18 and 24 months
    b. Indicators of readiness: walks, sits, and squats well, has voluntary control of bowel and urinary function, regular bowel movements, can communicate wetness or bowel movement, can remove clothes, wants to please caregivers, imitates
    c. Daytime bladder control by 2–3 years
    d. Nighttime bladder control by 3–4 years
C. Cognitive tasks
1. Follows simple directions by 2 years.
2. Begins to use short sentences at 18 months to 2 years.
3. Can remember and repeat 3 numbers by 3 years.

4. Knows own name by 12 months; refers to self, gives first name by 24 months; gives full name by 3 years.
5. Able to identify geometric forms by 18 months.
6. Achieves object permanence; is aware that objects exist even if not in view.
7. Uses "magical" thinking; believes own feelings affect events (e.g., anger causes rain).
8. Uses ritualistic behavior; repeats skills to master them and to decrease anxiety.
9. May develop dependency on "transitional object" such as blanket or stuffed animal.

D. Nutrition
1. Caloric requirement is approximately 100 calories/kg/day.
2. Increased need for calcium, iron, and phosphorus.
3. Needs 16–24 oz milk/day.
4. Appetite decreases.
5. Able to feed self.
6. Negativism may interfere with eating.
7. Initial dental examination at 3 years.

E. Safety
1. Turn pot handles toward back of stove.
2. Teach swimming and water safety; supervise near water.
3. Supervise play outdoors.
4. Avoid large chunks of meat, particularly hotdogs.
5. Do not allow child to walk around with objects such as lollipops in mouth.
6. Know when and how to use ipecac.
7. Car seat safety: children sit in forward facing car seat only after age is greater than 1 year and weight is greater than 20 lb. All car seats placed in rear seat of car. No car seats should be placed in front of the passenger side air bag.

F. Play
1. Predominantly "parallel play" period.
2. Imitation of adults often part of play.
3. Begins imaginative and make-believe play.
4. Provide toys appropriate for increased locomotive skills: push toys, rocking horse, riding toys or tricycles; swings and slide.
5. Give toys to provide outlet for aggressive feelings: work bench, toy hammer and nails, drums, pots, pans.
6. Provide toys to help develop fine motor skills, problem-solving abilities: puzzles, blocks; finger paints, crayons.

G. Fears: separation anxiety
1. Learning to tolerate and master brief periods of separation is important developmental task.
2. Increasing understanding of object permanence helps toddler overcome this fear.
3. Potential patterns of response to separation

    a. Protest: screams and cries when mother leaves; attempts to call her back.

    b. Despair: whimpers, clutches transitional object, curls up in bed, decreased activity, rocking.

    c. Denial: resumes normal activity but does not form psychosocial relationships; when mother returns, child ignores her.

  4. Bedtime may represent desertion.

Preschooler (3 to 5 years)

A. Physical tasks

  1. Slower growth rate continues

    a. Weight: increases 4–6 lb (1.8–2.7 kg) a year

    b. Height: increases 2½ inches (5–6.25 cm) a year

    c. Birth length doubled by 4 years

  2. Vital signs decrease slightly

    a. Pulse 90–100

    b. Respirations 24–25/minute

    c. Blood pressure: systolic 85–100 mmHg: diastolic 60–70 mmHg

  3. Permanent teeth may appear late in preschool period; first permanent teeth are molars, behind last temporary teeth.

  4. Gross motor development

    a. Walks up stairs using alternate feet by 3 years.

    b. Walks down stairs using alternate feet by 4 years.

    c. Rides tricycle by 3 years.

    d. Stands on 1 foot by 3 years.

    e. Hops on 1 foot by 4 years.

    f. Skips and hops on alternate feet by 5 years.

    g. Balances on 1 foot with eyes closed by 5 years.

    h. Throws and catches ball by 5 years.

    i. Jumps off 1 step by 3 years.

    j. Jumps rope by 5 years.

  5. Fine motor development

    a. Hand dominance is established by 5 years.

    b. Builds a tower of blocks by 3 years.

    c. Ties shoes by 5 years.

    d. Ability to draw changes over this time

      1) copies circles, may add facial features by 3 years.

      2) copies a square, traces a diamond by 4 years.

      3) copies a diamond and triangle, prints letters and numbers by 5 years.

    e. Handles scissors well by 5 years.

B. Psychosocial tasks

  1. Becomes independent

    a. Feeds self completely.

    b. Dresses self.

    c. Takes increased responsibility for actions.

      2. Aggressiveness and impatience peak at 4 years then abate; by 5 years child is eager to please and manners become more evident.

      3. Gender-specific behavior is evident by 5 years.

      4. Egocentricity changes to awareness of others; rules become important; understands sharing.

C. Cognitive development

      1. Focuses on one idea at a time; cannot look at entire perspective.

      2. Awareness of racial and sexual differences begins.

          a. Prejudice may develop based on values of parents.

          b. Manifests sexual curiosity.

          c. Sexual education begins.

          d. Beginning body awareness.

      3. Has beginning concept of causality.

      4. Understanding of time develops during this period.

          a. Learns sequence of daily events.

          b. Is able to understand meaning of some time-oriented words (day of week, month, etc.) by 5 years.

      5. Has 2000-word vocabulary by 5 years.

      6. Can name four or more colors by 5 years.

      7. Is very inquisitive.

D. Nutrition

      1. Caloric requirement is approximately 90 calories/kg/day.

      2. May demonstrate strong taste preferences.

      3. More likely to taste new foods if child can assist in the preparation.

E. Safety

      1. Safety issues similar to toddler

      2. Education of children concerning potential dangers important during this period

      3. Car safety: children 20–40 lb and younger than age 4 should ride in car safety seat. Children over 40 lb and between ages 4 and 8 should ride in a booster seat in the rear of the car.

F. Play

      1. Predominantly "associative play" period.

      2. Enjoys imitative and dramatic play.

          a. Imitates same-sex role functions in play.

          b. Enjoys dressing up, dollhouses, trucks, cars, telephones, doctor and nurse kits.

      3. Provide toys to help develop gross motor skills: tricycles, wagons, outdoor gym; sandbox, wading pool.

      4. Provide toys to encourage fine motor skills, self-expression, and cognitive development: construction sets, blocks, carpentry tools; flash cards, illustrated books, puzzles; paints, crayons, clay, simple sewing sets.

      5. Television, when supervised, can provide a quiet activity; some programs have educational content.

6. Imaginary playmates common during this period.
    a. More prevalent in bright children
    b. Help child deal with loneliness and fears
    c. Abandoned by school age
G. Fears
    1. Greatest number of imagined and real fears of childhood during this period.
    2. Fears concerning body integrity are common.
        a. Child is able to imagine an event without experiencing it.
        b. Observing injuries or pain in others can precipitate fear.
        c. Magical and animistic thinking allows children to develop many illogical fears (fear of inanimate objects, the dark, ghosts).
    3. Exposing child to feared object in a safe situation may provide a degree of conditioning; child should progress at own rate.

School-Age (6 to 12 years)

A. Physical tasks
    1. Slow growth continues.
        a. Height: 2 inches (5 cm) per year
        b. Weight: doubles over this period
        c. At age 9, both sexes same size; age 12, girls bigger than boys
    2. Dentition
        a. Loses first primary teeth at about 6 years.
        b. By 12 years, has all permanent teeth except final molars.
    3. Bone growth faster than muscle and ligament development; very limber but susceptible to bone fractures during this time.
    4. Vision is completely mature; hand-eye coordination develops completely.
    5. Gross motor skills: predominantly involving large muscles; children are very energetic, develop greater strength, coordination, and stamina.
    6. Develops smoothness and speed in fine motor control.
B. Psychosocial tasks
    1. School occupies half of waking hours; has cognitive and social impact.
        a. Readiness includes emotional (attention span), physical (hearing and vision), and intellectual components.
        b. Teacher may be parent substitute, causing parents to lose some authority.
    2. Morality develops
        a. Before age 9 moral realism predominates: strict superego, rule dominance; things are black or white, right or wrong.
        b. After age 9 autonomous morality develops: recognizes differing points of view, sees ''gray'' areas.

3. Peer relationships
   a. Child makes first real friends during this period.
   b. Is able to understand concepts of cooperation and compromise (assist in acquiring attitudes and values); learns fair play vs competition.
   c. Help child develop self-concept.
   d. Provide feeling of belonging.
4. Enjoys family activities.
5. Has some ability to evaluate own strengths and weaknesses.
6. Has increased self-direction.
7. Is aware of own body; compares self to others; modesty develops.

C. Cognitive development
   1. Period of industry
      a. Is interested in exploration and adventure.
      b. Likes to accomplish or produce.
      c. Develops confidence.
   2. Concept of time and space develops.
      a. Understands causality.
      b. Masters concept of conservation: permanence of mass and volume; concept of reversibility.
      c. Develops classification skills: understands relational terms; may collect things.
      d. Masters arithmetic and reading.

D. Nutrition
   1. Caloric needs diminish in relation to body size: 85 kcal/kg.
   2. "Junk" food may become a problem; excess sugar, starches, fat.
   3. Obesity is a risk in this age group.
   4. Nutrition education should be integrated into school program.

E. Safety
   1. Incidence of accidents is decreased when compared with younger children.
   2. Motor vehicle accidents most common cause of severe injury and death.
   3. Other common activities associated with injuries include sports (skateboarding, rollerskating, etc.).
   4. Education and supervision are key elements in prevention.
      a. Proper use of equipment
      b. Risk-taking behavior

5. Car safety: children weighing over 40 lb and younger than age 8 should ride in a booster seat placed in the rear of the car. Children over age 8 can use shoulder/lap belt combination in rear seat of the car. Children younger than age 12 should not sit in the front passenger seat or in front of an air bag.

F. Play

1. Rules and ritual dominate play; individuality not tolerated by peers; knowing rules provides sense of belonging; "cooperative play."
2. Team play: games or sports
   a. Help learn value of individual skills and team accomplishments.
   b. Help learn nature of competition.
3. Quiet games and activities: board games, collections, books, television, painting
4. Athletic activities: swimming, hiking, bicycling, skating

G. Fears: more realistic fears than younger children; include death, disease or bodily injury, punishment; school phobia may develop, resulting in psychosomatic illness.

Adolescent (12 to 19 years)

A. Physical tasks

1. Fast period of growth
2. Vital signs approach adult norms
3. Puberty
   a. Follows same pattern for all races and cultures.
   b. Is related to hormonal changes.
   c. Results in growth spurt, change in body structure, development of secondary sex characteristics, and reproductive maturity.
   d. Girls: height increases approximately 3 inches/year; slows at menarche; stops around age 16.
   e. Boys: growth spurt starts around age 13; height increases 4 inches/year; slows in late teens.
   f. Boys double weight between 12 and 18, related to increased muscle mass.
   g. Body shape changes
      1) boys become leaner with broader chest.
      2) girls have fat deposited in thighs, hips, and breasts; pelvis broadens.
   h. Apocrine glands cause increased body odor.
   i. Increased production of sebum and plugging of sebaceous ducts causes acne.
4. Sexual development: girls
   a. Menarche
      1) onset about 2 years after first of pubescent changes
      2) average age 12½ years
      3) first 1–2 years: menses irregular, infertile

        b. Menstrual cycle: controlled by complex interaction of hormones.

        c. Development of secondary sex characteristics and sexual functioning under hormonal control (see Table 4-21).

        d. Breast development is first visible sign of puberty.

            1) bud stage: areola around nipple is protuberant.

            2) breast development is complete around the time of first menses.

    5. Sexual development: boys

        a. Development of secondary sex characteristics, sex organs and function under hormonal control (see Table 4-21).

        b. Enlargement of testes is first sign of sexual maturation; occurs at approximately age 13, about 1 year before growth spurt.

        c. Scrotum and penis increase in size until age 18.

        d. Reaches reproductive maturity about age 17, with viable sperm.

        e. Nocturnal emission: a physiologic reflex to ejaculate buildup of semen; natural and normal; occurs during sleep (child should not be made to feel guilty; needs to understand that this is not enuresis).

        f. Masturbation increases (also a normal way to release semen).

        g. Pubic hair continues to grow and spread until mid 20s.

        h. Facial hair; appears first on upper lip.

        i. Voice changes due to growth of laryngeal cartilage.

        j. Gynecomastia: slight hypertrophy of breasts due to estrogen production; will pass within months but causes embarrassment.

B. Psychosocial tasks

    1. Early adolescence: ages 12–14 years

        a. Starts with puberty.

        b. Physical body changes result in an altered self-concept.

        c. Tends to compare own body to others.

        d. Early and late developers have anxiety regarding fear of rejection.

        e. Fantasy life, daydreams, crushes are all normal, help in role play of varying social situations.

        f. Is prone to mood swings.

        g. Needs limits and consistent discipline.

    2. Middle adolescence: ages 15–16 years

        a. Is separate from parents (except financially).

        b. Can identify own values.

        c. Can define self (self-concept, strengths and weaknesses).

        d. Involved with peer group; conforms to values/fads.

        e. Has increased heterosexual interest; communicates with opposite sex; may form "love" relationship.

        f. Sex education continues.

3. Late adolescence: ages 17–19 years
    a. Achieves greater independence.
    b. Chooses a vocation.
    c. Participates in society.
    d. Finds an identity.
    e. Finds a mate.
    f. Develops own morality.
    g. Completes physical and emotional maturity.
C. Cognitive development
    1. Develops abstract thinking abilities.
    2. Is often unrealistic.
    3. Is capable of scientific reasoning and formal logic.
    4. Enjoys intellectual abilities.
    5. Is able to view problems comprehensively.
D. Nutrition
    1. Nutritional requirements peak during years of maximum growth: age 10–12 in girls, 2 years later in boys.
    2. Appetite increases.
    3. Inadequate diet can retard growth and delay sexual maturation.
    4. Food intake needs to be balanced with energy expenditure.
    5. Increased needs include calcium for skeletal growth; iron for increased muscle mass and blood cell development; zinc for development of skeletal and muscle tissue and sexual maturation.
E. Safety
    1. Accidents are leading cause of death: motor vehicle accidents, sports injuries, firearms accidents.
    2. Safety measures include education about proper use of equipment and caution concerning risk taking.
    3. Drug and alcohol use may be a serious problem during this period.
    4. Adolescent characteristics of poor impulse control and recklessness make prevention complex.
F. Activities: group activities predominate (sports are important); activities involving opposite sex by middle adolescence.
G. Fears
    1. Threats to body image: acne, obesity
    2. Injury or death
    3. The unknown

■ ANALYSIS

Nursing diagnoses for problems of growth and development may include
A. Altered thought processes
B. Knowledge deficit (specify)
C. Disturbance in self-esteem
D. Social isolation

E. High risk for violence
F. Altered family process
G. Ineffective family coping
H. Altered health maintenance
I. Altered parenting

■ PLANNING AND IMPLEMENTATION
Goals

A. Child will achieve appropriate developmental level for age.
B. Family/child will adapt successfully to developmental changes.
C. Family/child will cope successfully with crises of illness and hospitalization.
D. Family/child will cope successfully with issues related to death and dying.

Interventions for the Ill or Hospitalized Child
Communicating with Children

A. Speak in quiet, pleasant tones.
B. Bend down to meet child on own level.
C. Use words appropriate to age/communication ability; do not use cliches.
D. Do not explain more than is necessary.
E. Always explain what you are going to do and give the reason for it.
F. Be honest; do not lie about whether something will hurt.
G. Do not make a promise you know you cannot keep.
H. Observe nonverbal behavior for clues to level of understanding.
I. Do not threaten; and when necessary, punish the act, not the child ("I like you, but not what you did.").
J. Never shame a child by using terms like baby or sissy.
K. Allow child to show feelings (hurt and anger); provide therapeutic play, pounding or throwing toys; allow child to cry; encourage drawing and creative writing.
L. Provide time to talk; encourage a trusting environment where the child can talk without embarrassment and confide without fear.
M. Provide support to child and parents/family.
N. Teach parents to anticipate next stage of development.
O. If teaching with a child is interrupted, start over from the beginning.
P. Promote independence; allow the child to perform as many self-care activities as possible.
Q. Do not compare child's progress to that of anyone else.
R. Provide praise at every opportunity.
S. Instead of asking what something is, ask child to give it a name or tell you about it.

T. Allow choices where possible, but do not use yes/no questions unless you can accept a "no" answer ("It is time for your medication now; do you want it with milk or juice?" versus "Do you want your medication now?").

U. Involve parents in child's care.

V. Keep routines as much like home as possible (on admission, ask parents about routines such as toileting, eating, sleeping, and names for bowel movements and urination).

W. Allow parents time and opportunities to ask questions and express themselves.

X. If parents cannot stay with child, encourage them to bring in a favorite toy, pictures of family members, or to make a tape to be played for the child.

Play

A. Play is a way to solve problems, become enculturated, express creativity, decrease stress in the environment, prepare for different situations, sublimate sensations, enhance fine and gross motor development as well as social development.

B. Make play appropriate for mental age and physical/disease state (e.g., appropriate for oxygen tents, isolation, hearing or vision defects).

C. Use multisensory stimulation.

D. Provide toys safe for mental age (no points, sharp edges, small parts, loud noises, propelled objects).

E. Offer play specific to age group.
   1. Toddler: enjoys repetition; solitary play, parallel play.
   2. Preschooler: likes to role play and make believe; associative play.
   3. School-age: likes group, organized activities (to enhance sharing); cooperative play, group goals with interaction.

Preparation for Procedures

A. Allow child to play with equipment to be used.

B. Demonstrate procedure first on a doll.

C. Teach child skills that will be needed after the procedure and provide time to practice (crutches, blow bottles).

D. Show the child pictures of staff garb, special treatment room, special machines to be used, etc., before the procedure.

E. Describe sensations the child may experience during or after the procedure and what child will have to do.

F. Listen carefully to child to detect misconceptions or fantasies.

G. With younger children, the preparatory information should be simple and as close to the time of the procedure as possible.

H. Parents can often be helpful in preparing child for procedures, but need to be prepared as well.
   1. May need different explanation, away from child.
   2. Should have opportunity to ask questions about what will happen to child.

I. School-age children and adolescents may not wish parents to be present during procedure.
   1. Child's desires should be confirmed.
   2. Parents need to be assured that this is not rejection by child.
J. Inadequate preparation leads to heightened anxiety that may result in regressive behavior, uncooperativeness, or acting out.

■ EVALUATION

A. Child maintains normal developmental level during hospitalization.
B. Parents participate in care of child during hospitalization.

■ GROWTH AND DEVELOPMENT ISSUES
Health Promotion

A. Immunization schedule (see Table 1-1).
B. Types of immunity.
C. Considerations concerning immunization schedule
   1. If the immunization schedule is interrupted it is not necessary to reinstitute the entire series. Immunization should occur on the next visit as if the usual interval has elapsed.
   2. If immunization status is unknown, children should be considered susceptible and appropriate immunizations administered
   3. For children not immunized during the first year of life and who are less than 7 years old the same immunizations are given but following different time schedule.
   4. For children 7 years old and older who are not immunized, Td rather than DTaP is administered.
   5. Preterm infants are immunized according to chronological, not corrected age.
   6. Minor illnesses are not contraindications to immunization.
D. Contraindications for immunization
   1. Severe allergic reaction to a vaccine contraindicates further doses of that vaccine.
   2. Anaphylactic reaction to a vaccine additive contraindicates the use of vaccines containing that substance (e.g., eggs, neomycin, streptomycin).
   3. Immunocompromised persons should not receive live vaccines.
   4. Immunizations should be delayed after recent transfusion with passive immunity agents (e.g., gamma globulin).
E. Tuberculin testing
   1. The tuberculin skin test is the only practical tool for diagnosing tuberculosis infection.

TABLE 1-1 2004 Recommended Primary Immunization Schedule*

Age	Immunization	Comment
Birth-2 months	Hepatitis B #1	Given IM; recommended before discharge from hospital after birth; can be delayed ONLY if mother is hepatitis B surface antigen negative
1–4 months	Hepatitis B #2	
6–18 months	Hepatitis B #3	
2, 4, and 6 months	DTaP	Diptheria, tetanus, acellular pertussis; given IM
	Hib	*Haemophilus influenzae* type b conjugate vaccine; also available in combination with DTaP; given IM
	PCV	Pneumococcal conjugate vaccine; for all infants up to age 23 months and chronically ill up to 59 months; not given to healthy children after 24 months; given IM
2, 4, and 6–18 months	IPV	Inactivated polio vaccine; given SC
12–15 months	MMR #1	Measles, mumps, rubella; given SC
	PCV	
	Hib	
12–18 months	Varicella	Given SC; if given after age 13 years, two doses are required, given at least 4 weeks apart
15–18 months	DTaP	
4–6 years	DTaP booster	No pertussis fraction of DTaP after age 7
	IPV	

Continued

Table 1-1   Continued

Age	Immunization	Comment
	MMR #2	At least 4 weeks should elapse between MMR #1 and #2
11–12 years	Td	At least 5 years should elapse since prior DTaP; booster Td every 10 years
yearly, beginning at 6 months	Influenza	Recommended yearly; intranasal version may be given to children ≥ age 5; injected version given IM; two doses required in children ≤8 years who have not had prior influenza vaccination

Note: From http://www.cispimmunize.org; also see http://www.aap.org
Recommendations are issued at least yearly.
Nonimmunized children are immunized by the AAP/ACIP catch-p schedule.

2. Tuberculin testing may be done at the same visit at which an immunization is being given.
3. Routine testing is no longer recommended. Testing is always indicated for individuals with known contact with a person with tuberculosis disease.
4. Positive reaction signifies infection with *Mycobacterium tuberculosis.*
5. Positive reaction indicates need for further evaluation.
6. Children from other countries who have received BCG vaccine against tuberculosis may show positive skin test.
F. Common childhood communicable diseases (see Table 1-2).

Challenges of Parenting

A. Failure to Thrive (FTT)
    1. General information
        a. A condition in which a child fails to gain weight and is persistently less than the 5th percentile on growth charts.
        b. When related to nonorganic cause, it is usually due to a disrupted maternal-child relationship.
        c. Other pathology (especially absorption problems and hormonal dysfunction) must be ruled out before a disorder can be diagnosed as FTT.
        d. Growth and developmental delay usually improve with appropriate stimulation.

TABLE 1-2   Communicable Childhood Diseases

Disease	Characteristics	Immunization
Diphtheria	A respiratory disease caused by bacteria. Bacteria forms a pseudomembrane across the trachea causing respiratory distress; also produces an exotoxin that causes myocarditis and neurologic problems.	Included in DTaP up to 6 years, then in Td*, repeated every 10 years throughout life.
Pertussis (whooping cough)	Respiratory disease caused by bacteria; life threatening in young children. Severe paroxysmal cough results in severe respiratory distress; complications include seizures, pneumonia, encephalopathy and death.	Included in DTaP; not given after 6 years because of risk from associated side effects. Do not give pertussis vaccine if child has active neurologic disorder.
Tetanus (lockjaw)	Neurologic disorder caused by bacterial exotoxin affects motor neurons, causing rigidity and spastic muscles; first symptom is stiffness of the jaw (trismus). No immunity is conferred after having the disease; associated mortality 25–50%.	Included in DTaP up to 6 years; included in Td* every 10 years throughout life. May be given with a puncture wound if the wound is dirty and no immunization has been given in 5 years, or if wound is clean but more than 10 years have elapsed since previous immunization.
Measles (rubeola)	Viral infection producing harsh cough, maculopapular rash, photophobia, and Koplik spots; complications may include pneumonia, bacterial superinfections and encephalitis. Incubation period is 8 to 12 days. Care includes keeping room darkened and providing antipruritic measures.	Maternal antibodies last for at least a year, then included in MMR* given at 12 to 15 months. Do not give to pregnant women or immunocompromised persons.

Continued

Table 1-2   Continued

Disease	Characteristics	Immunization
German measles (rubella)	Viral infection causing lymphadenopathy and pink maculopapular rash; very mild disease, no specific care needed; complications may include arthralgia or arthritis, especially if occurring in young adults. Greatest danger is if pregnant woman contracts the disease; causes serious congenital anomalies.	Included in MMR*
Mumps (parotitis)	Viral infection causing swelling of the salivary glands with painful swallowing. Ice collar may help relieve discomfort. Complications include orchitis (usually unilateral) if disease occurs after puberty, aseptic meningitis, encephalitis.	Included in MMR*
Poliomyelitis (polio)	Viral infection, 95% of infected clients have no symptoms. Virus multiplies in the GI tract and enters the bloodstream to affect the CNS, resulting in paralysis in less than 2% of infected.	IPV*
Chickenpox (varicella)	Most common communicable childhood disease, caused by the varicella zoster virus. Causes rash that starts on the trunk and spreads. Rash starts as vesicles,	Short-term protection from maternal antibodies. Varicella vaccine.

which then erupt and crust over.

Highly contagious from 2 days prior to rash to 6 days after rash erupts; incubation period 21 days.

Once lesions have crusted or scabbed over they are no longer contagious.

Care is directed at comfort measures.

*For immunization schedule and additional information about vaccine see Table 1-1

2. Assessment findings
   a. Sleep disturbances; rumination (voluntary regurgitation and reswallowing)
   b. History of parental isolation and social crisis with inadequate support systems
   c. Physical exam reveals delayed growth and development (decreased vocalization, low interest in environment) and characteristic postures (child is stiff or floppy, resists cuddling)
   d. Disturbed maternal-infant interaction may be demonstrated in feeding techniques, amount of stimulation provided by mother, ability of mother to respond to infant's cues
3. Nursing interventions
   a. Provide consistent care.
   b. Teach parents positive feeding techniques.
      1) provide quiet environment.
      2) follow child's rhythm of feeding.
      3) maintain face-to-face posture with child.
      4) talk to child encouragingly during feeding.
   c. Involve parents in care.
      1) provide supportive environment.
      2) give positive feedback.
      3) demonstrate and reinforce responding to child's cues.
   d. Refer to appropriate community agencies.
B. Child abuse
   1. General information
      a. Physical, emotional, or sexual abuse of children: may result from intentional and nonaccidental actions; or may be from intentional and nonaccidental acts of omission (neglect).
      b. In sexual abuse, 80% of children know their abuser.

    c. Problem usually related to parents' limited capacity to cope with, provide for, or relate to a child and/or to each other.

    d. Adults who abuse were often themselves victims of child abuse; although abuser may care about child, pattern of response to frustration and discipline is to be abusive.

    e. Occurs in all socioeconomic groups.

    f. Only 10% of abusers have serious psychologic disturbances, but most have low self-esteem, little confidence, low tolerance for frustration.

    g. Abuse is most common among toddlers as they exercise autonomy and parents may sense loss of power.

2. Assessment findings

    a. History may be indicative of child abuse.

        1) history inconsistent with injury

        2) delay in seeking medical attention

        3) history changes with repetition

        4) no explanation for injury

    b. Skin injuries (bruises, lacerations, burns) are most common; may show outline of instrument used and may be in varying stages of healing.

    c. Musculoskeletal injuries, fractures (especially chip or spiral fractures), sprains, dislocations are also common; X-rays may show multiple old fractures.

    d. Signs of central nervous system (CNS) injuries include subdural hematoma, retinal hemorrhage (shaken baby syndrome).

    e. Abdominal injuries may include lacerated liver, ruptured spleen.

    f. Observation of parents and child may reveal interactional problems.

        1) Does parent respond to child's cues?

        2) Does parent comfort child?

        3) Does child respond to parent with fear?

3. Nursing interventions

    a. In emergency room: tend to physical needs of child first; determination of existence of abuse must wait until child's condition is stable.

    b. Report suspected child abuse to appropriate agency.

    c. Provide a role model for parents in terms of communication, stimulation, feeding, and daily care of child.

    d. Encourage parents to be involved in child's care.

    e. Encourage parents to express feelings concerning abuse, hospitalization, and home situation.

        1) feelings of fear and guilt should be acknowledged.

        2) provide reassurance.

    f. Provide family education concerning child care, especially safety and nutrition needs, discipline, and age-appropriate stimulation.

    g. Initiate referrals for long-term follow-up (community agencies, pediatric and mental health clinics, self-help groups).

C. Learning disabilities
  1. General information
    a. A heterogeneous group of disorders manifested by significant difficulties in acquisition and use of listening, speaking, writing, reasoning, or math skills
    b. Presumed to be due to CNS dysfunction
    c. Children of average or above-average IQ
    d. Affects all aspects of learning, not just academics
    e. Boys affected 6 times more often than girls
    f. Categories include
        1) receptive/sensory: perceptual problem (dyslexia, visual misperception)
        2) integrative: difficulty processing information (analysis, organization, sequencing, abstract thought)
        3) expressive: motor dysfunction (aphasia, writing or drawing difficulties, difficulty in sports or games)
        4) diffuse: combination of above
  2. Assessment findings
    a. Poor attention span
    b. Poor grades, normal IQ
    c. Low general information scores on standardized IQ tests
    d. Decreased participation in extracurricular activities or hobbies
    e. Low self-esteem due to multiple failures
    f. Diagnostic tests: specific testing to confirm diagnosis and determine type of defect
  3. Medical management: psychostimulants may be prescribed to reduce hyperactivity and frustration and to increase attention span and self-control; side effects include anorexia.
  4. Nursing interventions
    a. Environmental manipulation for behavior management
        1) limit external stimuli.
        2) maintain predictable routines.
        3) enforce limits on behavior.
    b. Teaching strategies tailored for child's specific defects
        1) repeat directions often.
        2) elicit feedback from child.
        3) give time to ask questions.
        4) keep teaching sessions short.
        5) do not give nonessential information.
D. Sudden infant death syndrome (SIDS)
  1. General information
    a. Sudden death of any young child that is unexpected by history and in which thorough postmortem examination fails to demonstrate adequate cause of death
    b. Cannot be predicted; cannot be prevented (unexpected and unexplained)

   c. Peak age: 3 months; 95% by 6 months
   d. Usually occurs during sleep; there is no struggle and death is silent
   e. Diagnosis made at autopsy
   f. Although cause of death is not known, suffocation and DTaP reactions are *not* causes of SIDS
 2. Assessment findings
   a. Factors associated with increased SIDS risk: prematurity, low birth weight, multiple births, siblings of SIDS victims, maternal substance abuse
   b. Infants with neurologic problems and abnormal respiratory function at higher risk
   c. Co-sleeping with parents, prone sleep position, soft bedding associated with higher risk
 3. Nursing interventions
   a. Nursing care is directed at supporting parents/family; parents usually arrive at emergency department.
   b. Provide a room for the family to be alone if possible, stay with them; prepare them for how infant will look and feel (baby will be bruised and blanched due to pooling of blood until death was discovered; also will be cold).
   c. Let parents say good-bye to baby (hold, rock).
   d. Reinforce that death was not their fault.
   e. Provide appropriate support referrals: clergy, notification of significant others, local SIDS program, visiting nurse.
   f. Explain how parents can receive autopsy results.
   g. Notify family physician or pediatrician.

■ DEATH AND DYING
Overview
Parental Response to Death

A. Major life stress event
B. Initially parents experience grief in response to potential loss of child
  1. Acknowledgment of terminal disease is a struggle between hope and despair with resultant awareness of inevitable death.
  2. Parents will be at different stages of grief at different times and constantly changing.
C. Parental response is related to age of child, cause of death, available social support, and degree of uncertainty; response might include denial, shock, disbelief, guilt.
D. Parents often confronted with major decisions such as home care versus hospital care, use of investigational drugs, and continuation of life supports.
E. May have long-term disruptive effects on family system
  1. Stress may result in divorce.
  2. May contribute to behavioral problems or psychosomatic symptoms in siblings.
F. Bereaved parents experience intense grief of long duration.

Child's Response to Death

A. Child's concept of death depends on mental age.
   1. Infants and toddlers
      a. Live only in present.
      b. Are concerned only with separation from mother and being alone and abandoned.
      c. Can sense sadness in others and may feel guilty (due to magical thinking).
      d. Do not understand life without themselves.
      e. Can sense they are getting weaker.
      f. Healthy toddlers may insist on seeing a significant other long after that person's death.
   2. Preschoolers
      a. See death as temporary; a type of sleep or separation.
      b. See life as concrete; they know the word ''dead'' but do not understand the finality.
      c. Fear separation from parents; want to know who will take care of them when they are dead.
      d. Dying children may regress in their behavior.
   3. School-age
      a. Have a concept of time, causality, and irreversibility (but still question it).
      b. Fear pain, mutilation, and abandonment.
      c. Will ask directly if they are dying.
      d. See death as a period of immobility.
      e. Interested in the death ceremony; may make requests for own ceremony.
      f. Feel death is punishment.
      g. May personify death (bogey man, angel of death).
      h. May know they are going to die but feel comforted by having parents and loved ones with them.
   4. Adolescents
      a. Are thinking about the future and knowing they will not participate.
      b. May express anger at impending death.
      c. May find it difficult to talk about death.
      d. Have an accurate understanding of death.
      e. May wish to write something for friends and family, make things to leave, or make a tape.
      f. May wish to plan own funeral.

Nursing Implications

Communicating with Dying Child

A. Use the child's own language.
B. Do not use euphemisms.

C. Do not expect an immediate response.

D. Never give up hope.

Care Guidelines at Impending Death

A. Do not leave child alone.

B. Do not whisper in the room (increases fears).

C. Know that touching child is important.

D. Let the child and family talk and cry.

E. Continue to read favorite stories to child or play favorite music.

F. Let parents participate in care as far as they are emotionally capable.

G. Be aware of the needs of siblings who are in the room with the family.

REVIEW QUESTIONS

1. The nurse has assessed four children of varying ages; which one requires further evaluation?

   1. A 7-month-old who is afraid of strangers.

   2. A 4-year-old who talks to an imaginary playmate.

   3. A 9-year-old with enuresis.

   4. A 16-year-old male who had nocturnal emissions.

2. The nurse is caring for a 5-year-old child who has leukemia and is now out of remission and not expected to survive. The child says to his mother, "Will you take care of me when I am dead the way you do now?" The child's mother asks the nurse how to answer her child. The nurse's response should be based on which of the following understandings of the child's behavior?

   1. The child is denying that he has a terminal illness.

   2. The child may be hallucinating.

   3. Children of this age do not understand the finality of death.

   4. Most 5-year-old children have a great fear of mutilation.

3. The nurse is talking with the mother of a 1-year-old child in well-baby clinic. Which statement the mother makes indicates a need for more instruction in keeping the child safe?

   1. "I have some syrup of ipecac at home in case my child ever needs it."

   2. "I put all the medicines on the highest shelf in the kitchen."

   3. "We have moved all the valuable vases and figurines out of the family room."

   4. "My husband put the gates up at the top and bottom of the stairs."

4. A baby was born 6 weeks prematurely and is now 2 months old, and her mother brings her to the clinic for her checkup. Administration of DTaP will depend on

   1. the presence of sufficient muscle mass.
   2. whether the vaccines are live or inactive.
   3. the Denver Developmental Screening results.
   4. calculating her age by subtracting six weeks from the due date.

5. A 12-month-old is brought in for her well-child checkup. All of the immunizations are up to date. The child's mother asks the nurse what immunizations her child will receive today. The nurse's best response is that the child is due for her

   1. first dose of MMR.
   2. second dose of Hib.
   3. third dose of DtaP.
   4. final dose of IPV.

6. The presence of what condition would necessitate a change in the standard immunization schedule for a child?

   1. Allergy to eggs.
   2. Immunosuppression.
   3. Congenital defects.
   4. Mental retardation.

7. A 2-year-old is brought to the pediatric clinic with an upper respiratory infection. After assessing the child, the nurse suspects this child may be a victim of child abuse. Physical signs that almost always indicate child abuse are

   1. diaper rash.
   2. bruises on the lower legs.
   3. asymmetrical burns on the legs.
   4. welts or bruises in various stages of healing.

8. Which parent-child interaction does NOT warrant further assessment when child abuse is suspected? The parent who

   1. appears tired and disheveled.
   2. is hypercritical of the child.
   3. pushes the frightened child away.
   4. expresses far more concern than the situation warrants.

9. When child abuse is suspected, the nurse knows that abusive burns will

    1. have a number of scars.
    2. have identifiable shapes.
    3. display an erratic pattern.
    4. be on one side of the body.

10. The nurse is testing reflexes in a 4-month-old infant as part of the neurologic assessment. Which of the following findings would indicate an abnormal reflex pattern and an area of concern in a 4-month-old infant?

    1. Closes hand tightly when palm is touched.
    2. Begins strong sucking movements when mouth area is stimulated.
    3. Hyperextends toes in response to stroking sole of foot upward.
    4. Does not extend and abduct extremities in response to loud noise.

11. The mother of a 4-month-old infant asks the nurse when she can start feeding her baby solid food. Which of the following should the nurse include in teaching this mother about the nutritional needs of infants?

    1. Infant cereal can be introduced by spoon when the extrusion reflex fades.
    2. Solid foods should be given as soon as the infant's first tooth erupts.
    3. Pureed food can be offered when the infant has tripled his birth weight.
    4. Infant formula or breast milk provides adequate nutrients for the first year.

12. The nurse is assessing a 6-month-old infant during a well-child visit. The nurse makes all of the following observations. Which of the following assessments made by the nurse is an area of concern indicating a need for further evaluation?

    1. Absence of Moro reflex.
    2. Closed posterior fontanel.
    3. Three pound weight gain in 2 months.
    4. Moderate head lag when pulled to sitting position.

13. The nurse is giving anticipatory guidance regarding safety and injury prevention to the parents of an 18-month-old toddler. Which of the following actions by the parents indicates understanding of the safety needs of a toddler?

    1. Supervise the child in outdoor, fenced play areas.
    2. Teach the child swimming and water safety.
    3. Use automobile booster seat with lap belt.
    4. Allow child to cross the street with 4-year-old sibling.

14. The community health nurse is making a newborn follow-up home visit. During the visit the 2-year-old sibling has a temper tantrum. The parent asks the nurse for guidance in dealing with the toddler's temper tantrums. Which of the following is the most appropriate nursing action?

    1. Help the child understand the rules.
    2. Leave the child alone in his bedroom.
    3. Suggest that the parent ignore the child's behavior.
    4. Explain that the toddler is jealous of the new baby.

15. The parent of a 3-year-old child brings the child to the clinic for a well-child checkup. The history and assessment reveals the following findings. Which of these assessment findings made by the nurse is an area of concern and requires further investigation?

    1. Unable to ride a tricycle.
    2. Has ability to hop on one foot.
    3. Uses gestures to indicate wants.
    4. Weight gain of 4 pounds in last year.

16. The parents of a 4-year-old child tell the nurse that the child has an invisible friend named "Felix." The child blames "Felix" for any misbehavior and is often heard scolding "Felix," calling him a "bad boy." The nurse understands that the best interpretation of this behavior is which of the following?

    1. A delay in moral development.
    2. Impaired parent-child relationship.
    3. A way for the child to assume control.
    4. Inconsistent parental discipline strategies.

17. The nurse is caring for a 5-year-old child who is in the terminal stages of acute leukemia. The child refuses to go to sleep and is afraid that his parents will leave. The nurse recognizes that the child suspects he is dying and is afraid. Which of the following questions about death is most likely to be made by a 5-year-old child?

    1. "What does it feel like when you die?"
    2. "Who will take care of me when I die?"
    3. "What will my friends do when I die?"
    4. "Why do children die if they're not old?"

18. The parents of an 8-year-old child bring the child into the clinic for a school physical. The nurse makes all of the following assessments. Which assessment finding is an area of concern and needs further investigation?

1.   Complains of a stomach ache on test days at school.

2.   Has many evening rituals and resists going to bed at night.

3.   Refers to self as being too dumb and too small during the exam.

4.   Has lost three deciduous teeth and has the central and lateral incisors.

19. The nurse is performing a neurologic assessment on an 8-year-old child. As part of this neurologic assessment the nurse is assessing how the child thinks. Which of the following abilities best illustrates that the child is developing concrete operational thought?

1.   Able to make change from a dollar bill.

2.   Describes a ball as both red and round.

3.   Tells time in terms of after breakfast and before lunch.

4.   Able to substitute letters for numbers in simple problems.

20. The nurse is caring for a 10-year-old child during the acute phase of rheumatic fever. Bed rest is part of the child's plan of care. Which of the following diversional activities is developmentally appropriate and meets the health needs of this child in the acute phase of rheumatic fever?

1.   Using handheld computer video games.

2.   Sorting and organizing baseball cards in a notebook.

3.   Playing basketball with a hoop suspended from the bed.

4.   Using art supplies to make drawings about the hospital experience.

21. The nurse is caring for a 13-year-old who has been casted following spinal instrumentation surgery to correct idiopathic scoliosis. The nurse is helping the teen and family plan diversional activities while the teen is in the cast. Which of the following activities would be most appropriate to support adolescent development while the teen is casted?

1.   Take the teen shopping at the mall in a wheelchair.

2.   Plan family evenings playing a variety of board games.

3.   Have teen regularly attend special school activities for own class.

4.   Encourage siblings to spend time with teen watching television and movies.

22. A 2-month-old infant is in the clinic for a well-baby visit. Which of the following immunizations can the nurse expect to administer?

1.   TD, Varicella, IPV.

2.   DTaP, Varicella.

3.   DTaP, MMR, Menomune.

4.   DTaP, Hib, IPV, HBV.

23. An 18-month-old child with a history of falling out of his crib has been brought to the emergency room by the parents. Examination of the child reveals a skull fracture and multiple bruises on the child's body. Which of the following findings obtained by the nurse is most suggestive of child abuse?

    1. Poor personal hygiene of the child.
    2. Inability of the parents to comfort the child.
    3. Conflicting explanations about the accident from the parents.
    4. Cuts and bruises on the child's lower legs in various stages of healing.

24. The nurse is discussing the risk of sudden infant death syndrome (SIDS) in infants with the parents whose second baby died of SIDS 6 months ago. The parents express fear that other children will die from SIDS since they have already had one baby die. Which of the following statements made by the parents indicate their understanding of the relationship of future children and the risk of SIDS?

    1. "Any new baby will be on home monitoring for one year to prevent SIDS."
    2. "There is a 99% chance that we will not have another baby die of SIDS."
    3. "Genetic testing is available to determine the likelihood of another baby dying from SIDS."
    4. "There is medicine that can be used to stimulate the heart rate while the baby is sleeping."

ANSWERS AND RATIONALES

1. 3. A 9-year-old should not be wetting the bed. This child may have physiologic or psychologic problems.

2. 3. Preschool children do not understand the finality of death. They often view it as a long sleep. It is common for preschoolers to ask who will take care of them when they die. Preschool children may know the word "dead" but do not really comprehend what it means.

3. 2. At 1 year of age babies are, or soon will be, climbing on everything. Putting medicines on the highest shelf is not sufficient. All medicines should be put in a locked cabinet.

4. 1. DtaP is given intramuscularly; therefore, administration is dependent on the presence of sufficient muscle mass, which may not be present in the infant who was born prematurely.

5. 1. Current recommendations call for measles, mumps, and rubella combined vaccine (MMR) to be given at 12–15 months.

6. **2.** Immunosuppressed clients may need alteration in immunization protection as live virus vaccines may overwhelm them.

7. **4.** Injuries at various stages of healing are symptomatic of child abuse.

8. **1.** Being tired and disheveled gives no information about the quality of the parent-child interaction. It may be a normal state for a busy parent.

9. **2.** Burns typical of child abuse have symmetrical shapes and resemble the shape of the item used to burn the child.

10. **1.** The palmar grasp is present at birth. The palmar grasp lessens by age 3 months and is no longer reflexive. The infant is able to close hand voluntarily.

11. **1.** Infant cereal is generally introduced first because of its high iron content. The infant is able to accept spoon feeding at around 4 to 5 months when the tongue thrust or extrusion reflex fades.

12. **4.** By 4 to 6 months, head control is well established. There should be no head lag when infant is pulled to a sitting position by the age of 6 months.

13. **1.** The child has great curiosity and has the mobility to explore. Toddlers need to be supervised in play areas. Play areas with soft ground cover and safe equipment need to be selected.

14. **3.** The best approach toward extinguishing attention-seeking behavior is to ignore it as long as the behavior is not inflicting injury.

15. **3.** This behavior indicates a delay in language and speech development. The child may not be able to hear. The child should have a vocabulary of about 900 words and use complete sentences of three to four words.

16. **3.** Imaginary friends are a normal part of development for many preschool children. These imaginary friends often have many faults. The child plays the role of the parent with the imaginary friend. This becomes a way of assuming control and authority in a safe situation.

17. **2.** The greatest fear of preschool children is being left alone and abandoned. Preschool children still think as though they are alive and need to be taken care of.

18. **3.** The school-age years are very important in the development of a healthy self-esteem. These statements by the 8-year-old child indicate a risk for development of a sense of inferiority and need further assessment.

19. **1.** This ability illustrates the concept of conservation, which is one of the major cognitive tasks of school-age children.

20. **2.** The middle childhood years are times for collections. The collections of middle to late school-age children become orderly, selective, and neatly organized in scrapbooks. This quiet activity supports the development of

industry and concrete operational thought as well as the physical restrictions related to the rheumatic fever.

21. **3.** Early adolescents have a strong need to fit in and be accepted by their peers. Attending school activities helps the teen continue peer relationships and develop a sense of belonging.

22. **4.** Healthy infants at 2 months of age receive diphtheria, tetanus, and pertussis (DTaP); hemophilus influenza (Hib); polio vaccine (IPV); and hepatitis B virus (HBV).

23. **3.** Incompatibility between the history and the injury is probably the most important criterion on which to base the decision to report suspected abuse.

24. **2.** Whether subsequent siblings of the SIDS infant are at risk is unclear. Even if the increased risk is correct, families have a 99% chance that their subsequent child will not die of SIDS.

2

Multisystem Stressors

■ GENETIC DISORDERS

A. Genes are functional units of heredity, capable of replication, mutation, and expression.
B. Teratology is the branch of embryology that deals with the study of abnormal development and congenital malformations.
   1. *Congenital disorders:* present at birth, although may not be noticeable until later; may be caused by genetic factors, nongenetic factors, or a combination.
   2. *Genetic disorders:* caused by a single aberrant gene or a deviation in chromosome structure or number.
C. In humans there are normally 46 chromosomes (23 pairs) that contain the genes.
   1. *Genotype:* the gene constitution of an individual
   2. *Phenotype:* the outward visible physical appearance/expression of a person's genes (color, size, allergies)
   3. *Karyotype:* the number and pattern of chromosomes in a cell
   4. *Allele:* one or two or more forms of a gene that controls expression of specific characteristic (e.g., genes for eye color)
      a. *Mendel's law:* for each hereditary property we receive 2 genes, 1 from each parent; 1 is dominant and expressed; 1 is recessive and not expressed.
      b. *Homozygous:* alleles for characteristic are identical; both dominant (DD) or both recessive (dd).
      c. *Heterozygous:* alleles are different (Dd).
D. Normal cell division
   1. *Meiosis:* cell division that produces gametes, each with a haploid set of chromosomes (one-half the number of the parent cell); this is reductional division, occurs in the ova and sperm.
   2. *Mitosis:* cell division that produces two cells (daughter cells), each with a full complement of chromosomes, identical to the composition of the parent cell.

CHAPTER OUTLINE

Genetic Disorders

Fluid and Electrolyte, Acid-Base Balances

Accidents, Poisonings, and Ingestion

Principles of Inheritance

Traits that are controlled by genes located on autosomes are inherited according to dominant or recessive patterns. Most cases of autosomal inheritance in humans involve traits controlled by one gene.

Autosomal Dominant

A. General information
1. Allele responsible for the trait (or disease) is dominant.
2. Only one parent needs to pass on the gene (child may be heterozygous for trait).
3. Examples of inherited diseases; Huntington's chorea, myotonic muscular dystrophy, night blindness, osteogenesis imperfecta, neurofibromatosis.

B. Genetic counseling: advise parents that if one of them has a disease inherited through autosomal dominant pattern, there is a 50% chance with each pregnancy that the child will have the disease/disorder.

Autosomal Recessive

A. General information
1. Allele responsible for trait (or disease) will not result in expression if the other allele in the pair is dominant.
2. Both parents must pass on the gene(s) (child is homozygous for trait).
3. Examples of inherited diseases: cystic fibrosis, PKU, sickle cell anemia, albinism, Tay-Sachs.

B. Genetic counseling: advise parents that if both are heterozygous for the trait then
1. There is a 25% chance with each pregnancy of having a child with the disease/disorder.
2. There is a 50% chance with each pregnancy of having a child who is a carrier of the disease but who will not have the symptoms.
3. There is a 25% chance with each pregnancy of having a child who will neither have the disease nor be a carrier.

Sex-Linked (X-Linked) Inheritance

A. General information
1. Inheritance of characteristics located on X and Y chromosomes
2. Only known genetic locus on the Y chromosome is associated with determination of male sex.
3. X chromosome carries other traits in addition to determination of female sex.
4. Sex-linked inheritance in males: even a recessive defective gene on X chromosome can manifest itself in males because there is no opposing normal gene on Y chromosome.

5. Sex-linked inheritance in females: recessive defective gene can be masked by a normal dominant gene.
6. Examples of sex-linked inherited disorders: color blindness, baldness, hemophilia A and B, Duchenne's muscular dystrophy.

B. Genetic counseling
1. If a woman is a carrier for a sex-linked disorder and her partner does not have the disorder
   a. There is a 50% chance with each pregnancy that her son will have the disorder.
   b. There is a 50% chance her daughter will become a carrier.
2. If a man has a sex-linked disorder, all his daughters will be carriers but none will manifest the disease.
3. For sex-linked disorders, there are no carrier states in males.

Chromosome Alterations

A. General information: deviations from normal chromosome complement may be numeric or structural.
1. *Mutation:* spontaneous alteration in genetic material not present in previous generation
2. *Nondisjunction:* failure of a pair of chromosomes to separate during meiosis; results in numeric change called trisomy (47 chromosomes); can be passed on by either parent (one parent would pass 24 chromosomes)
3. *Translocation:* the transfer of all or part of a chromosome to another location on the same chromosome or to a different chromosome after chromosome breakage
4. *Mosaicism:* the presence in the same individual of two or more genotypically different cell lines

B. Genetic counseling: varies depending on the origin of the alteration
1. Random risk: chromosome alterations caused by environmental agents are not likely to occur in subsequent pregnancies. Therefore, the risk of the same defect recurring is no more than for any person in the general population.
2. High risk: at least one parent carries a chromosomal aberration or mutant gene and passes it on to the offspring (e.g., if a parent is a balanced translocation carrier, the risk of a child being affected is 1 in 4)
3. Moderate risk: largest group; includes multifactorial disorders. Risk recurrence in these disorders is empiric, based not on genetic theory but on prior experience and observation.

Assessment

History

A. Careful, detailed history is the basis of genetic counseling; can help confirm diagnosis and establish recurrence risk in multifactorial disorders.

B. Family history (pattern of affected family members) is recorded in form of pedigree chart or family tree.
  1. Information about affected child and immediate family: history of this pregnancy and all previous pregnancies, including stillbirths and abortions; information about siblings
  2. Information about maternal relatives
     a. Mother's siblings
     b. Outcome of maternal grandmother's pregnancies
     c. Health status of maternal relatives
  3. Information about paternal relatives: same as maternal

Laboratory/Diagnostic Tests

A. Amniocentesis
  1. Examination of amniotic fluid to screen for
     a. Some inborn errors of metabolism
     b. Chromosomal abnormalities
     c. Some CNS disorders (spina bifida)
     d. Sex of infant in sex-related disorders
  2. Indications
     a. One parent is chromosome mosaic or has balanced translocation.
     b. Mother is age 35 or older.
     c. Both parents are heterozygous for an autosomal recessive disorder.
     d. Mother is carrier of an X-linked disorder.
     e. Couple already has an affected child.
B. Karyotyping (chromosomal analysis)
  1. Confirms or refutes probable diagnosis of chromosomal abnormality.
  2. Identifies whether individual is a carrier of chromosomal abnormality.
  3. Determines infant's sex if necessary.
C. Determination of fetal status

Analysis

Nursing diagnoses for the family/individual with a genetic disorder may include
A. Disturbed thought processes
B. Deficient knowledge (specify)
C. Risk for altered parenting
D. Grief (anticipatory)

Planning and Implementation

Goals

A. Child will achieve maximum potential for cognitive and motor development.
B. Family will develop effective coping strategies.

Interventions

A. Provide community health agency referral.
B. Support family in identification of appropriate stimulation programs for child.
C. Communicate with and provide support for parents.
D. Offer genetic counseling (see Principles of Inheritance, page 444).

Evaluation

A. Optimum level of motor and cognitive development is attained.
B. Self-care is performed at satisfactory level.
C. Family is able to function appropriately.
D. Parents demonstrate ability to meet child's physical and developmental needs.
E. Parents derive comfort/satisfaction from parenting affected child.

Chromosome Disorder

Down Syndrome

A. General information
  1. One of the most common causes of mental retardation; incidence: about 1 in 600 live births
  2. Caused by an extra chromosome 21 (total 47)
    a. Most cases associated with nondisjunction; incidence increased with maternal, and to some degree paternal, age; incidence in women over age 35 markedly increased
    b. Also associated with translocation; hereditary type, incidence not increased with parental age
B. Assessment findings
  1. Head and face
    a. Small head, flat facial profile, broad flat nose
    b. Small mouth, normal-size protruding tongue
    c. Upward slanting palpebral fissure
    d. Low-set ears
  2. Extremities
    a. Short, thick fingers and hands
    b. Simian creases (single crease across palms)
    c. Muscle weakness, lax joints
  3. Associated anomalies and disorders
    a. Congenital heart defects (40% incidence)
    b. GI structural defects
    c. Increased incidence of leukemia
    d. Increased incidence of respiratory infection
    e. Visual defects: strabismus, myopia, nystagmus, cataracts
    f. Obesity in older children
  4. Retardation usually moderate, IQ 50–70

C. Nursing interventions: see also Mental Retardation
   1. Provide parent education concerning
      a. Increased susceptibility to respiratory infection
      b. Nutritional needs, feeding techniques
      c. Medication administration if necessary
      d. Protection from injury due to hypotonia, atlanto-axial instability (weak neck)
      e. Needs of siblings
   2. Promote developmental progress
   3. Provide genetic counseling.

■ FLUID AND ELECTROLYTE, ACID-BASE BALANCES
General Principles and Variations from Adult

A. Percent body water compared to total body weight
   1. Premature infant: 90% water
   2. Infant: 75-80% water
   3. Child: 64% water
B. Infant also has a higher percentage of water in extracellular fluid compared to adults (therefore, infant has less fluid reserve).
C. Renal function
   1. Concentrating ability of kidney does not reach adult levels until approximately age 2; specific gravity of infant's urine is 1.003.
   2. Glomerular filtration rate does not reach adult levels until approximately age 2.
   3. Average urine output
      a. Infant: 5-10 ml/hour
      b. 1-10 years: 10-25 ml/hour
      c. 35 ml/hour thereafter
D. Metabolic rate in children is 2-3 times that of adults; children therefore have an increased need for nutrients and fluids, and an increased amount of waste to excrete.
E. Fluid is not conserved; there is less reserve, and children more prone to fluid volume deficit than adults; $\frac{1}{2}$ of infant's extracellular fluid is exchanged each day compared with only $\frac{1}{5}$ of adult's.
F. Children have faster respiratory rate than adults, causing more water loss through breathing.
G. Infants have a greater body surface area per kg body weight than adults, therefore fluid loss through skin (evaporation) is greater in children.

Assessment
Health History

A. Ascertain age, recent weight, usual feeding habits/patterns, amount and type of daily intake.
B. Determine usual voiding/stooling habits and volume of urine/stool output.

C. Identify any recent illnesses or medications taken.
D. Ascertain usual activity level.

Physical Examination

A. Measure present weight and vital signs.
B. Observe general appearance.
   1. Muscle tone
   2. Reflex responses
   3. Activity level
C. Inspect skin and mucous membranes for turgor, color, temperature.
D. Head and face
   1. Inspect fontanels, eye orbits.
   2. Ascertain presence of tears, saliva.
E. Abdomen/genitalia
   1. Auscultate for bowel sounds, peristaltic waves.
   2. Inspect for diaper rash, urine stream.

Laboratory/Diagnostic Tests

A. Blood studies
   1. Hbg and hct
   2. Sodium, potassium, chloride, calcium, magnesium
   3. pCO_2 and CO_2
   4. pH
B. Urine studies: specific gravity, glucose, ketones, osmolarity, pH
C. Stool studies: culture, reducing substances, blood, sodium, potassium, pH

Analysis

Nursing diagnoses for children with fluid/electrolyte and acid-base imbalances may include
A. Diarrhea
B. Pain
C. Deficient fluid volume
D. Imbalanced nutrition
E. Impaired oral mucous membrane
F. Impaired skin integrity
G. Ineffective tissue perfusion
H. Impaired urinary elimination

Planning and Implementation

Goals

A. Child will have normal hydration status.
B. Parents will demonstrate knowledge of child's disorder, prescribed treatment, and prevention of complications.

Interventions

A. Maintain strict I&O.
   1. Weigh diapers.
   2. Monitor urine specific gravity.
   3. Hematest stools.
B. Take daily weights.
C. Keep NPO for bowel rest.
D. Administer IV fluids.
   1. Maintenance plus replacement
   2. Generally use hypotonic solutions (0.25 NSS, 0.33 NSS, or 0.45 NSS)
E. Provide pacifier for infant.
F. Reintroduce oral fluids slowly.
   1. In children under 2 years use Pedialyte, a balanced electrolyte solution.
   2. In children over 2 use weak tea, flat soda.
   3. Do not use
      a. Broth (high sodium)
      b. Milk/formula (high solute)
      c. Water, glucose water, Jell-O (no electrolytes)

Evaluation

A. Child has adequate hydration status.
   1. Adequate I&O
   2. Normal stooling pattern
   3. Good skin turgor
   4. Normal vital signs
   5. Normal serum laboratory values
B. Parents participate in care, demonstrate understanding of signs and symptoms of disorder and treatment.

Disorders

Dehydration

A. The most common fluid and electrolyte disturbance in infants and children
B. Osmotic factors, particularly sodium, control the movement of fluid between extracellular and intracellular compartments and influence the types of dehydration
   1. *Isotonic dehydration: most common*
      a. Plasma sodium level is normal (130–150 mEq/liter).
      b. Water and electrolyte lost in proportionate amounts; net loss is isotonic.
      c. Major loss is from extracellular fluid; loss of circulating blood volume.
      d. Shock may develop if losses are severe.
   2. *Hypotonic dehydration*
      a. Plasma sodium level is less than 130 mEq/liter.

    b. Electrolyte deficit exceeds water deficit.

    c. May occur when fluid and electrolyte losses are replaced with plain or glucose water.

    d. Fluid lost from extracellular compartment; also moves from extracellular to intracellular compartment.

    e. Signs of decreased fluid appear sooner with smaller fluid losses than in isotonic dehydration.

    f. Shock is a frequent finding.

3. *Hypertonic dehydration*

    a. Plasma sodium exceeds 150 mEq/liter.

    b. Water loss exceeds electrolyte loss; may occur when fluid and electrolyte losses are replaced with large amount of solute (hypertonic formula).

    c. Fluid shifts from the intracellular to the extracellular compartments.

    d. Physical signs of dehydration may be less apparent.

    e. Neurologic symptoms (e.g., seizures) may occur.

Diarrhea

A. General information

  1. A change in consistency and frequency of stool

  2. Very common in young children

  3. Caused by bacteria and viruses, parasites, poisons, inflammation, malabsorption, allergies, abnormal bowel motility, and anatomic alterations

  4. Infants can easily lose 5% of their body weight in 1 day

  5. Intestinal fluids are alkaline; large loss causes metabolic acidosis

  6. Also causes bicarbonate and potassium loss

  7. Body may use its own fat for energy, leading to ketosis

B. Assessment findings

  1. History of frequent stools; child may complain of or indicate abdominal cramping by guarding, weight loss; child may be lethargic and irritable

  2. Decreased urine output, decreased tears and saliva, dry mucous membranes, dry skin with poor tissue turgor

  3. In children less than 18 months, may find depressed anterior fontanel

  4. Soft eyeballs with sunken appearance

  5. Ashen skin color; cold extremities

  6. High-pitched cry

  7. Increased pulse rate and decreased blood pressure

  8. Diagnostic tests

    a. Hct elevated if dehydrated

    b. Serum sodium and potassium decreased

    c. BUN elevated if renal circulation is decreased

    d. CBC will show increased bands if caused by bacterial infection

    e. Low pH and positive sugar with disaccharide intolerance

    f. Stool culture will identify specific microorganism

    g. Leukocytes in stool if caused by enteroinvasive organisms

C. Nursing interventions

  1. Keep NPO to rest bowel, if ordered.

  2. Administer IV fluid therapy as ordered.

  3. Resume oral feedings slowly; regular diet is recommended.

  4. Provide skin care to prevent/treat excoriation of diaper area.

  5. Test all stool and chart results.

  6. Isolation may be ordered with infectious cause.

Vomiting

A. General information

  1. Common symptom during childhood; usually not a cause for concern

  2. Differs from spitting up (dribbling of undigested formula, often with burping)

  3. If prolonged may result in metabolic alkalosis or aspiration

B. Assessment findings: in addition to vomiting, child may have fever, abdominal pain, and distension.

C. Nursing interventions

  1. Assist with identification and treatment of underlying cause.

    a. Assess for accompanying diarrhea that may indicate gastroenteritis.

    b. Determine if others in family/school/etc., are also sick; may indicate food poisoning.

    c. Assess for history of anxiety-producing life events.

    d. Assess amount and force of vomitus; forceful, projectile vomiting may indicate pyloric stenosis

    e. Determine frequency and character of vomitus (color, whether formula or food, presence of bile or blood), relationship to feeding (new foods, overeating).

  2. Prevent complications: monitor fluid/electrolyte and acid-base status

  3. Administer antiemetics if ordered; trimethobenzamide HCl (Tigan) and promethazine HCl (Phenergan) recommended for children.

■ ACCIDENTS, POISONINGS, AND INGESTION

A. Accidents are the main cause of death in children over the age of 1 year.

B. 90% of accidents are preventable.

C. Interaction among host (the child), agent (the principal cause), and environment ($^2/_3$ of accidents occur in the home); safeguard the host while the agent and environment are made safer.

D. Methods of prevention

  1. Childproofing the environment

  2. Educating parents and child

NURSING ALERT

Three indications of a child in respiratory distress from choking are:

1. They cannot speak
2. They become cyanotic
3. They collapse

---

    3. Legislation (e.g., seat belts, safe toys)
    4. Anticipatory guidance
    5. Understanding and applying growth and development principles
        a. Infant: totally dependent on adults for maintenance of safe environment
        b. Toddler: more mobile, impatient; urge to investigate and imitate; climbing, running, jumping
        c. Preschooler: very curious, exploring neighborhood, running, climbing, riding bikes; can accept and respond to teaching but still needs protection
        d. School-age and adolescent: taking dares, sports injuries, peer pressure, learning to drive

E. Precipitating factors
    1. Arguments or tension in the home
    2. Change in routines
    3. Tired child/tired parents
    4. Inadequate babysitting
    5. Hungry child
    6. Illness in immediate family member

F. Potential outcomes include temporary incapacitation, permanent disfigurement, and death

Specific Disorders

Pediatric Poisonings

A. General information
    1. Toddlers and suicidal adolescents most often involved
    2. Deaths have declined due to continued efforts in prevention and the establishment of poison control centers
    3. Modes of exposure: ocular, skin, ingestion (vast majority)
    4. Types of substances ingested: drugs, household products (cleaning agents), garden supplies, plants and berries
    5. Most ingestions are acute in nature and accompanied by a history of invasion of the medicine chest or cabinet where household cleaners are kept
    6. Chronic ingestions result in accumulation of toxic substance, such as lead

NURSING ALERT

Risk factors for poisonings are:

- Curiosity due to developmental age
- Lack of understanding of danger
- Lack of age-appropriate supervision

DELEGATION TIP

M anagement of poisoning episodes including administering the directed antidote may be delegated to all ancillary personnel and to parents calling the poison control center.

B. General assessment findings
   1. Signs vary depending on substance ingested
   2. May evidence bradycardia; tachycardia; tachypnea; slow depressed respiration; hypotension or hypertension; hypothermia or hyperpyrexia
   3. Confusion, disorientation, coma, ataxia, seizures
   4. Miosis, mydriasis, nystagmus
   5. Jaundice, cyanosis
   6. Child may have a distinctive odor: hydrocarbons, alcohol, garlic, sweat
C. General interventions
   1. Resuscitate child and stabilize condition: establish patent airway and provide measures to restore circulation as indicated.
   2. Prevent absorption.
      a. Determine what, when, and how much was ingested; will frequently not be able to identify substance.
      b. Induce emesis. Best within 1 hour of ingestion.
         1) indicated in all cases *except* caustic material ingestion, or in a child who is comatose, experiencing seizures, or lacking gag reflex
         2) drug of choice is syrup of ipecac.
            a) administer 30 ml for adolescents, 15 ml for children 1–12 years, 10 ml for children under 1 year.
            b) follow with 100–300 ml water.
            c) if no response in 20–30 minutes, repeat dose once.
            d) produces vomiting almost 100% of the time.
      c. Gastric lavage: may also be used to prevent absorption

CLIENT TEACHING CHECKLIST

| nstruct parents to keep the phone number of the poison control center by all the telephones in the house and not to initiate any intervention without the center's direction.

    1) use largest nasogastric (NG) or orogastric tube possible.
        2) aspirate gastric contents.
        3) use water or $\frac{1}{2}$ normal saline.
        4) continue until return is clear.
    d. Activated charcoal: minimizes absorption of toxins by binding them on its surface
        1) administer after vomiting with ipecac treatment
        2) administer 5–10 g for each gram of drug or chemical ingested.
        3) mix charcoal with water or diet soda to make a syrup that can be given by mouth or NG tube.
    e. Cathartic: may be used after emesis or lavage to speed elimination of ingested substance; recommended agents are sodium or magnesium sulfate.
  3. Provide treatment and prevention information to parents.
    a. Parents should always be instructed to save container, vomitus, spills on clothing for analysis.
    b. Teach parents about safety practices that will decrease chances of accidental poisonings; educate as to use of drugs, labeling, storage, and handling of household products, importance of child-resistant safety packaging.
    c. Stress importance of having syrup of ipecac in the home and on trips (30 ml can be purchased over-the-counter) and instruct parents on proper administration.
    d. Advise parents to keep poison control center phone number readily available.
    e. Incorporate anticipatory guidance related to developmental stage of child.
    f. Discuss general first aid measures with parents.

Salicylate Poisoning

A. General information
  1. Toxicity begins at doses of 150–200 mg/kg.
  2. Products include not only aspirin but oil of wintergreen and analgesic cold medicines.
  3. Peak effect of aspirin is 2–4 hours and effects may last 8 hours.

    4. Ingestion may be accidental or due to therapeutic overdosing.

    5. Salicylate ingestion causes

        a. Acid-base alterations

        b. Respiratory alkalosis

        c. Metabolic acidosis

        d. Impaired glucose metabolism

        e. An inhibition of prothrombin formation

B. Assessment findings

    1. Hyperventilation, confusion, loss of consciousness

    2. Hyperpnea, hyperpyrexia, dehydration

    3. CNS depression, vomiting, lethargy

    4. Coma, respiratory failure, circulatory collapse

C. Nursing interventions

    1. Assist with emergency management

    2. Administer fluid therapy

    3. Monitor vital signs, BP, urine specific gravity, I&O

    4. Monitor temperature, provide tepid sponging or cooling mattress

    5. Provide emotional support to child and family

    6. Administer vitamin K

Acetaminophen Ingestion

A. General information

    1. Has become a commonly used analgesic-antipyretic

    2. Little associated morbidity or mortality in accidental ingestion

    3. Major risk is severe hepatic damage

B. Assessment findings

    1. Vague and nonspecific initially; nausea, vomiting, anorexia, sweating

    2. Jaundice, liver tenderness, increase in liver enzymes, abdominal pain

    3. Progression to hepatic failure

C. Nursing interventions

    1. Emesis or lavage; do *not* use activated charcoal (will bind antidote).

    2. Administer antidote (acetylcysteine [Mucomyst]): lessens hepatic damage if given within 16 hours of ingestion.

Lead Poisoning

A. General information

    1. Increased blood lead levels resulting from ingestion and absorption of lead-containing substances

    2. Most common source is lead-based paint (used in houses prior to 1950)

    3. Toddlers and preschoolers most often affected; many have pica (tendency to eat nonfood substances)

    4. Lead value of more than 10 µg/dl is considered a health hazard

    5. Acute symptoms usually appear once level is 70 µg/dl

6. Lead is absorbed through the GI tract and pulmonary system; it is then deposited in bone, soft tissue, and blood; excretion occurs via urine, feces, and sweat; toxic effects are due to enzyme inhibition.
7. Low dietary iron and calcium may enhance toxic effects.
8. Widespread screening programs have diminished severe effects.

B. Assessment findings
1. Abdominal complaints including colicky pain, constipation, anorexia, vomiting, weight loss
2. Pallor, listlessness, fatigue
3. Clumsiness, irritability, loss of coordination, ataxia, seizures
4. Encephalopathy
5. Identification of lead in the blood
6. Erythrocyte protoporphyrin (EP) levels increased

C. Nursing interventions
1. Prevention
   a. Nutrition—adequate iron and calcium in diet
   b. Environment—damp mop and damp wipe floors, windowsills, cover over flaking paint, handwashing before meals, baths
2. Chelating agents
   a. Succimer (chemet)—oral
   b. Dimercaprol (BAL)—IM
   c. Disodium calcium edetate (calcium EDTA)—IV or IM
   d. IM agents—multiple injections—pain
      1) rotate sites
      2) warm soaks
      3) topical analgesia (EMLA cream)
   e. All chelating agents
      1) maintain hydration (chelation is toxic to kidneys).
      2) measure intake and output.
      3) monitor lead levels.
3. Provide nutritional counseling.
4. Aid in eliminating environmental conditions that led to lead ingestion.

Lyme Disease

A. General information
1. Caused by the spirochete *Borrelia burgdorferi*
2. Transmitted by a deer tick, requires 24-hour tick attachment
3. Most prevalent during summer and early fall
4. Symptoms usually involve the skin, nervous system, and joints
5. Incubation period is 3 to 32 days

B. Medical management
1. Blood tests available, but lack sensitivity and specificity, therefore diagnosis is often based on clinical and epidemiologic data.

2. Antibiotic treatment: if early infection, given for 10–21 days. If neurologic or arthritic symptoms occur, combined treatment for longer duration may be necessary.

C. Assessment findings

1. Divided into stages on the basis of chronologic relationship to the tick bite

   a. Stage I: Skin rash (erythema migrans) starting 3–32 days past tick bite and lasting about 3 weeks. Most common on thighs, buttock, axilla. Systemic symptoms of malaise, fatigue, headache, stiff neck, fever, arthralgia.

   b. Stage II: Symptoms of late disease may occur months to years after the initial disease. Includes neurologic symptoms such as facial palsies, sensory losses, focal weaknesses, cardiac rhythm abnormalities, and increased arthritis complaints involving multiple joints.

D. Nursing interventions

1. Medication administration
2. Prevention

   a. Avoid high-risk areas such as woody, grassy areas

   b. If walking in such areas, wear long pants, long-sleeved shirt, high socks, and sneakers

   c. Use insect repellents for skin and clothing

   d. After every potential exposure, check carefully for ticks

   e. Remove tick by pulling straight out with tweezers

REVIEW QUESTIONS

1. The mother of an 8-year-old brings her child to the physician because the child has a "funny red circle" on his leg. The mother reports that the child went on a camping trip last weekend. The physician draws blood to rule out Lyme disease and prescribes doxycycline for the child. The child's mother asks why an antibiotic is prescribed for a tick bite. The nurse's response is based on which of the following understandings?

   1. Lyme disease weakens the person so they are susceptible to infections.

   2. Lyme disease is caused by a spirochete that is sensitive to doxycycline.

   3. Doxycycline will kill the tick, which may still be in the child.

   4. Antibiotics are given to cure the infection at the site of the tick bite.

2. The mother of a 3-year-old child calls her nurse neighbor in a panic state, saying that the child swallowed most of a bottle of aspirin. The nurse determines that the child is still alert. In addition to calling the poison control center, the nurse should

1. induce vomiting in the child.
2. observe the child carefully until the ambulance arrives.
3. immediately start CPR.
4. give the child lots of milk to drink.

3. An 8-month-old infant was admitted to the hospital with severe diarrhea and dehydration.Fluid replacement therapy was initiated. Which observation the nurse makes indicates an improvement in the infant's status?
   1. Fontanels are depressed.
   2. Infant has gained 3 oz since yesterday.
   3. Skin remains pulled together after being gently pinched and released.
   4. The infant's hematocrit is greater today than yesterday.

4. A 17-year-old has Down syndrome. He is 57 inches tall and weighs 155 pounds. In planning his care, it is most important for the nurse to take into consideration
   1. his mental age.
   2. his chronologic age.
   3. his bone age.
   4. growth chart percentiles.

5. Down syndrome is caused by
   1. an autosomal recessive defect.
   2. an extra chromosome.
   3. a sex-linked defect.
   4. a dominant gene.

6. A 10-day-old baby is admitted with 5% dehydration. The nurse is most likely to note which of the following signs?
   1. Tachycardia.
   2. Bradycardia.
   3. Hypothermia.
   4. Hyperthermia.

7. The nurse is asked why infants are more prone to fluid imbalances than adults. The response is
   1. adults have a greater body surface area.
   2. adults have a greater metabolic rate.
   3. infants have functionally immature kidneys.
   4. infants ingest a lesser amount of fluid per kilogram.

8. A 10-month-old weighs 10 kg and has voided 100 ml in the past 4 hours. The nurse determines normal urine output based on the fact that normal urine output is
   1. 1–2 ml/kg/hour.
   2. 3–5 ml/kg/hour.
   3. 7–9 ml/kg/hour.
   4. 10 ml/kg/hour.

9. A 3-month-old is NPO for surgery. The nurse attempts to comfort him by
   1. administering acetaminophen.
   2. encouraging parents to leave so the child can rest.
   3. offering pacifier.
   4. giving 10 cc Pedialyte.

10. An 11-year-old is admitted for treatment of lead poisoning. The nurse includes which of the following in the plan of care?
    1. Oxygen.
    2. Strict intake and output.
    3. Heme-occult stool testing.
    4. Calorie counts.

11. A 2-month-old is admitted with diarrhea. What is the best room assignment for the nurse to make?
    1. Semi-private room with no roommate.
    2. Private room with no bathroom.
    3. Semi-private room with 10-year-old who has acute lymphocytic leukemia.
    4. Open ward.

12. The nurse is discussing safety measures to prevent poisoning with the mother of a 1-year-old. The nurse knows the mother understands safety precautions when she states,
    1. ''I have child protection locks on my cabinet under the sink.''
    2. ''My child is not potty-trained, so the bathroom is safe.''
    3. ''I keep all poisons and cleaners above the fridge.''
    4. ''I don't think I have any poisons in my house.''

13. A mother calls her local emergency room (ER) and tells the nurse, ''My 4-year-old just swallowed a bottle of aspirin. What should I do?'' After verifying that the child is still awake and alert, the triage nurse would give what advice to the mother?

1. Call 911, then give one glass milk to protect the esophagus.
2. Call 911, then give syrup of ipecac.
3. Bring child to local pediatrician.
4. Call a poison control center.

14. A 16-year-old admits to her mother that she tried to commit suicide by swallowing a bottle of Tylenol (acetaminophen) 16 hours ago. Her mother brings the girl to the ER. The nurse implements treatment of choice, which is
    1. ipecac syrup.
    2. activated charcoal.
    3. mucomyst.
    4. milk and observation.

15. The nurse would include which of the following nursing diagnoses for a 10-year-old client with stage I Lyme disease?
    1. Decreased cardiac output.
    2. Impaired mobility.
    3. Altered cerebral tissue perfusion.
    4. Alteration in skin integrity.

ANSWERS AND RATIONALES

1. **2.** Lyme disease is caused by a spirochete that is sensitive to antibiotics.

2. **1.** Since the child is still alert, the nurse should administer syrup of ipecac to induce vomiting. If the child were not conscious, lavage would be done upon arrival at the emergency department.

3. **2.** A weight gain would suggest greater circulating volume. Blood has weight.

4. **1.** Children with Down syndrome have some degree of mental retardation and care must be geared to their mental age.

5. **2.** In Down syndrome there is an extra chromosome on the 21st pair, which is why the disease is also called trisomy 21.

6. **1.** Tachycardia is associated with dehydration.

7. **3.** Infant kidneys are unable to concentrate or dilute urine, to conserve or secrete sodium, or to acidify urine.

8. **1.** Normal urine output is 1–2 ml/kg/hour.

9. **3.** Non-nutritive sucking will help console and pacify him.

10. 2. CaNaEDTA (treatment for lead poisoning) is nephrotoxic and strict intake and output records need to be kept.

11. 2. A bathroom is irrelevant with an infant in diapers. A private room is necessary.

12. 3. All cleaners and poisons should be kept in high locked cabinets.

13. 4. Phone numbers for poison control centers are located in the blue pages of phone books nationwide.

14. 3. Mucomyst is the treatment of choice to bind with acetaminophen and help reduce levels.

15. 4. Stage I consists of tick bite followed by small erythematous papules that may be described as burning.

3

The Neurosensory System

■ VARIATIONS FROM THE ADULT

Brain and Spinal Cord

Size and Structure

A. Rapid head growth in early childhood: brain is 25% of adult weight at birth, 75% at 2½ years, and 90% at 6 years.

B. Head growth results from development of nerve tracts within the brain and an increase in nerve fibers, not an increase in the number of neurons.

C. Infant's skull is not a rigid structure.
   1. Bones of skull are not fused until 18 months.
   2. Head circumference will increase with increase in intracranial volume in infants.
   3. Sutures may separate if there is significant gradual increase in intracranial volume up to age 12.

D. Fontanels ("soft spots"): areas of head not covered by skull
   1. Anterior fontanel
      a. Diamond-shaped opening at junction of parietal and frontal bones
      b. Closes between 9 and 18 months
   2. Posterior fontanel
      a. Triangular-shaped opening at junction of occipital and parietal bones
      b. Closes by 2 months
   3. Should feel flat and firm
   4. May be sunken with severe dehydration
   5. Will bulge with increased intracranial pressure (ICP)

Function

A. Cortical functions (e.g., fine motor coordination) are incompletely developed at birth.

B. The autonomic nervous system (ANS) is intact but immature.
   1. Infant has limited ability to control body temperature
   2. Infant's heart rate very sensitive to parasympathetic stimulation

C. Infant's behavior primarily reflexive
   1. Neurologic exam consists of evaluating reflexes
   2. Babinski's reflex normal in infant; disappears after child begins to walk
D. Peripheral neurons not myelinated at birth
   1. Myelination occurs in later infancy
   2. Motor skill development depends on myelinization
E. Infant usually demonstrates a dominance of flexor muscles; extremities will be flexed even when infant is sleeping
F. Small tremors are normal findings during first few months of life: not considered seizure activity if occurring in response to environmental stimuli, if they are not accompanied by abnormal eye movements, and if movements cease with passive flexion

Eye and Vision

A. Vision changes as the eye and eye muscles undergo physiologic change.
B. Visual function becomes more organized.
   1. Binocular vision developed by 4 months
   2. Maturation of eye muscles by 1 year
      a. Nystagmus common in infant
      b. Strabismus (eyes out of alignment when fixating on an object): due to imbalance in extraocular muscles, common up to 6 months, abnormal after 6 months
   3. Visual acuity changes
      a. 16 weeks: 20/50 to 20/100
      b. 1 year: 20/50+
      c. 2 years: 20/40
      d. 3 years: 20/30
      e. 4 years: nearly 20/20

Ear and Hearing

A. Hearing is fully developed at birth.
B. Abnormal physical structure of ears may indicate genetic problems (low-set ears often associated with renal problems or mental retardation).

■ ASSESSMENT

History

A. Most important part of neurologic evaluation
B. Family history: seizure disorders, degenerative neurologic diseases, mental retardation, sensory defects
C. History of pregnancy: maternal illness, placental dysfunction, fetal movements, nuchal cord, intrapartal fetal distress, prematurity, meconium staining, Apgar scores

D. Child's health history: delayed motor or speech development, hypotonia, seizures, childhood illnesses

E. Parental concerns: development, vision, hearing

Physical Examination

A. Inspect size and shape of head: note fontanels in infants, chart head circumference on growth chart.

B. Observe posture and activity: note flexed posture versus hypotonia or opisthotonos, symmetry of movement of extremities, excessive tremors or twitching, abnormal eye movements, ineffective suck or swallow, high-pitched cry.

C. Observe respiratory pattern: note apnea, ataxic breathing, asymmetric or paradoxic chest movement.

D. Determine developmental level with DDST.

E. Vision tests
  1. Binocularity
     a. Corneal light reflex test: performed by shining a light at the bridge of the nose as the child looks straight ahead; light reflex should fall at the same point in both pupils; deviation indicates strabismus
     b. Cover/uncover test: Ask child to fix on an object. Cover one eye, assess uncovered eye movement. Uncover eye, assess that eye for movement. Repeat by covering the other eye. Normal response— no movement of either eye in response to cover/uncover maneuver.
  2. Visual acuity
     a. Snellen E chart or Blackbird cards for preschoolers
     b. Snellen alphabet chart for older children
  3. Peripheral vision
  4. Color vision

F. Auditory tests
  1. Audiometry: perception of sound
  2. Tympanometry: conduction of sound in middle ear
  3. Crib-o-gram: neonatal motor response to sound
  4. Conduction tests
  5. Newborn hearing screening: auditory evoked response

Laboratory/Diagnostic Tests

A. Same neurologic tests that are used in adults are used in children.

B. Child should be carefully prepared and informed of what to expect during the test.

C. Sedation may be required for tests requiring child to be immobile for extended period.

D. Positioning and immobilization is crucial to the success of lumbar puncture.

■ ANALYSIS

Nursing diagnoses for the child with a disorder of the nervous system may include

A. Impaired physical mobility
B. Disturbed thought process
C. Disturbed sensory perceptions
D. Deficient knowledge
E. Pain
F. Compromised or disabled family coping
G. Risk for injury
H. Impaired verbal communication
 I. Risk for impaired skin integrity

■ PLANNING AND IMPLEMENTATION

Goals

A. Child will be protected from injury.
B. Child will be free from signs and symptoms of increased ICP.
C. Normal respiratory function will be maintained.
D. Optimum developmental level will be achieved.
E. Family will be able to care for child at home.

Interventions

Care of the Child with Increased Intracranial Pressure

A. General information
    1. Intracranial volume and pressure can increase as a result of
        a. Increased brain volume (cerebral edema, tumor)
        b. Increased cerebral blood volume (hematoma or hemorrhage)
        c. Increased cerebrospinal fluid (CSF) volume (hydrocephalus)
    2. Herniation of brain tissue: most serious complication of increased ICP; may result in life-threatening deterioration of vital functions
B. Medical management
    1. Directed towards reducing intracranial volume and controlling underlying disorder
    2. Drug therapy
        a. Osmotic diuretics (mannitol, glycerol) to reduce acute brain edema; for short-term use only
        b. Corticosteroids (dexamethasone) to reduce brain swelling
            1) may be used for longer periods than osmotic diuretics
            2) antacids may be given concomitantly to prevent gastric irritation
    3. Fluid restriction, hyperventilation, temperature regulation may all be used to control increased ICP
    4. Surgery: if increased ICP caused by obstruction to CSF, shunt procedures may be performed

C. Assessment findings
   1. Infants
       a. Lethargy, poor feeding, anorexia, vomiting, or irritability
       b. High-pitched cry
       c. Tense, bulging fontanel; increased head circumference; separation of cranial sutures
   2. Children
       a. Anorexia, nausea, vomiting, irritability, or lethargy
       b. Headache, blurred vision, papilledema
       c. Separation of cranial sutures
   3. Late signs
       a. Altered LOC
       b. Pupil dilation and sluggish response to light
       c. Tachycardia then bradycardia
       d. Altered respiratory rate then apnea
       e. Elevation in BP, increased pulse pressure
       f. Unstable temperature
D. Nursing interventions
   1. Administer medications as ordered.
       a. With osmotic diuretics, monitor fluid and electrolyte balance carefully.
       b. With corticosteroids, monitor for signs of gastric bleeding.
   2. Monitor hydration status carefully.
       a. Administer IV fluids as ordered, assess carefully for fluid overload.
       b. Assess for fluid and electrolyte imbalances.
       c. Monitor for hypovolemic shock if on strict fluid restriction.
   3. Assist with hyperventilation if ordered; monitor arterial blood gases (ABGs)
   4. Assist with reduction of body temperature as needed.
       a. Administer antipyretics as ordered.
       b. Use sponge baths, hypothermia pads as necessary.
   5. Monitor LOC and behavioral/mental changes carefully.
   6. Elevate head of bed 30–45° unless contraindicated (e.g., possible spinal injury); keep neck in neutral alignment and avoid flexion.
   7. Arrange nursing care activities to minimize stimulation and keep environment as quiet as possible.
   8. Prepare for shunt surgery (see below) if needed.

■ EVALUATION

A. Head growth progresses normally, fontanels are flat, and seizure activity is controlled.
B. Child maintains an appropriate activity level.
C. Child is placed in an appropriate special program or school, if needed.
D. Parents demonstrate ability to perform treatments and administer appropriate medications.

■ DISORDERS OF THE NERVOUS SYSTEM
Disorders of the Brain and Spinal Cord
Hydrocephalus

A. General information
1. Increased amount of CSF within the ventricles of the brain
2. May be caused by obstruction of CSF flow or by overproduction or inadequate reabsorption of CSF
3. May result from congenital malformation or be secondary to injury, infection, or tumor
4. Classification
   a. Noncommunicating: flow of CSF from ventricles to subarachnoid space is obstructed.
   b. Communicating: flow is not obstructed, but CSF is inadequately reabsorbed in subarachnoid space, or excess CSF is produced.
B. Assessment findings: depend on age at onset, amount of CSF in brain
1. Infant to 2 years: enlarging head size; bulging, nonpulsating fontanels; downward rotation of eyes; separation of cranial sutures; poor feeding, vomiting, lethargy, irritability; high-pitched cry and abnormal muscle tone
2. Older children: changes in head size less common; signs of increased ICP (vomiting, ataxia, headache) common; alteration in consciousness and papilledema late signs
3. Diagnostic tests
   a. Serial transilluminations detect increases in light areas
   b. CT scan shows dilated ventricles as well as presence of mass; with dye injection shows course of CSF flow
C. Nursing interventions: provide care for the child with increased ICP and for the child undergoing shunt procedures.

Shunts

A. General information
1. Insertion of a flexible tube into the lateral ventricle of the brain
2. Catheter is then threaded under the skin and the distal end positioned in the peritoneum (most common type) or the right atrium; a subcutaneous pump may be attached to ensure patency
3. Shunt drains excess CSF from the lateral ventricles of the brain in communicating or noncommunicating hydrocephalus; fluid is then absorbed by the peritoneum or enters the general circulation via the right atrium
B. Nursing interventions
1. Provide routine pre-op care with special attention to monitoring neurologic status.

NURSING ALERT

Folic acid deficiency in the mother is a suspected etiology of the problem.

---

    2. Provide post-op care.
       a. Maintain patency of the shunt.
          1) position child off the operative site.
          2) pump the shunt as ordered.
          3) observe for signs of infection of the incision.
          4) observe for signs of increased ICP.
          5) position the child with head slightly elevated or as ordered.
    3. Instruct parents regarding
       a. Wound care, positioning of infant, and how to pump the shunt
       b. Signs of infection
       c. Signs of increased ICP
       d. Need for repeated shunt revisions as child grows or if shunt becomes blocked or infected
       e. Expected level of developmental functioning
       f. Availability of support groups and community agencies

Spina Bifida (Myelodysplasia)

A. General information
    1. Failure of posterior vertebral arches to fuse during embryologic development
    2. Incidence: 2 in 1,000 infants in the United States
    3. Although actual cause is unknown, frequency of the defect is increased if a sibling has had a neural tube defect; radiation, viral, and environmental factors; and maternal folic acid deficiency have been suggested as causative.
    4. Site of the defect varies
       a. Approximately 85% of the defects in the spine involve the lower thoracic lumbar or sacral area.
       b. Defects in the upper thoracic and cervical regions make up the remaining 15%.
    5. Folic acid supplementation can decrease risk.

B. Types
    1. *Spina bifida occulta*
       a. Spinal cord and meninges remain in the normal anatomic position.
       b. Defect may not be visible, or may be identified by a dimple or a tuft of hair on the spine.
       c. Child is asymptomatic or may have slight neuromuscular deficit.
       d. No treatment needed if asymptomatic; otherwise treatment aimed at specific symptoms.

2. *Spina bifida cystica*
   a. *Meningocele*
      1) sac (meninges) filled with spinal fluid protrudes through opening in spinal canal; sac is covered with thin skin
      2) no nerves in sac
      3) no motor or sensory loss
      4) good prognosis after surgery
   b. *Myelomeningocele/meningomyelocele*
      1) same as meningocele except there are spinal nerves in the sac (herniation of dura and meninges).
      2) child will have sensory/motor deficit below site of the lesion.
      3) 80% of these children have multiple handicaps.
C. Medical management
   1. Surgery
      a. Closure of the sac within 48 hours of birth to prevent infection and preserve neural tissue
      b. Shunt procedure if accompanying hydrocephalus
      c. Orthopedic procedures to correct defects of hips, knees, or feet
   2. Drug therapy
      a. Antibiotics for prevention of infections.
      b. Anticholinergic drugs to increase bladder capacity and lower intravesicular pressure.
   3. Immobilization (casts, braces, traction) for defects of the hips, knees, or feet
D. Assessment findings
   1. Examine the defect for size, level, tissue covering, and CSF leakage.
   2. Motor/sensory involvement may include
      a. Voluntary movement of lower extremities
      b. Withdrawal of lower extremities or crying after pinprick
      c. Paralysis of lower extremities
      d. Joint deformities
      e. Hydrocephalus
      f. Evaluate bowel and bladder function. Neurogenic bowel and bladder occur in up to 90% of the children.
   3. Diagnostic tests
      a. Prenatal
         1) ultrasound image of the pregnant uterus shows fetal spinal defect and sac
         2) amniocentesis: increased alphafetoprotein (AFP) level prior to 18th week of gestation
      b. Postbirth
         1) X-ray of spine shows vertebral defect; CT scan of skull may show hydrocephalus
         2) myelogram shows extent of neural defect
         3) encephalogram may show hydrocephalus

CLIENT TEACHING CHECKLIST

D iscuss with the family the possibility of developing a bowel regime and a clean catheterization schedule; also discuss with the family the signs of shunt infection and malfunction.

---

       4) urinalysis, culture and sensitivity (C&S) may identify organism and indicate appropriate antibacterial therapy

       5) BUN may be increased

       6) creatinine clearance rate may be decreased

E. Nursing interventions

   1. Prevent trauma to the sac.

      a. Cover with sterile dressing soaked with normal saline.

      b. Position infant prone or side-lying.

      c. Keep the area free from contamination by urine or feces. A protective barrier drape may be necessary.

      d. Inspect the sac for intactness or signs of infection.

      e. Administer antibiotics as ordered.

   2. Prevent complications.

      a. Observe for signs of hydrocephalus, meningitis, joint deformities.

      b. Clean intermittent urinary catheterization to manage neurogenic bladder.

      c. Administer medications to prevent urinary complications as ordered.

      d. Perform passive ROM exercises to lower extremities.

   3. Provide adequate nutrition: adapt diet and feeding techniques according to the child's position.

   4. Provide sensory stimulation.

      a. Adjust objects for visual stimulation according to child's position.

      b. Provide stimulation for other senses.

   5. Provide emotional support to parents/family.

   6. Provide client teaching and discharge planning to parents concerning

      a. Wound care

      b. Physical therapy, range of motion exercises

      c. Signs of complications

      d. Medication regimen: schedule, dosage, effects, and side effects

      e. Feeding, diapering, positioning

      f. Availability of appropriate support groups/community agencies/ genetic counseling

Reye's Syndrome

A. General information
   1. An acute encephalopathy with fatty degeneration of the liver
   2. Reye's syndrome is a true pediatric emergency: cerebral complication may reach an irreversible state
   3. Increased ICP secondary to cerebral edema is major factor contributing to morbidity and mortality
   4. Early recognition and prompt management reducing mortality
   5. Etiology unknown
B. Medical management
   1. Proper initial staging essential.
   2. Treatment is supportive, based on stage of coma and level of blood ammonia.
   3. Treatment should take place in a pediatric intensive care unit.
C. Assessment findings
   1. Child appears to be recovering from a viral illness, such as influenza or chickenpox, during which salicylates have been administered; symptoms then appear that follow a definite pattern, which has led to clinical staging.
      a. Stage I: sudden onset of persistent vomiting, fatigue, listlessness
      b. Stage II: personality and behavior changes, disorientation, confusion, hyperreflexia
      c. Stage III: coma, decorticate posturing
      d. Stage IV: deeper coma, decerebrate rigidity
      e. Stage V: seizures, absent deep tendon reflexes, respiratory reflexes, flaccid paralysis
   2. Pathophysiologic changes include
      a. Increased free fatty acid level
      b. Hyperammonemia due to reduction of enzyme that converts ammonia to urea
      c. Impaired liver function
      d. Structural changes of mitochondria in muscle and brain tissue
      e. Significant swelling of the brain
D. Nursing interventions (depend on stage)
   1. Stage I: assess hydration status: monitor skin turgor, mucous membranes, I&O, urine specific gravity; maintain IV therapy.
   2. Stages I–V: assess neurologic status: monitor LOC, pupils, motor coordination, extremity movement, orientation, posturing, seizure activity.
   3. Stages II–V
      a. Assess respiratory status: note changing rate and pattern, presence of circumoral cyanosis, restlessness, agitation.
      b. Assess circulatory status: frequent vital signs, note neck vein distension, skin color and temperature, abnormal heart sounds.
      c. Support child/family.
         1) explain all treatments and procedures.
         2) incorporate family members in treatment as applicable.

> **3)** organize regular family and client-care conferences.
> **4)** use support services as needed.
>
> **d.** Provide additional parental and community education to ensure early recognition and treatment.

Seizure Disorders

A. General information

1. *Seizures:* recurrent sudden changes in consciousness, behavior, sensations, and/or muscular activities beyond voluntary control that are produced by excess neuronal discharge
2. *Epilepsy:* chronic recurrent seizures
3. Incidence higher in those with family history of idiopathic seizures
4. Cause unknown in 75% of epilepsy cases
5. Seizures may be symptomatic or acquired, caused by
   - **a.** Structural or space-occupying lesion (tumors, subdural hematomas)
   - **b.** Metabolic abnormalities (hypoglycemia, hypocalcemia, hyponatremia)
   - **c.** Infection (meningitis, encephalitis)
   - **d.** Encephalopathy (lead poisoning, pertussis, Reye's syndrome)
   - **e.** Degenerative diseases (Tay-Sachs)
   - **f.** Congenital CNS defects (hydrocephalus)
   - **g.** Vascular problems (intracranial hemorrhage)
6. Pathophysiology
   - **a.** Normally neurons send out messages in electrical impulses periodically, and the firing of individual neurons is regulated by an inhibitory feedback loop mechanism
   - **b.** With seizures, many more neurons than normal fire in a synchronous fashion in a particular area of the brain; the energy generated overcomes the inhibitory feedback mechanism
7. Classification (Table 3-1)
   - **a.** Generalized: initial onset in both hemispheres, usually involves loss of consciousness and bilateral motor activity
   - **b.** Partial: begins in focal area of brain and symptoms are related to a dysfunction of that area; may progress into a generalized seizure, further subdivided into simple partial or complex partial

B. Medical management

1. Drug therapy (refer to Anticonvulsants)
   - **a.** Phenytoin (Dilantin)
     - **1)** often used with phenobarbital for its potentiating effect
     - **2)** inhibits spread of electrical discharge
     - **3)** side effects include gum hyperplasia, hirsutism, ataxia, gastric distress, nystagmus, anemia, sedation
   - **b.** Phenobarbital: elevates the seizure threshold and inhibits the spread of electrical discharge
2. Surgery: to remove the tumor, hematoma, or epileptic focus

TABLE 3-1   Types of Seizures

Type of Seizure	Clinical Findings
Generalized seizures	
Major motor seizure (grand mal)	May be preceded by aura; tonic and clonic phases.
	Tonic phase: limbs contract or stiffen; pupils dilate and eyes roll up and to one side; glottis closes, causing noise on exhalation; may be incontinent; occurs at same time as loss of consciousness; lasts 20–40 seconds.
	Clonic phase: repetitive movements, increased mucus production; slowly tapers.
	Seizure ends with postictal period of confusion, drowsiness.
Absence seizure (petit mal)	Usually nonorganic brain damage present; must be differentiated from daydreaming.
	Sudden onset, with twitching or rolling of eyes; lasts a few seconds.
Myoclonic seizure	Associated with brain damage, may be precipitated by tactile or visual sensations.
	May be generalized or local.
	Brief flexor muscle spasm; may have arm extension, trunk flexion.
	Single group of muscles affected; involuntary muscle contractions; myoclonic jerks.
Akinetic seizure (tonic)	Related to organic brain damage.
	Sudden brief loss of postural tone, and temporary loss of consciousness.
Febrile seizure	Common in 5% of population under 5, familial, nonprogressive; does not generally result in brain damage.
	Seizure occurs only when fever is rising. EEG is normal 2 weeks after seizure.

Continued

Table 3-1 Continued

Type of Seizure	Clinical Findings
Partial seizures	
Psychomotor seizure	May follow trauma, hypoxia, drug use. Purposeful but inappropriate, repetitive motor acts.
	Aura present; dreamlike state.
Simple partial seizure	Seizure confined to one hemisphere of brain.
	No loss of consciousness.
	May be motor, sensory, or autonomic symptoms.
Complex partial seizure	Begins in focal area but spreads to both hemispheres.
	Impairs consciousness.
	May be preceded by an aura.
Status epilepticus	Usually refers to generalized grand mal seizures.
	Seizure is prolonged (or there are repeated seizures without regaining consciousness) and unresponsive to treatment.
	Can result in decreased oxygen supply and possible cardiac arrest

C. Assessment findings
  1. Clinical picture varies with type of seizure (see Table 3-1)
  2. Diagnostic tests
     a. Blood studies to rule out lead poisoning, hypoglycemia, infection, or electrolyte imbalances
     b. Lumbar puncture to rule out infection or trauma
     c. Skull X-rays, CT scan, or ultrasound of the head, brain scan, arteriogram, or pneumoencephalogram to detect any pathologic defects
     d. EEG may detect abnormal wave patterns characteristic of different types of seizures
        1) child may be awake or asleep; sedation is ordered and child may be sleep deprived the night before the test
        2) evocative stimulation: flashing strobe light, clicking sounds, hyperventilation

> ### DELEGATION TIP
>
> nstruct ancillary personnel on emergency seizure precautions and encourage them to implement these precautions while calling for help. They should also monitor for breathing and initiate CPR if necessary.

D. Nursing interventions
    1. During seizure activity
        a. Protect from injury.
            1) prevent falling, gently support head.
            2) decrease external stimuli; do not restrain.
            3) do not use tongue blades (they add additional stimuli).
            4) loosen tight clothing.
        b. Keep airway open.
            1) place in side-lying position.
            2) suction excess mucous.
        c. Observe and record seizure.
            1) note any preictal aura.
                a) affective signs: fear, anxiety
                b) psychosensory signs: hallucinations
                c) cognitive signs: ''déjà-vu'' symptoms
            2) note nature of the ictal phase.
                a) symmetry of movement
                b) response to stimuli; LOC
                c) respiratory pattern
            3) note postictal response: amount of time it takes child to orient to time and place; sleepiness.
    2. Provide client teaching and discharge planning concerning
        a. Care during a seizure
        b. Need to continue drug therapy
        c. Safety precautions/activity limitations
        d. Need to wear Medic-Alert identification bracelet or carry identification card
        e. Potential behavioral changes and school problems
        f. Availability of support groups/community agencies
        g. How to assist the child in explaining disorder to peers

Cerebral Palsy (CP)

A. General information
    1. Neuromuscular disorder resulting from damage to or altered structure of the part of the brain responsible for controlling motor function
    2. Incidence: 1.5–5 in 1,000 live births

NURSING ALERT

M any clients have increased caloric requirements due to increased activity and movement .

   3. May be caused by a variety of factors resulting in damage to the CNS; possible causes include
      a. Prenatally: genetic, altered neurologic development, or infection, trauma, or anoxia to mother (toxemia, rubella, accidents, chorioamnionitis)
      b. Perinatally: during the birth process (drugs at delivery, precipitate delivery, fetal distress, breech deliveries with delay)
      c. Postnatally: kernicterus or head trauma (child falls out of crib or is hit by a car)
B. Medical management
   1. Drug therapy
      a. Antianxiety agents
      b. Skeletal muscle relaxants
      c. Local nerve blocks
   2. Physical/occupational therapy
   3. Speech/audiology therapy
   4. Surgery: muscle- and tendon-releasing procedures
C. Assessment findings: disease itself does not progress once established; progressive complications, however, cause changes in signs and symptoms
   1. Spasticity: exaggerated hyperactive reflexes (increased muscle tone, increase in stretch reflex, scissoring of legs, poorly coordinated body movements for voluntary activities)
      a. Occurs with pyramidal tract lesion
      b. Found in 40% of all CP
      c. Results in contractures
      d. Also affects ability to speak: altered quality and articulation
      e. Loud noise or sudden movement causes reaction with increased spasm
      f. No parachute reflex to protect self when falling
   2. Athetosis: constant involuntary, purposeless, slow, writhing motions
      a. Occurs with extrapyramidal tract (basal ganglia) lesion
      b. Found in 40% of all CP
      c. Athetosis disappears during sleep; therefore, contractures do not develop
      d. Movements increase with increase in physical or emotional stress
      e. Also affects facial muscles

3. Ataxia: disturbance in equilibrium; diminished righting reflex (lack of balance, poor coordination, dizziness, hypotonia)
   a. Occurs with extrapyramidal tract (cerebellar) lesion
   b. Found in 10% of all CP
   c. Muscles and reflexes are normal
4. Tremor: repetitive rhythmic involuntary contractions of flexor and extensor muscles
   a. Occurs with extrapyramidal tract (basal ganglia) lesion
   b. Found in 5% of all CP
   c. Interferes with performance of precise movements
   d. Often a mild disability
5. Rigidity: resistance to flexion and extension resulting from simultaneous contraction of both agonist and antagonist muscle groups
   a. Occurs with extrapyramidal tract (basal ganglia) lesion
   b. Found in 5% of all CP
   c. Diminished or absent reflexes
   d. Potential for severe contractures
6. Associated problems
   a. Mental retardation: the majority of CP clients are of normal or higher than average intelligence, but are unable to demonstrate it on standardized tests; 18–50% have some form of mental retardation
   b. Hearing loss in 13% of CP clients
   c. Defective speech in 75% of CP clients
   d. Dental anomalies (from muscle contractures)
   e. Orthopedic problems from contractures or inability to mobilize
   f. Visual disabilities in 28% due to poor muscle control
   g. Seizures
   h. Disturbances of body image, touch, perception
   i. Feelings of worthlessness
D. Nursing interventions
   1. Obtain a careful pregnancy, birth, and childhood history.
   2. Observe the child's behavior in various situations.
   3. Assist with activities of daily living (ADL), help child to learn as many self-care activities as possible; CP clients cannot do any task unless they are consciously aware of each step in the task; careful teaching and demonstration is essential.
   4. Provide a safe environment (safety helmet, padded crib).
   5. Provide physical therapy to prevent contractures and assist in mobility (braces if necessary).
   6. Provide client teaching and discharge planning concerning
      a. Nature of disease: CP is a nonfatal, noncurable disorder
      b. Need for continued physical, occupational, and speech therapy
      c. Care of orthopedic devices
      d. Provision for child's return to school
      e. Availability of support groups/community agencies

Tay-Sachs Disease

A. General information
1. Degenerative brain disease, caused by absence of hexosaminidase A from all body tissues
2. Autosomal recessive inheritance
3. Occurs predominantly in children of Eastern European Jewish ancestry
4. A fatal disease; death usually occurs before age 4
B. Assessment findings
1. Progressive lethargy in a previously healthy 2- to 6-month-old infant
2. Loss of developmental accomplishments
3. Loss of visual acuity
4. Hyperreflexia, decerebrate posturing, dysphagia, malnutrition, seizures
5. Diagnosis confirmed by classic cherry-red spot on the macula and by enzyme measurements in serum, amniotic fluid, or white cells
C. Nursing interventions
1. Support parents at time of diagnosis; help them cope with feelings of anger and guilt.
2. Assist parents in planning long-term care for the child.
3. Provide genetic counseling and psychologic follow-up as needed.

Disorders of the Eye

Blindness

A. Causes
1. Genetic disorders: Tay-Sach's disease, inborn errors of metabolism
2. Maternal infections during pregnancy: TORCH syndrome
3. Perinatal: prematurity, retrolental fibroplasia
4. Postnatal: trauma, childhood infections
B. Medical management: treatment of causative disorders
C. Assessment findings
1. Vacant stare; obvious failure to look at objects
2. Rubbing eyes, tilting head, examining objects very close to the eyes
3. Does not reach for objects (over 4 months)
4. Does not smile when mother smiles (over 3 months) but does smile in response to mother's voice
5. Crawls or walks into furniture (over 12 months)
6. Does not respond to the motions of others
7. No concept of the look of an object, no concept of color or reflection of self
8. Other senses become more keenly developed to compensate
9. Unable to copy the actions of others; delayed motor milestones in accomplishing tasks but are not mentally handicapped
10. Various degrees (20/200 O.U. and worse)
D. Nursing interventions
1. For hospitalized child, find out parents' usual method of care.

2. Encourage infant to be active; use multisensory stimulation (rocking, water play, musical toys, touch).
3. From ages 2–5 arrange environment for maximum autonomy and safety (e.g., avoid foods with seeds and bones).
4. Speak before you touch the child, announce what you plan to do.
5. Do not rearrange furniture without first telling child.
6. For a partially sighted child
   a. Encourage child to sit in front of classroom.
   b. Speak directly to child's face; do not look down or turn back.
   c. Use large print and provide adequate nonglare lighting.
   d. Use contrasting colors to help locate areas.
7. Provide client teaching and discharge planning concerning
   a. General child care, with adaptations for safety and developmental/functional level
   b. Availability of support groups/community agencies
   c. Special education programs
   d. Interaction with peers: assist child as necessary

Conjunctivitis

A. General information: infection of membrane covering anterior surface of eye globe and inner surface of eyelid due to multiple causes (bacterial, viral, allergic)
B. Medical management: ophthalmic antibiotics, steroids, anesthetics
C. Assessment findings: weeping eye, reddened conjunctiva, sensitivity to light, eyelid stuck shut with exudate
D. Nursing interventions
   1. Administer medications as ordered: apply ophthalmic antibiotic ointments from inner to outer canthus (do not let container touch eye).
   2. Provide client teaching and discharge planning concerning measures to prevent spread of infection
      a. Very contagious if bacterial or viral; no school until antibiotics have been taken for 24–48 hours
      b. Should not share pillows, tissues, toys
      c. Good hand-washing technique
      d. Medication regimen: schedule, dosage, desired and side effects

Disorders of the Ear

Deafness

A. Causes
   1. Conductive: interference in transmission from outer to middle ear from chronic otitis media, foreign bodies
   2. Sensorineural: dysfunction of the inner ear; damage to cranial nerve VIII (from rubella, meningitis, drugs)

B. Medical management
  1. Treatment of causative disorders
  2. Speech/auditory therapy
  3. Hearing aids
  4. Surgery, depending on the cause
      a. Cochlear implant for neural deafness
C. Assessment findings
  1. Infant
      a. Fails to react to loud noises (does have a Moro reflex, but not to noise)
      b. Makes no attempt to locate sound
      c. Remains in babbling stage or ceases to babble
      d. Fails to develop speech
      e. Startled by sudden appearances
  2. All children
      a. Respond only when speaker's lips are visible
      b. Cannot concentrate for long on visual images; constantly scan the surroundings for change
      c. May have slow motor development
      d. Appear puzzled or withdrawn, or strain to hear
      e. Use high volume on TV/radio
  3. Audiologic testing
      a. Slight hearing deficit: difficulty hearing faint sounds, very little interference in school, no speech defect, benefits from favorable seating
      b. Mild hearing deficit: can understand conversational speech at 3-5 feet when facing the other person, decreased vocabulary, may miss half of class discussions
      c. Marked hearing deficit: misses most of conversation, hears loud noises, needs special education for language skills
D. Nursing interventions
  1. Speak slowly, not more loudly.
  2. Face child.
  3. Get child's attention before talking; let child see you before performing any care.
  4. Get feedback from child to make sure child has understood.
  5. Decrease outside noises that could interfere with child's ability to discern what you are saying.
  6. Be careful not to cover your mouth with hands.
  7. Teach language through visual cues, touch, and kinesthetics.
  8. Use body demonstrations or use doll play.
  9. Provide appropriate stimulation (puppets and musical toys are inappropriate).
  10. Provide client teaching and discharge planning concerning
      a. General child care, with adaptation for safety and developmental/functional levels

    b. Availability of support groups/community agencies

    c. Special education programs

    d. Care and use of hearing aids, cochlear implant equipment

    e. Interaction with peers: assist child as needed

Otitis Media

A. General information

    1. Bacterial or viral infection of the middle ear

    2. More common in infants and preschoolers as the ear canal is shorter and more horizontal than in older children; also found in children with cleft lip/palate

    3. Blockage of eustachian tube causes lymphedema and accumulation of fluid in the middle ear

B. Medical management

    1. Drug therapy

        a. Systemic and otic antibiotics

        b. Analgesics/antipyretics

    2. Surgery: myringotomy, with or without insertion of tubes (incision into the tympanic membrane to relieve the pressure and drain the fluid)

C. Assessment findings

    1. Dysfunction of eustachian tube

    2. Ear infection usually related to respiratory infection

    3. Increased middle ear pressure; bulging tympanic membrane

    4. Pain; infant pulls or touches ear frequently

    5. Irritability; cough; nasal congestion

    6. Diagnostic tests: C&S of fluid reveals causative organism

D. Nursing interventions

    1. Administer antibiotics as ordered, for a full 10-day course. When administering ear drops pull earlobe up and back for children older than 3 years and down and back if younger.

    2. Administer acetaminophen for fever and discomfort.

    3. Administer decongestants to relieve eustachian tube obstruction as ordered.

    4. Provide care for child with a myringotomy tube insertion (day surgery)

        a. Child should wear earplugs when swimming, showering, or having hair washed; do not permit diving.

        b. Be aware that tubes may fall out for no reason.

    5. Provide client teaching and discharge planning concerning

        a. Medication administration

        b. Post-op care, depending on the type of surgery

REVIEW QUESTIONS

1. An infant who was born with a myelomeningocele with accompanying hydrocephalus has had a shunt procedure to alleviate the hydrocephalus. The baby should be placed in which of the following positions?
   1. Trendelenburg.
   2. Supine.
   3. Lithotomy.
   4. Prone.

2. The nurse is caring for an infant who is born with hydrocephalus and has a shunt inserted. Which of the following signs indicates that the shunt is functioning properly?
   1. The sunset sign.
   2. A bulging anterior fontanel.
   3. Decreasing daily head circumference.
   4. Widened suture lines.

3. A 13-year-old has been diagnosed as having epilepsy. A positive sign that the child is taking his Dilantin properly is
   1. hair growth on his upper lip.
   2. absence of seizures.
   3. lowered hemoglobin and hematocrit.
   4. drowsiness.

4. A 3-year-old is admitted with a diagnosis of viral meningitis. During an initial assessment the nurse would expect to find
   1. headache, fever, and petechiae.
   2. seizures, lethargy, and hypothermia.
   3. pallor, anorexia, and bulging fontanels.
   4. fever, irritability, and nuchal rigidity.

5. To meet the sensory need of a child with viral meningitis, nursing strategies should include
   1. minimizing bright lights and noise.
   2. promoting active range of motion.
   3. increasing environmental stimuli.
   4. avoiding physical contact with family members.

6. When addressing the emotional needs of the parents of a young child with meningitis, the primary focus should be on

1. assuming all responsibility for physical care of the child.

2. providing reassurance that the symptoms will resolve within the week.

3. reinforcing information about the child's condition and plan of treatment.

4. explaining the importance of an optimistic outlook when interacting with their child.

7. Discharge teaching for the parents of a child who had viral meningitis should include

   1. engaging a tutor to assist with learning problems.

   2. administering the prescribed antibiotic.

   3. notifying the physician if the child's fever or headache persists more than a few days after discharge.

   4. encouraging the child to resume normal activities immediately.

8. A 6-year-old is brought to the emergency department unconscious after being hit by a car. The most helpful information for the nurse performing the neurological examination is the nurse's knowledge of

   1. normal growth and development.

   2. the child's usual behavior and status.

   3. the child's past medical history.

   4. the child's growth and developmental progress during infancy.

9. The nurse is assessing a child who has a head injury for the occulocephalic reflex (doll's eyes). The nurse understands that the doll's eye reflex is present if the child's eyes

   1. move in the same direction in which his head is turned.

   2. move in the direction opposite to which his head is turned.

   3. remain midline when his head is turned.

   4. move to the medial aspect of the orbit when his head is turned.

10. The pupils of a child with a head injury are dilated and react sluggishly. This is indicative of

    1. barbiturate overdosage.

    2. damage to the diencephalon.

    3. damage to the sympathetic system.

    4. damage to the parasympathetic system.

11. A 4-year-old female is admitted to the pediatric intensive care unit (PICU) after suffering a severe closed head injury following a car accident. An intracranial

pressure (ICP) monitor is in place and reveals an ICP of 40 mmHg. In an effort to lower the ICP, the nurse knows the *best* position for the client would be

1. supine with the head turned to the right.
2. supine with the head turned to the left.
3. supine with the head midline.
4. side-lying on the right with the head turned to the left.

12. A 5-year-old female is admitted to the PICU after being hit by a car while riding her bike. She sustained a severe closed head injury and has an ICP monitor in place. Her ICP is 40 mmHg and mannitol is ordered. What is the rationale for administering mannitol for a child with an increased ICP?

1. It will produce a rise in the intravascular osmolality, resulting in a shift of free water from the interstitial and cellular spaces to the intravascular space, thus decreasing the ICP.
2. It will produce a decrease in the intravascular osmolality, resulting in a shift of free water from the interstitial and cellular spaces to the intravascular space, thus decreasing the ICP.
3. It will produce a rise in the intravascular osmolality, resulting in a shift of free water from the intravascular space to the cellular space, thus decreasing the ICP.
4. It will produce a decrease in the intravascular osmolality, resulting in a shift of free water from the interstitial space to the cellular space, thus decreasing the ICP.

13. An infant who has a ventriculoperitoneal (VP) shunt in place for treatment of hydrocephalus is hospitalized for potential shunt malfunction. When developing the plan of care, which of the following assessment findings would the nurse list as a *positive* sign of shunt malfunction?

1. Overriding sutures.
2. Bulging, tense anterior fontanel.
3. Flat, soft anterior fontanel.
4. Consistent head circumference.

14. A male newborn was just admitted to the pediatric floor with a myelomeningocele. When developing the preoperative plan of care, the nurse lists "high risk for infection of and trauma to the nonepithelialized lesion" as the diagnosis of most concern. The *most effective* strategy to prevent infection and trauma to the lesion would be to

1. leave the lesion uncovered and open to the air and place the baby supine.
2. cover the lesion with sterile, saline-soaked gauze and place the baby prone.

3. apply lotion to the lesion and place the baby on his side.

4. cover the lesion with dry sterile gauze and place the baby supine.

15. The nurse has been giving instructions to parents on measures to prevent Reye's syndrome. When questioning the parents on a safe medication to provide to their child during a viral illness, which choice indicates that they understand steps toward Reye's syndrome prevention?

1. Pepto-Bismol.

2. Acetaminophen (Tylenol).

3. Children's aspirin.

4. Adult aspirin.

16. The nurse is caring for a 5-year-old boy with a known seizure disorder. On entering his room, the nurse sees that he is experiencing a generalized, tonic-clonic seizure. The *first* intervention for the nurse would be to

1. immediately leave the room to retrieve intravenous (IV) phenobarbital.

2. place a metal spoon between his teeth to prevent him from biting his tongue.

3. position him on his side to maintain a patent airway.

4. try to hold the client down.

17. When assessing a client who is taking hydantoin (Dilantin), the nurse would recognize which of the following findings as side effects?

1. Drowsiness and irritability.

2. Slurred speech and increased salivation.

3. Hair loss and tremor.

4. Gum hyperplasia and nystagmus.

18. A 12-year-old girl with cerebral palsy has severe language deficits and poor muscle coordination.However, she can voluntarily turn her head from side to side and her mother reports that she has normal intelligence. The nurse is concerned with the child's ability to call when help is needed. Considering the child's abilities, which of the following would be the *best* way for her to call the nurse?

1. Kick the side rails of the bed.

2. Scream loudly.

3. Press the call bell with her fingers.

4. Press a large, padded call bell with her cheek.

19. When teaching a child measures to prevent spread of conjunctivitis, the nurse would recognize that *further* instruction is necessary when the child states the following,

1. "It is important that I wash my hands regularly."
2. "I can use a tissue to clean my eyes, but must throw it away immediately."
3. "I need to use my own washcloth and towel, not my sister's."
4. "My Dad said he would carry a handkerchief with him so I could wipe my eyes with it during the day."

20. A woman brings her daughter to the pediatric clinic because she is concerned that the child has otitis media. On examination, the nurse would recognize which of the following findings as the *most common* positive sign of otitis media?
    1. Temperature of 39°C and loss of appetite.
    2. Pearly gray tympanic membrane and rhinorrhea.
    3. Pain on pressure on the tragus and edema within the canal.
    4. Feeling of "fullness" in the ear and a popping sensation during swallowing.

ANSWERS AND RATIONALES

1. **4.** Pressure must be kept off the spinal sac.
2. **3.** With improved draining of the CSF, the head circumference should become smaller.
3. **2.** Phenytoin (Dilantin) is an antiepileptic drug that controls seizures. Absence of seizures indicates the client is taking the medication properly.
4. **4.** The clinical symptoms of viral (aseptic) meningitis include fever, irritability, and stiffness of the neck (nucchal rigidity). Other symptoms include drowsiness, photophobia, weakness, painful extremities, and sometimes seizures. Aseptic meningitis usually resolves within 2 weeks.
5. **1.** Photophobia and hypersensitivity to environmental stimuli are common clinical manifestations of meningeal irritation and infection. Comfort measures include providing an environment that is quiet and has minimal stressful stimuli.
6. **3.** Successful coping in times of anxiety and stress requires that the nurse be available to provide information that validates parental right to know and participation in their child's care.
7. **3.** Parents should be instructed to contact the physician if the child's symptoms worsen or persist. The child recovering from viral meningitis should show signs of feeling better a week after discharge.
8. **2.** The child's usual behavior and level of development is what provides critical baseline information about his pretrauma neurological condition.

9. **2.** The occulocephalic reflex occurs if, when the head of an unconscious child is turned rapidly in one direction, the eyes move in the opposite direction.

10. **4.** When dilated pupils react sluggishly to light or are nonreactive, it is an indication that there has been damage to the parasympathetic nervous system, which controls the pupillary constriction response.

11. **3.** The client's head must be kept in midline to facilitate venous return. Clients with a severe closed head injury have low intracranial compliance and turning of the head may result in an increase of ICP of 10-15 mmHg. The head of bed (i.e., 30°) should be determined individually for each client based on the ICP and cerebral perfusion pressure (CPP) as well as the clinical appearance.

12. **1.** A shift in fluid from the interstitial and cellular space to the intravascular space will occur with a rise in intravascular osmolality, the fluid will then be diuresed resulting in a decreased ICP.

13. **2.** This is a common sign of shunt malfunction. The best way to assess an infant's fontanel is when the infant is upright and calm. In this position, a fontanel that is bulging and firm to light palpation is considered abnormal.

14. **2.** The lesion must be kept moist with sterile, saline-soaked gauze. The prone position should be maintained preoperatively to prevent tension on the lesion and minimize trauma.

15. **2.** Acetaminophen does not contain salicylates, which have been suspected as an ingredient that can lead to Reye's syndrome.

16. **3.** The first priority is to maintain a patent airway. The best position for the client during a seizure is on his side.

17. **4.** Hydantoin (Dilantin) may cause gum hyperplasia and nystagmus. Other side effects include hirsutism, ataxia, diplopia, anorexia, nausea, nervousness, and folate deficiency.

18. **4.** She is able to control her head movements voluntarily. A large padded call bell could easily be pressed when she turns her head to the side.

19. **4.** The eye should be wiped with disposable tissues after a single use and no other individual should be exposed to items that come in contact with the infected eye.

20. **1.** Common signs of otitis media include fever (as high as 40°C), postauricular and cervical lymph gland enlargement, rhinorrhea, vomiting, diarrhea, loss of appetite, and red tympanic membrane. Infants become irritable, hold their ears, and roll their head from side to side. Young children verbally complain of pain. A concurrent respiratory or pharyngeal infection may also be present.

4

The Cardiovascular System

■ VARIATIONS FROM THE ADULT

Fetal Circulation

A. Fetal circulation differs from adult circulation in several ways and is designed to ensure a high-oxygen blood supply to the brain and myocardium.

B. Characteristics
   1. Placenta is the source of oxygen for the fetus.
   2. Fetal lungs receive less than 10% of the blood volume; lungs do not exchange gas.
   3. Right atrium of fetal heart is the chamber with the highest oxygen concentration.

C. Pattern of altered blood flow and facilitating structures
   1. Blood is carried from the placenta through the umbilical vein and enters the inferior vena cava through the ductus venosus.
   2. This permits most of the highly oxygenated blood to go directly to the right atrium, bypassing the liver.
   3. This right atrial blood flows directly into the left atrium through the foramen ovale, an opening between the right and left atria.
   4. From the left atrium, blood flows into the left ventricle and aorta, through the subclavian arteries, to the cerebral and coronary arteries, resulting in the brain and heart receiving the most highly oxygenated blood.
   5. Deoxygenated blood returns from the head and arms through the superior vena cava, enters the right atrium, and passes into the right ventricle.
   6. Blood from the right ventricle flows into the pulmonary artery, but because fetal lungs are collapsed, the pressure in the pulmonary artery is very high.
   7. Because pulmonary resistance is high, most of the blood passes into the distal aorta through the ductus arteriosus, which connects the pulmonary artery and the aorta distal to the origin of the subclavian arteries.
   8. From the aorta, blood flows to the rest of the body.

Normal Circulatory Changes at Birth

A. When the umbilical cord is clamped or severed, the blood supply from the placenta is cut off, and oxygenation must then take place in the newborn's lungs.

B. As the lungs expand with air, the pulmonary artery pressure decreases and circulation to lungs increases.

C. Structural changes

1. Ductus venosus: after the umbilical cord is severed, flow through the ductus venosus decreases and eventually ceases; it constricts within 3–7 days after birth and eventually becomes ligamentum venosum.

2. Foramen ovale
   a. Functional closure of this valvelike opening occurs when pressure in the left atrium exceeds pressure in the right.
   b. Expansion of the pulmonary artery causes a drop in pulmonary artery pressure and in right atrial and ventricular pressure.
   c. At the same time there is increased pulmonary blood flow to the left atrium and increased aortic pressure (from clamping of the umbilical cord), which in turn raises left ventricular and left atrial pressure.
   d. Anatomic closure of the foramen ovale occurs within the first weeks after birth with the deposit of fibrin.

3. Ductus arteriosus
   a. Increase in aortic blood flow increases aortic pressure and decreases right-to-left shunt through the ductus arteriosus; shunt becomes bidirectional.
   b. Increased pulmonary blood flow increases arterial oxygen, causing vasoconstriction of ductus arteriosus within hours of birth.
   c. Functional closure occurs when this constriction causes cessation of blood flow, usually 24 hours after birth.
   d. Anatomic closure occurs when there is growth of fibrous tissue in the lumen of the ductus arteriosus, by 1–3 weeks.

Abnormal Circulatory Patterns after Birth

A. Normal blood flow in the child may be disrupted as a result of abnormal openings between the pulmonary and systemic circulations.

B. Any time there is a defect connecting systemic and pulmonary circulation, blood will go from high to low pressure (the path of least resistance).

1. Normally pressure is higher in the systemic circulation, so blood will be shunted from systemic to pulmonary (left to right).

2. An obstruction to pulmonary blood flow, however, may cause increased pressure proximal to the site of the obstruction.

3. With an obstruction to pulmonary blood flow, as well as an opening between ventricles, the blood flow may be right to left (if right-sided pressure exceeds left-sided pressure).

NURSING ALERT

C hildren with congenital heart defects are often asymptomatic if the defect is small.

■ ASSESSMENT
Overview

A. Approximately 40,000 babies are born with congenital heart disease (CHD) in the United States yearly.
B. One-third of these babies will be seriously ill at birth, one-third will have problems detected during childhood or later, and one-third never have problems.
C. Etiology is multifactional.

History

A. Family history: parental history of CHD, congenital defects in siblings, history of genetic problems in family.
B. History of pregnancy: rubella, viral infections, medications, X-ray exposure, alcohol ingestion, cigarette smoking.
C. Child's health history
   1. Presenting problem: symptoms may include
      a. Feeding problems: fatigue, irritability, tachypnea, profuse sweating
      b. Failure to thrive
      c. Respiratory difficulties: tachypnea, difficulty breathing, frequent respiratory infections
      d. Color changes: pallor, cyanosis (persistent or intermittent)
      e. Activity intolerance
      f. All presenting symptoms must be explored within a developmental framework
   2. Past medical history: rheumatic fever; associated chromosomal abnormalities (e.g., Down syndrome)

Physical Examination

A. Plot height and weight on growth chart; measure respiratory rate and rhythm; inspect for chest enlargement or asymmetry.
B. Inspect for presence of cyanosis: lips, mucous membranes, extremities.
C. Inspect for clubbing of fingers (thought to be caused by increased capillary formation and soft tissue fibrosis).
D. Observe for distended veins.
E. Palpate/percuss quality and symmetry of pulses, size of liver and spleen, presence of thrill over heart during expiration.

F. Auscultate for heart rate and rhythm.
G. Auscultate for abnormal heart sounds and murmurs; murmurs are caused by abnormal flow of blood between chambers or vessels; classified as
   1. Innocent: no anatomic or physiologic abnormality
   2. Functional: no anatomic defect, but may be caused by a physiologic abnormality
   3. Organic: caused by a structural abnormality
H. Measure blood pressure in both arm and thigh.
   1. In infants under 1 year, arm and thigh blood pressure should be the same.
   2. In children over 1 year, systolic pressure in leg is usually higher by 10–40 mmHg.
   3. A wide pulse pressure (greater than 50 mmHg) or a narrow pulse pressure (less than 10 mmHg) may be associated with a heart defect.
I. Select proper blood pressure cuff size.
   1. Too small a cuff can give a falsely elevated BP reading
   2. Bladder inside the cuff should be two-thirds the length of the upper arm

Laboratory/Diagnostic Tests

A. Chest X-ray
B. Cardiac fluoroscopy
C. Magnetic resonance imaging (MRI)
D. Electrocardiogram
E. Echocardiography
F. Hematologic testing: polycythemia is often associated with cyanotic heart defects
G. Cardiac catheterization
   1. Femoral vein often used for access
   2. Catheter threaded into right side of the heart since septal defects permit entry into the left side
   3. Nursing care: pretest
      a. Child's preparation should be based on developmental level, level of understanding, and past experience.
      b. Use doll play and pictures as appropriate.
      c. Describe sensations child will feel in simple terms.
      d. Administer medications as ordered.
   4. Nursing care: posttest
      a. Check extremity distal to the catheterization site for color, temperature, pulse, capillary refill.
      b. Keep extremity distal to the catheterization site extended for 6 hours.
      c. Check pressure dressing over catheterization site for bleeding.

    d. Monitor heart rate for signs of bradycardia, tachycardia, and dysrhythmia.

    e. Monitor for transient temperature elevation due to physiologic dehydration (NPO, contrast media).

    f. Monitor urine output and blood pressure.

■ ANALYSIS

Nursing diagnoses for the child with a disorder of the cardiovascular system may include

A. Delayed growth and development

B. Risk for injury: physiologic

C. Imbalanced nutrition: less than body requirements

D. Fear/anxiety

E. Risk for infection

F. Deficient knowledge

G. Decreased cardiac output

H. Excess fluid volume

■ PLANNING AND IMPLEMENTATION
Goals

A. Tissue will be adequately oxygenated.

B. Child will achieve normal growth and development milestones.

C. Child will be free from symptoms of complications of heart disease.

D. Parents will understand child's condition.

E. Parents will be able to care for child at home.

Interventions
Care of the Child with Heart Failure (HF)

A. General information

    1. Usually due to a surgically correctable structural abnormality of the heart that results in increased blood volume and pressure or increased pulmonary blood flow

    2. A symptom complex reflecting the heart's inability to meet the metabolic demands of the body

B. Medical management

    1. Directed toward improvement of cardiac function and energy conservation

    2. Drug therapy

        a. Digitalis to improve myocardial contractility and slow the heart rate

        b. ACE inhibitors to decrease cardiac afterload

        c. Diuretics to decrease total body water and to increase urine output

        d. Potassium supplement if diuretic is potassium depleting

     3. High-caloric formula or nasogastric feedings may be required to meet nutritional needs

C. Assessment findings

     1. Tachycardia, gallop rhythm, cardiomegaly, decreased peripheral pulses, and mottling of the extremities

     2. Tachypnea, retractions, grunting, nasal flaring, cough, cyanosis, orthopnea

     3. Hepatomegaly, edema, distended neck and peripheral veins, decreased urine output

     4. Failure to thrive, decreased exercise tolerance

D. Nursing interventions

     1. Decrease energy expenditure

          a. Frequent rest periods

          b. Small, frequent feedings

          c. Minimize crying

          d. Prevent cold stress

     2. Provide adequate nutrition

          a. Estimate daily caloric requirement

          b. Use soft nipple

          c. Consider gavage feeding if necessary

     3. Monitor fluid status

          a. I&O, specific gravity

          b. Daily weight

     4. Administer medications as ordered

          a. Digoxin

               1) check dosage with another RN

               2) give 1 hour before feeding or 2 hours after feeding

               3) take apical pulse for 1 minute; if bradycardia is present, hold dose and contact physician

               4) monitor serum potassium levels; if less than 3.5 mEq/L, may be contraindicated

               5) monitor therapeutic effects; therapeutic serum digoxin levels range from 0.8 to 2.0 µg/L.

               6) monitor for toxicity: nausea, anorexia, vomiting, lethargy, bradycardia

               7) parent/child teaching

          b. ACE inhibitors—also monitor BP

          c. Diuretic

               1) intake and output

               2) daily weight

               3) monitor side effects: dehydration, electrolyte imbalance especially hypokalemia (potentiates digoxin and may lead to toxicity)

               4) parent/child teaching

5. Provide adequate rest
6. Prevent infections
7. Promote growth and development
8. Reduce respiratory distress
   a. Position in semi- or high-Fowler's position
   b. Knee-chest position for children with tetralogy of Fallot

■ EVALUATION

A. Child demonstrates optimal cardiac status.
   1. Normal color
   2. No respiratory distress
   3. Increased exercise tolerance
   4. Satisfactory growth
B. Child has no evidence of complications.
C. Parents demonstrate ability to care for child, perform necessary treatments, and administer prescribed medications.

■ DISORDERS OF THE CARDIOVASCULAR SYSTEM
Congenital Heart Defects

See Figure 4-1.

Classification

A. Defects associated with increased pulmonary blood flow
   1. Left-to-right shunting of blood across a septal defect or blood vessel (higher left side heart pressure)
   2. Pulmonary overcirculation and increased work of ventricles, possible right ventricular hypertrophy
   3. Risk for heart failure
   4. Usually acyanotic
   5. Examples: atrial septal defect, ventricular septal defect, patent ductus arteriosus, atrioventricular canal (also called endocardial cushion defect)
B. Defects associated with decreased pulmonary blood flow
   1. Right-to-left shunting of blood due to presence of a defect and obstruction of pulmonary blood flow (obstructed pulmonary flow leads to higher right side heart pressure)
   2. Some or most blood does not enter the pulmonary circulation and does not pick up oxygen in the lungs; instead, blood is shunted to the left side of the heart
   3. Deoxygenated as well as oxygenated blood circulated to the body
   4. Cyanosis and hypoxemia present
   5. Example: tetralogy of Fallot

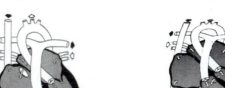

Atrial Septal Defect   Ventricular Septal Defect

Patent Ductus Arteriosus   Coarctation of the Aorta   Transposition of Great Arteries

Truncus Arteriosus   Tetralogy of Fallot

FIGURE 4-1   Congenital heart abnormalities

C. Defects causing obstruction to cardiac chamber outflow
   1. Narrowing of outflow tract from heart to blood vessels
   2. Increased work of heart as it strains to push blood out
   3. Risk for heart failure and poor cardiac output
   4. Examples: coarctation of the aorta, pulmonic stenosis, aortic stenosis
D. Defects associated with mixing of saturated and desaturated blood
   1. Oxygenated and deoxygenated blood mixes in heart chambers
   2. Increased pulmonary blood flow due to defect
   3. Hypoxemia and cyanosis present, often severe
   4. Risk for poor cardiac output and risk for heart failure (HF).

5. Examples: transposition of the great vessels (also called transposition of the great arteries), truncus arteriosus, hypoplastic left heart syndrome

Increased Pulmonary Blood Flow

A. General information and medical management
1. Atrial septal defect (ASD): opening between right and left atria with left-to-right shunting of blood
    a. 15% of congenital heart defects
    b. Manifestations dependent on age and size and location of defect.
    c. Small lesions may be asymptomatic until childhood.
    d. Dyspnea, tachycardia, growth failure, HF may be present. Systolic pulmonary ejection murmur present.
    e. Surgical repair includes patching of defect—open heart/cardiopulmonary bypass procedure. Some defects plugged during cardiac catheterization.
2. Ventricular septal defect (VSD): opening in ventricular septum with left-to-right shunting of blood
    a. 25% of congenital heart defects.
    b. Manifestations dependent on age, size of defect, and degree of pulmonary vascular resistance. Usually found in infancy.
    c. Small lesions may be asymptomatic; may close spontaneously.
    d. With large lesions, higher pressure in ventricles results in high degree of shunting.
    e. Risk for right ventricular hypertrophy, HF, bacterial endocarditis, pulmonary problems.
    f. Dyspnea, tachycardia, growth failure, HF, frequent respiratory infections common. Harsh systolic murmur at lower left sternal border present.
    g. Surgical repair includes suturing or patching of defect using open heart/cardiopulmonary bypass procedure, usually done in infancy. Primary (complete) repair is preferred.
    h. Occasionally, surgical palliation with pulmonary artery banding for severely ill infants, with complete repair when infant is more stable. Banding decreases blood flow through pulmonary artery: decreases pressure difference between right and left ventricles to decrease left-to-right shunting of blood across defect.
3. Patent ductus arteriosus (PDA): failure of fetal ductus arteriosus to close after birth
    a. 10% of congenital heart defects in term infants, more common in preterm infants.
    b. Blood vessel connecting pulmonary artery and aorta.
    c. Higher pressure in aorta results in left-to-right shunting of blood from aorta to pulmonary circulation.

      d. Manifestations depend on size of defect. Small lesions may be asymptomatic.

      e. Risk for HF.

      f. May have bounding pulses and visible precordial pulsations (especially preterm infants). Continuous machine-like murmur at upper left sternal border.

      g. Administration of indomethacin may close defect in preterm infants.

      h. If indomethacin fails, or if not a preterm infant, surgical ligation of vessel (closed heart procedure) or mechanical occlusion of vessel.

   4. Atrioventricular canal (AV canal): combination septal defect resulting in large opening between right and left atria and ventricles and defects of valves.

      a. Most common cardiac defect in children with Down syndrome.

      b. High degree of left-to-right shunting of blood.

      c. Heart failure commonly develops. Pulmonary flow murmurs and valvular murmurs present.

      d. Open heart/cardiopulmonary bypass surgical repair.

B. Assessment findings in conditions with increased pulmonary blood flow

   1. Poor feeding, anorexia

   2. Growth failure, poor weight gain

   3. Respiratory difficulties: tachypnea, dyspnea, orthopnea, coughing, wheezing, hoarseness, grunting, nasal flaring, retractions, frequent respiratory infections

   4. Exercise intolerance, fatigue, lethargy, excessive sweating with feeding or activity

   5. Signs/symptoms of heart failure

   6. Cardiac murmur

C. Nursing interventions

   1. Prepare child/family for diagnostic studies, surgery.

   2. Administer medications as ordered. See HF.

   3. Ensure adequate nutrition.

      a. Anticipate infant hunger to prevent crying and increased oxygen demands.

      b. Small, frequent feedings/small frequent, nutritious meals if child.

      c. Feed infants in semi-upright position.

      d. Soft nipple to decrease fatigue during infant feedings. Gavage feedings may be necessary.

      e. Burp frequently during bottle and breast feedings.

      f. Observe for tolerance of feedings if high-calorie formula or breast milk fortifier used: vomiting, diarrhea.

      g. Assist breastfeeding mothers.

      h. Monitor growth.

   4. Monitor vital signs.

5. Provide rest.
    a. Quiet age-appropriate play if HF present.
    b. Cluster care to provide periods of undisturbed rest.
    c. Anticipate needs; prevent crying.
6. Position semi-upright if HF or respiratory difficulty present.
7. Prevent infections.
8. Meet age-appropriate developmental needs.
9. Bacterial endocarditis antibiotic prophylaxis for unrepaired ASD, VSD, PDA, and all other CHD before or after repair. Give prescribed antibiotic 1 hour before dental, genitourinary tract, and surgical procedures. Will be required throughout life.
10. Teach care to family.

Decreased Pulmonary Blood Flow

A. General information and medical management
    1. Tetralogy of Fallot (TOF)
        a. Most common CHD causing cyanosis and hypoxemia; 10% of all CHD.
        b. Four associated defects: pulmonary stenosis, VSD, overriding aorta (also called dextropositioned aorta), right ventricular hypertrophy.
        c. Pulmonary stenosis creates obstruction to outflow of blood from right ventricle to pulmonary artery, causing decreased pulmonary blood flow. Increased right ventricle pressure creates right-to-left shunt. Right-shifted aorta sits over VSD so blood from both right and left ventricles flows into aorta.
        d. Aorta carries mixed oxygenated and deoxygenated blood to body.
        e. Manifestations include low oxygen saturation, cyanosis, polycythemia, activity intolerance, fatigue, poor feeding, poor growth, harsh systolic murmur along left sternal border, hypercyanotic spells (also called TET spells), also signs of chronic hypoxia.
        f. Hypercyanotic spells: occur when oxygen demand exceeds supply.
            1) transient obstruction of pulmonary blood flow.
            2) increasing cyanosis, tachypnea, poor muscle tone, loss of consciousness.
            3) May progress to seizures, CVA, death. often precipitated by crying, feeding, defecation.
            4) treat by placing in knee-chest position, give oxygen, morphine, occasionally propranolol.
        g. Surgical repair includes open heart/cardiopulmonary bypass procedure to patch VSD and relieve stenosis. Palliative surgery to increase pulmonary blood flow includes anastomosis of right or left subclavian artery to pulmonary artery (Blalock-Taussig shunt).

B. Assessment findings in conditions with decreased pulmonary blood flow
 1. Low oxygen saturation
 2. Cyanosis
 3. Polycythemia (chronic hypoxemia results in increased production of RBCs)
 4. Clubbing of digits (chronic hypoxia)
 5. Poor feeding, anorexia, fatigue, activity intolerance, growth failure, weak cry
 6. Squatting: increases systemic vascular resistance and improves pulmonary blood flow (not seen frequently due to early repair of cardiac defects)
 7. Hypercyanotic (TET) spells
 8. Tachycardia, tachypnea, dyspnea
 9. Cardiac murmur
 10. Risk for emboli, bacterial endocarditis
C. Nursing interventions
 1. Squatting: observe only. No other intervention needed unless distress develops.
 2. Cluster care. Provide age-appropriate quiet activities. Promote uninterrupted rest.
 3. Provide oxygen as needed.
 4. Prevent crying; anticipate needs.
 5. Monitor vital signs.
 6. Support nutrition (see interventions for increased pulmonary blood flow).
 7. Prepare child/family for diagnostic tests and surgery.
 8. Administer medications as ordered.
 9. Bacterial endocarditis prophylaxis as above.
 10. For hypercyanotic spells, place in knee-chest position, administer oxygen, prepare to administer morphine.
 11. Meet age-appropriate developmental needs.
 12. Teach care to parents.

Obstruction to Outflow

A. General information and medical management
 1. Coarctation of the aorta: narrowing of a portion of aorta, usually near aortic arch beyond left subclavian artery
   a. Decreased blood flow to lower part of body, more blood shunted to arms and head.
   b. Manifestations dependent on degree of narrowing, include arm blood and pulse pressures greater than in legs, strong brachial and diminished femoral pulses, lower body cooler than upper. In older children, dizziness, headaches, fainting, epistaxis occur.
   c. Risk for heart failure, hypertension, rupture of aorta, CVA.
   d. Vascular surgery to remove narrowed portion or repair with graft.

2. Pulmonic stenosis: narrowed pulmonic valve opening
   a. Minor to moderate narrowing may be asymptomatic.
   b. Severe narrowing causes increased work of right ventricle and ventricular hypertrophy.
   c. Manifestations: cyanosis, systolic thrill, systolic ejection murmur at upper left sternal border.
   d. Repair includes balloon angioplasty to dilate stenosed area or surgical valvotomy.
3. Aortic stenosis: narrowed aortic valve
   a. Increased resistance to left ventricular blood outflow into aorta.
   b. Leads to left ventricular hypertrophy, left-sided heart failure.
   c. Manifestations include faint pulses, tachycardia, hypotension, poor feeding, exercise intolerance, aortic murmur.
   d. Repair: balloon angioplasty or valvotomy.
B. Assessment findings: HF, cardiac murmur; also see individual defects
C. Nursing interventions
   1. Monitor for hypotension.
   2. Monitor for HF.
   3. Monitor for cyanosis and hypoxemia in children with pulmonic stenosis.
   4. Prepare child and family for diagnostic/therapeutic procedures and surgery.
   5. Support nutrition as above.
   6. Promote rest as above.
   7. Administer medications as ordered.
   8. Bacterial endocarditis prophylaxis as above.
   9. Meet age-appropriate developmental needs.
   10. Teach care to parents.

Lesions with Mixing of Saturated and Desaturated Blood

A. General information and medical management
   1. Transposition of the great vessels (transposition of the great arteries): aorta emerges from right ventricle and pulmonary artery emerges from left ventricle.
      a. Essentially two independent circulations:
         1) unoxygenated blood from right ventricle exits to aorta, goes to body and returns to right atrium without flowing to lungs.
         2) oxygenated blood exits left ventricle to pulmonary arteries, goes to lungs, and returns to left atrium.
      b. Incompatible with life unless there is communication between left and right sides of heart (usually through foramen ovale or PDA).
      c. Manifestations include neonatal cyanosis, hypoxemia, systolic murmur.
      d. Treatment includes administration of Prostaglandin E to maintain patency of ductus arteriosus, balloon atrial septostomy (also called Rashkind procedure) during cardiac catheterization to improve mixing of blood in atria.

NURSING ALERT

C hildren with minimum communication are severely cyanotic and depressed at birth. Prostaglandin E1 is given to prevent closure of a patent ductus.

    e. Surgical repair: arterial switching procedure in newborn period or installation of atrial baffle to direct venous blood to left ventricle and oxygenated blood to right ventricle (Senning and Mustard procedures) in older children (rarely used).

2. Truncus arteriosus: failure of embryonic blood vessel to divide into aorta and pulmonary artery results in one large vessel positioned over both ventricles.

    a. Has associated large VSD.

    b. Both oxygenated and deoxygenated blood flow to systemic circulation; blood flow and pressure in pulmonary circulation are increased.

    c. Manifestations include cyanosis, growth failure, activity intolerance, heart failure.

    d. Treatment includes digoxin and diuretics for HF.

    e. Surgical repair includes open heart/cardiopulmonary bypass procedure to close VSD, incorporate trunk into left ventricle, grafting of right and left pulmonary arteries to right ventricle.

3. Hypoplastic left heart syndrome: poorly developed left side of heart, including hypoplastic left ventricle, aortic valve atresia or mitral valve atresia, narrowed ascending aorta and aortic arch.

    a. Some oxygenated blood flows from left atrium across foramen ovale to right atrium, enters pulmonary circulation, and flows across PDA into aorta.

    b. Clinical manifestations include progressive cyanosis, pallor, weak or absent pulses, HF, shock.

    c. Treatment includes administration of Prostaglandin E to maintain PDA, administration of medications to support blood pressure and cardiac function.

    d. Usually fatal without surgery or heart transplantation.

        1) Norwood procedure (palliative): connect pulmonary artery and aorta, create ASD, allows mixed blood to get to tissues.

        2) repair includes intracardiac redirection of blood flow (Fontan procedure) involving open heart/cardiopulmonary bypass technique.

        3) heart transplant may be performed.

B. Assessment findings in conditions with mixing of oxygenated and deoxygenated blood

1. Cyanosis and hypoxemia

2. Tachycardia, dyspnea, tachypnea

CLIENT TEACHING CHECKLIST

Instruct the family regarding:

- Home care requirements related to nutrition, rest, and oxygenation,
- Safe administration of medications (cardiac drugs and diuretics).

    3. Cardiac murmur
    4. Poor feeding, growth failure, activity intolerance, weak cry, lethargy
    5. Varying degrees of HF
    6. Polycythemia
    7. Clubbing of digits
    8. Risk for bacterial endocarditis, emboli, stroke
C. Nursing interventions
    1. Prepare child/family for diagnostic procedures and surgery.
    2. Assess vital signs and assess for poor cardiac output.
    3. Monitor infants receiving Prostaglandin E for apnea, hypotension, hypothermia.
    4. Cluster care to provide periods of uninterrupted rest.
    5. Provide oxygen as ordered.
    6. Prevent crying; anticipate needs.
    7. Support nutrition (see interventions for increased pulmonary blood flow).
    8. Bacterial endocarditis prophylaxis as above.
    9. Meet age-appropriate developmental needs.
    10. Teach care to parents.

Cardiac Surgery

A. General information
    1. Surgical correction of congenital defects within the heart, or surgery of the great vessels in the immediate area surrounding the heart
    2. Open-heart surgery (uses cardiopulmonary bypass): provides a relatively blood-free operative site; heart-lung machine maintains gas exchange during surgery
    3. Closed-heart surgery does not use cardiopulmonary bypass machine; indicated for ligation of a patent ductus arteriosus or coarctation of the aorta
B. Nursing interventions: preoperative
    1. Determine the child's level of understanding; have child draw a picture, tell you a story, or use doll play.
    2. Correct misunderstandings/teach the child about the surgery using diagrams and play therapy; use terms appropriate to developmental level.

3. Accompany the child to the operating and recovery rooms and the intensive care unit, explaining the various equipment; allow child to handle/experience it, if possible, and introduce staff and clients, depending on child's developmental/emotional levels.
4. Have child practice post-op procedures (turning, coughing, deep breathing, etc.).
5. Include parents in teaching sessions, but have separate sessions for the parents only.
6. Establish pre-op baseline data for vital signs, activity/sleep patterns, I&O.

C. Nursing interventions: postoperative
   1. Prevent injury/complications.
      a. Monitor vital signs and circulatory pressure readings frequently until stable. Monitor EKG.
      b. Assess neurologic status frequently.
      c. Observe surgical site for intactness/drainage.
   2. Promote gas exchange (client may be on mechanical ventilation).
      a. Position as ordered.
      b. Administer oxygen at prescribed rate.
      c. Provide humidification.
      d. Suction as necessary.
      e. Perform postural drainage and chest percussion as ordered.
      f. Turn, cough, and deep breathe hourly.
      g. Perform routine care of chest tubes and drainage system, depending on the type of surgery.
   3. Monitor I&O.
   4. Provide nutrition as ordered.
   5. Provide alternative means of communication if mechanical ventilation is used, e.g., picture cards.
   6. Provide psychologic support of the child/family.
   7. Allow activity as tolerated.
   8. Provide client teaching and discharge planning concerning
      a. Need for child/family to express feelings/fears
      b. Resumption of ADL
      c. Assisting child in dealing with peers/returning to school
      d. Referral for parents to support groups/community agencies

Acquired Heart Disease

Rheumatic Fever (RF)

A. General information
   1. An inflammatory disorder that may involve the heart, joints, connective tissue, and the CNS
   2. Peaks in school-age children; linked to environmental factors and family history of disorder

3. Thought to be an autoimmune disorder
   a. Preceded by an infection of group A beta-hemolytic streptococcus (usually a strep throat); the heart itself is not infected, however.
   b. Antigenic markers for strep toxin closely resemble markers for heart valves; this resemblance causes antibodies made against the strep to also attack heart valves.
4. Prognosis depends on degree of heart damage

B. Medical management
   1. Drug therapy
      a. Penicillin
         1) used in the acute phase
         2) used prophylactically for several years after the attack
         3) erythromycin substituted if child is sensitive to penicillin
      b. Salicylates: for analgesic, anti-inflammatory, antipyretic effect
      c. Steroids: for anti-inflammatory effect
   2. Decrease cardiac workload: bed rest until lab studies return to normal

C. Assessment findings
   1. Major symptoms (Jones' criteria)
      a. Carditis
         1) seen in 50% of clients
         2) Aschoff nodules (areas of inflammation and degeneration around heart valves, pericardium, and myocardium)
         3) valvular insufficiency of mitral and aortic valves possible
         4) cardiomegaly
         5) shortness of breath, hepatomegaly, edema
      b. Polyarthritis
         1) migratory, therefore no contractures develop
         2) most common in large joints, which become red, swollen, painful
         3) synovial fluid is sterile
         4) no arthralgia
      c. Chorea (Sydenham's chorea, St. Vitus' dance): CNS disorder characterized by abrupt, purposeless, involuntary muscular movements
         1) gradual, insidious onset: starts with personality change or clumsiness
         2) mostly seen in prepubertal girls
         3) may appear months after strep infection
         4) movements increase with excitement
         5) lasts 1–3 months

    d. Subcutaneous nodules
        1) usually a sign of severe disease
        2) occur with active carditis
        3) firm, nontender nodes on bony prominences of joints
        4) lasts for weeks
    e. Erythema marginatum: transient, nonpruritic rash starting with central red patches that expand; results in series of irregular patches with red, raised margins and pale centers (resemble giraffe spots)
  2. Minor symptoms
    a. Reliable history of RF, fever
    b. Recent history of strep infection
    c. Diagnostic tests: erythrocyte sedimentation rate (ESR) and antistreptolysin O (ASO) titer increased; changes on ECG
D. Nursing interventions
  1. Carditis
    a. Administer penicillin as ordered.
        1) used prophylactically to prevent future attacks of strep and further damage to the heart
        2) to be taken until age 20 or for 5 years after attack, whichever is longer
    b. Promote bed rest until ESR returns to normal.
  2. Arthritis: administer aspirin as ordered, change child's position in bed frequently.
  3. Chorea
    a. Decrease stimulation.
    b. Provide a safe environment: no forks with meals, assistance with mobility.
    c. Provide small, frequent meals; increased muscle activity causes increased kcal requirements.
  4. Nodules and rash: none.
  5. Alleviate child's anxiety about the ability of heart to continue to function.
  6. Prevent recurrent infection.
  7. Minimize boredom with age-appropriate sedentary play.
  8. Provide client teaching and discharge planning concerning
    a. Adaptation of home environment to promote bed rest (commode, call bell, diversional activities)
    b. Importance of prophylactic medication regimen
    c. Diet modification in relation to decreased activity/cardiac demands
    d. Avoidance of reinfections
    e. Home-bound education
    f. Availability of community agencies

REVIEW QUESTIONS

1. A 4-year-old with tetralogy of Fallot is seen in a squatting position near his bed. The nurse should
   1. administer oxygen.
   2. take no action if he looks comfortable but continue to observe him.
   3. pick him up and place him in Trendelenburg's position in bed.
   4. have him stand up and walk around the room.

2. A 2-month-old is suspected of having coarctation of the aorta. The cardinal sign of this defect is
   1. clubbing of the digits and circumoral cyanosis.
   2. pedal edema and portal congestion.
   3. systolic ejection murmur.
   4. upper extremity hypertension.

3. When assessing the apical heart rate in infants and toddlers, the point of maximal impulse (PMI) is
   1. between the third and fourth left intercostal space.
   2. between the fourth and fifth left intercostal space.
   3. at the fifth intercostal space to the right of the midclavicular line.
   4. in the aortic area.

4. A 2-week-old infant has a patent ductus arteriosus. Prior to administering digoxin the nurse should
   1. take the apical pulse for 30 seconds and multiply by 2.
   2. give the medication if his pulse is 92, but notify the physician.
   3. take the radial pulse for 1 full minute.
   4. give the medication after finding that the apical pulse is 135 beats/minute.

5. The nurse is planning care for a 2-week-old infant who has a congenital heart defect. Which of the following actions are appropriate? Select all that apply.
   1. _____ Using a soft "preemie" nipple for feedings.
   2. _____ Providing passive stimulation.
   3. _____ Allowing him to cry to promote increased oxygenation.
   4. _____ Placing him in orthopneic position.

6. A 10-year-old has been hospitalized for 2 weeks with rheumatic fever. The child's mother questions whether her other children can catch the rheumatic fever. The nurse's best response is

   1. "The fact that you brought your child to the hospital early enough will decrease the chance of your other children getting it."
   2. "It is caused by an autoimmune reaction and is not contagious."
   3. "You appear concerned that your child's disease is contagious.
   4. "Your other children should be taking antibiotics to prevent them from catching rheumatic fever."

7. A 10-year-old child is admitted with rheumatic fever. In addition to carditis, the nurse should assess the child for the presence of

   1. arthritis.
   2. bronchitis.
   3. malabsorption.
   4. oliguria.

8. An infant's blood pressure is reported to be very high. What is the most appropriate nursing action to take?

   1. Take it again in 20 minutes.
   2. Call the house officer.
   3. Measure the cuff width to the infant's arm.
   4. Prepare to give an antihypertensive.

9. Prior to discharge from the newborn nursery at 48 hours old, the nurse knows that murmurs are frequently assessed and are most often due to which factor?

   1. A ventricular septal defect.
   2. Heart disease of the newborn period.
   3. Transition from fetal to pulmonic circulation.
   4. Cyanotic heart disease.

10. A 10-year-old with a ventricular septal defect (VSD) is going to have a cardiac catheterization.Which of the following needs to be a high priority for the nurse to assess?

    1. Capillary refill.
    2. Breath sounds.
    3. Arrhythmias.
    4. Pedal pulses.

11. An infant with heart failure (HF) is admitted to the hospital. Which goal has the highest priority when planning nursing care?

    1. The infant will maintain an adequate fluid balance.
    2. The infant will have digoxin at the bedside.
    3. Skin integrity will be addressed.
    4. Administer medications on time.

12. An infant on the ward is receiving digoxin and diuretic therapy. The nurse knows that which of the following choices indicates no toxicity?

    1. Heart rate less than 100, no dysrhythmias.
    2. Heart rate of 80–100.
    3. Heart rate greater than 100, no dysrhythmias.
    4. Vomiting.

13. An infant with cardiac disease has been admitted to the nursery from the delivery room. Which finding helps the nurse to differentiate between a cyanotic and an acyanotic defect?

    1. Infants with cyanotic heart disease feed poorly.
    2. The pulse oximeter does not read above 93%.
    3. Infants with cyanotic heart disease usually go directly to the operating room.
    4. Cyanotic heart disease causes high fevers.

14. A child with tetralogy of Fallot has been admitted. What equipment is most important to have at the bedside?

    1. Morphine.
    2. A blood pressure cuff.
    3. A thermometer.
    4. An oxygen setup.

15. A 9-year-old boy has been transferred back to the floor after cardiac surgery. Which of the following does the nurse need to include in the plan of care to evaluate that the fluid needs are being appropriately met?

    1. Call if the heart rate falls below 60 per minute.
    2. Place a Foley catheter.
    3. Prepare to assist with an arterial line to monitor blood pressure.
    4. Calculate the daily maintenance fluid requirements and ensure correct delivery.

16. A 9-year-old girl with rheumatic fever is asking to play. Which diversional activity is the nurse likely to offer?

1. Walking to the gift store.

2. Coloring books and crayons.

3. A 300 piece puzzle.

4. A dancing contest.

17. A 10-year-old has been diagnosed with rheumatic fever and is now being discharged. What statement made by the parents shows an understanding of long-term care?

    1. "She will need penicillin each day."

    2. "She will need antibiotic prophylaxis when she has dental work."

    3. "We will have yearly checkups."

    4. "The murmur will always go away by adolescence."

ANSWERS AND RATIONALES

1. **2.** Squatting is a normal response in a child who has tetralogy of Fallot. This position increases pulmonary blood flow because it changes the relationship between systemic and pulmonary vascular resistance.

2. **4.** Coarctation of the aorta is characterized by upper extremity hypertension and diminished pulses in the extremities.

3. **1.** The heartbeat is most easily counted at the point of maximum impulse. From birth through toddlerhood it is located between the third and fourth left intercostal space.

4. **4.** The apical pulse is taken for one full minute and the medication is withheld if the pulse is less than 100 beats/minute.

5. **1.** Using a soft "preemie" nipple for feedings should be selected. This will help to reduce energy expenditure.
   Providing passive stimulation should be selected. This will help to reduce energy expenditure.
   Placing the child in orthopneic position should be selected. This will help promote oxygenation.

6. **2.** Rheumatic fever is an autoimmune reaction to a streptococcal infection and is limited to the person having the reaction. It is not a contagious disease.

7. **1.** A major symptom of rheumatic fever is arthritis.

8. **3.** The cuff should be approximately two-thirds the length of the humerus.

9. **3.** As the transition occurs, the murmurs may become loud, and then resolve.

10. **4.** The nurse needs to know the baseline pedal pulses.

11. 1. This is a major priority for HF clients.

12. 3. Infants' heart rates need to be greater than 100, with no rhythm disturbances.

13. 2. Cyanotic heart disease is unlikely to produce a reading above 93%.

14. 3. This is used emergently in a Tet spell.

15. 4. It is vital for pediatric nurses to know exactly how much fluid should be delivered each 24 hours to evaluate proper fluid needs.

16. 3. This will be quiet, yet stimulating.

17. 2. This will be necessary for many years.

5

The Hematologic System

■ VARIATIONS FROM THE ADULT

A. In the young child all the bone marrow is involved in blood cell formation.
B. By puberty, only the sternum, ribs, pelvis, vertebrae, skull, and proximal epiphyses of femur and humerus are involved.
C. During the first 6 months of life, fetal hemoglobin is gradually replaced by adult hemoglobin, and it is only after this that hemoglobin disorders can be diagnosed.

■ ASSESSMENT

History

A. Family history: genetic hematologic disorders, anemia, or jaundice
B. History of pregnancy: parents' blood types, anemia, infection or drug ingestion, course of labor and delivery
C. Child's health history
   1. Neonatal course: occurrence, duration, and treatment of jaundice; bleeding episodes; blood transfusions
   2. Accidents, operations, hospitalizations (any blood transfusions or unusual bleeding)
   3. Nutrition: dietary intake of iron and vitamin B_{12}; history of pica
   4. Ingestions: lead-based paint; drugs
   5. Ability to participate in age-appropriate activities

Physical Examination

A. General appearance
   1. Skin: note whether cyanotic, pale, ruddy, jaundiced; note bruises or petechiae, other evidences of hemorrhage; pain, swelling around joints.
   2. Neurologic status: note listlessness or fatigue, irritability, dizziness, or lightheadedness.
B. Measure vital signs; note tachycardia or tachypnea.

   C. Plot height and weight on growth chart.

   D. Inspect and palpate abdomen; note enlargement of liver and spleen, pain, or tenderness on palpation.

■ ANALYSIS

Nursing diagnoses for the child with a disorder of the hematologic system may include

A. Activity intolerance

B. Pain

C. Impaired gas exchange

D. Ineffective tissue perfusion: cardiopulmonary

E. Imbalanced nutrition

■ PLANNING AND IMPLEMENTATION
Goals

A. Child will have adequate tissue oxygenation.

B. Child will be free from complications associated with hematologic diseases.

C. Child will be free from pain, or have pain controlled.

D. Optimal growth and developmental level will be achieved.

E. Parents will participate in care of child.

■ EVALUATION

A. Serum values of hematologic components are normal.

B. Child is free from signs or symptoms of infection.

C. Child has no abnormal bleeding episodes.

D. Normal activity level is maintained without pain or fatigue.

E. Parents are able to describe symptoms of disease and complications.

F. Parents are able to administer medications and participate in child's care.

■ DISORDERS OF THE HEMATOLOGIC SYSTEM
Anemias
Iron Deficiency Anemia

A. General information: iron deficiency is most common cause of anemia in children; children whose diet consists mainly of cow's milk, which is low in absorbable iron, are especially vulnerable.

B. Assessment findings

   1. Pallor, fatigue, irritability

   2. History of iron-deficient diet

    3. Diagnostic tests
       a. RBC normal or slightly reduced
       b. Hgb below normal range for child
       c. Hct below normal
C. Nursing interventions
    1. Add iron to formula, food, or by vitamins by age 4–6 months.
       a. Oral iron
          1) give iron with citrus juice and on empty stomach (iron is best absorbed in an acidic environment).
          2) have child use straw if possible, since iron stains teeth and skin.
       b. Administer IM iron if ordered. Use z-track method.
    2. Provide iron-rich foods: meats, nuts, dried beans/legumes, dried fruit, dark-green leafy vegetables, whole grains, egg yolk, potatoes, shellfish.
D. Also see page 274.

Sickle-Cell Anemia

A. General information (see Figure 5-1)
    1. Most common inherited disorder in U.S. African American population; sickle cell trait found in 10% of African Americans.
    2. Autosomal recessive inheritance pattern.
    3. Individuals who are homozygous for the sickle cell gene have the disease (more than 80% of their hemoglobin is abnormal [HgbS]).
    4. Those who are heterozygous for the gene have sickle cell trait (normal hemoglobin predominates, may have 25–50% HgbS). Although sickle cell trait is not a disease, carriers may exhibit symptoms under periods of severe anoxia or dehydration.
    5. In this disease, the structure of hemoglobin is changed; the sixth rung of the beta chain changes glutamine for valine.
    6. HgbS (abnormal Hgb), which has reduced oxygen-carrying capacity, replaces all or part of the hemoglobin in the RBCs.
    7. When oxygen is released, the shape of the RBCs changes from round and pliable to crescent shaped, rigid, and inflexible.
    8. Local hypoxia and continued sickling lead to plugging of vessels.
    9. Sickled RBCs live for 6–20 days instead of 120, causing hemolytic anemia.
    10. Usually no symptoms prior to age 6 months; presence of increased level of fetal hemoglobin tends to inhibit sickling.
    11. Death often occurs in early adulthood due to occlusion or infection.
    12. *Sickle cell crisis*
       a. Vaso-occlusive (thrombocytic) crisis: most common type
          1) crescent-shaped RBCs clump together; agglutination causes blockage of small blood vessels.

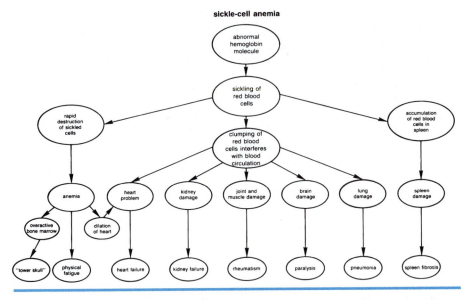

FIGURE 5-1   A series of damages and effects caused by sickle-cell anemia

      2) blockage causes the blood viscosity to increase, producing sludging and resulting in further hypoxia and increased sickling.

    b. *Splenic sequestration:* often seen in toddler/preschooler

      1) sickled cells block outflow tract resulting in sudden and massive collection of sickled cells in spleen.

      2) blockage leads to hypovolemia and severe decrease in hemoglobin and blood pressure, leading to shock.

B. Medical management: sickle cell crisis

  1. Drug therapy

    a. Urea: interferes with hydrophobic bonds of the HgbS molecules

    b. Analgesics/narcotics to control pain

    c. Antibiotics to control infection

  2. Exchange transfusions

  3. Hydration: oral and IV

  4. Bed rest

  5. Surgery: splenectomy

C. Assessment findings

  1. First sign in infancy may be "colic" due to abdominal pain (abdominal infarct)

  2. Infants may have dactylitis (hand-foot syndrome): symmetrical painful soft tissue swelling of hands and feet in absence of trauma (aseptic, self-limiting)

  3. Splenomegaly: initially due to hemolysis and phagocytosis; later due to fibrosis from repeated infarct to spleen

NURSING ALERT

A ny condition which creates the need for additional oxygen, such as dehydration, fever, and unnecessary exertion, can precipitate a sickle-cell crisis.

4. Weak bones or spinal defects due to hyperplasia of marrow and osteoporosis
5. Frequent infections, especially with *H. influenzae* and *D. pneumoniae*
6. Leg ulcers, especially in adolescents, due to blockage of blood supply to skin of legs
7. Delayed growth and development, especially delay in sexual development
8. CVA/infarct in the CNS
9. Renal failure: difficulty concentrating urine due to infarcts; enuresis
10. Heart failure due to hemosiderosis
11. Priapism: may result in impotence
12. Pain wherever vaso-occlusive crisis occurs
13. Development of collateral circulation
14. Diagnostic tests
    a. Hgb indicates anemia, usually 6–9 g/dl
    b. Sickling tests
       1) sickle cell test: deoxygenation of a drop of blood on a slide with a cover slip; takes several hours for results to be read; false negatives for the trait possible.
       2) Sickledex: a drop of blood from a finger stick is mixed with a solution; mixture turns cloudy in presence of HgbS; results available within a few minutes; false negatives in anemia clients or young infants possible.
    c. Hgb electrophoresis: diagnostic for the disease and the trait; provides accurate, fast results.
D. Nursing interventions: sickle cell crisis
    1. Keep child well hydrated and oxygenated.
    2. Avoid tight clothing that could impair circulation.
    3. Keep wounds clean and dry.
    4. Provide bed rest to decrease energy expenditure and oxygen use.
    5. Correct metabolic acidosis.
    6. Administer medications as ordered.
       a. Analgesics: acetaminophen, Ketoralac (NSAID), morphine (avoid aspirin as it enhances acidosis, which promotes sickling).
       b. Avoid anticoagulants (sludging is not due to clotting)
       c. Antibiotics
    7. Administer blood transfusions as ordered.
    8. Keep arms and legs from becoming cold.

NURSING ALERT

TP frequently occurs in children ages 2–5. Guard against injury by supervising activities and maintaining a safe environment.

9. Decrease emotional stress.
10. Provide good skin care, especially to legs.
11. Test siblings for presence of sickle cell trait/disease.
12. Provide client teaching and discharge planning concerning
    a. Pre-op teaching for splenectomy if needed
    b. Genetic counseling
    c. Need to avoid activities that interfere with oxygenation, such as mountain climbing, flying in unpressurized planes

Disorders of Platelets or Clotting Mechanism

Idiopathic Thrombocytopenic Purpura (ITP)

A. General information
   1. Increased destruction of platelets with resultant platelet count of less than 100,000/mm³ characterized by petechiae and ecchymoses of the skin
   2. Exact cause unknown; may be an autoimmune mechanism; onset sudden, often preceded by a viral illness
   3. The spleen is the site for destruction of platelets; spleen is not enlarged
B. Medical management
   1. Drug therapy: steroids, immunosuppressive agents, anti-D antibody
   2. Platelet transfusion
   3. Surgery: splenectomy
C. Assessment findings
   1. Petechiae: spider-web appearance of bleeding under skin due to small size of platelets
   2. Ecchymosis
   3. Blood in any body secretions, bleeding from mucous membranes, nosebleeds
   4. Diagnostic tests: platelet count decreases, anemia
D. Nursing interventions
   1. Control bleeding
      a. Administer platelet transfusions as ordered.
      b. Apply pressure to bleeding sites as needed.
      c. Position bleeding part above heart level if possible.
   2. Prevent bruising.

3. Provide support to client and be sensitive to change in body image.
4. Protect from infection.
5. Measure normal circumference of extremities for baseline.
6. Administer medications orally, rectally, or IV, rather than IM; if administering immunizations, give subcutaneously (SC) and hold pressure on site for 5 minutes.
7. Administer analgesics (acetaminophen) as ordered; avoid aspirin.
8. Provide care for the client with a splenectomy.
9. Provide client teaching and discharge planning concerning
    a. Pad crib and playpen, use rugs wherever possible.
    b. Provide soft toys.
    c. Sew pads in knees and elbows of clothing.
    d. Provide protective headgear during toddlerhood.
    e. Use soft Toothettes instead of bristle toothbrushes.
    f. Keep weight to low normal to decrease extra stress on joints.
    g. Use stool softeners to prevent straining.
    h. Avoid contact sports; suggest swimming, biking, golf, pool.

Hemophilia

A. General information
    1. A group of bleeding disorders where there is a deficit of one of several factors in clotting mechanism
    2. Sex-linked, inherited disorder; classic form affects males only
    3. Types
        a. *Hemophilia A:* factor VIII deficiency (75% of all hemophilia)
        b. *Hemophilia B (Christmas disease):* factor IX deficiency (10–12% of all hemophilia)
        c. *Hemophilia C:* factor XI deficiency (autosomal recessive, affects both sexes)
    4. Only the intrinsic system is involved; platelets are not affected, but fibrin clot does not always form; bleeding from minor cuts may be stopped by platelets.
    5. If individual has less than 20–30% of factor VIII or IX, there is an impairment of clotting and clot is jelly-like.
    6. Bleeding in neck, mouth, and thorax requires immediate professional care.

B. Assessment findings
1. Prolonged bleeding after minor injury
   a. At birth after cutting of cord
   b. Following circumcision
   c. Following IM immunizations
   d. Following loss of baby teeth
   e. Increased bruising as child learns to crawl and walk
2. Bruising and hematomas but no petechiae
3. Peripheral neuropathies (due to bleeding near peripheral nerves): pain, paresthesias, muscle atrophy
4. Hemarthrosis
   a. Repeated bleeding into a joint results in a swollen and painful joint with limited mobility
   b. May result in contractures and possible degeneration of joint
   c. Knees, ankles, elbows, wrists most often affected
5. Diagnostic tests
   a. Platelet count normal
   b. Prolonged coagulation time: PTT increased
   c. Anemia
C. Nursing interventions
1. Control acute bleeding episode.
   a. Apply ice compress for vasoconstriction.
   b. Immobilize area to prevent clots from being dislodged.
   c. Elevate affected extremity above heart level.
   d. Provide manual pressure or pressure dressing for 15 minutes; do not keep lifting dressing to check for bleeding status.
   e. Maintain calm environment to decrease pulse.
   f. Avoid sutures, cauterization, aspirin: all exacerbate bleeding.
   g. Administer hemostatic agents as ordered.
      1) fibrin foam
      2) topical application of adrenalin/epinephrine to promote vasoconstriction
2. Provide care for hemarthrosis.
   a. Immobilize joint and control acute bleeding.
   b. Elevate joint in a slightly flexed position.
   c. Avoid excessive handling of joint.
   d. Administer analgesics as ordered; pain relief will minimize increases in pulse rate and blood loss.
   e. Aspirin should not be given because it inhibits platelet function.
   f. Instruct to avoid weight bearing for 48 hours after bleeding episode if bleeding is in lower extremities.
   g. Provide active or passive ROM exercises after bleeding has been controlled (48 hours), as long as exercises do not cause pain or irritate trauma site.

CLIENT TEACHING CHECKLIST

To minimize throat discomfort teach parents to offer the child:

- drinks such as milk shakes
- fruit ice
- cool bland foods
- Warm saline gargles
- analgesics

---

3. Administer factor VIII concentrate, or DDAVP as ordered
4. Provide client teaching and discharge planning concerning
   a. Prevention of trauma (see Idiopathic Thrombocytopenic Purpura)
   b. Genetic counseling
      1) when mother is carrier: 50% chance with each pregnancy for sons to have hemophilia, 50% chance with each pregnancy for daughters to be carriers
      2) when father has hemophilia, mother is normal: no chance for children to have disease, but all daughters will be carriers
   c. Availability of support/counseling agencies

Disorder of White Blood Cells

Infectious Mononucleosis

A. General information
   1. Viral infection that causes hyperplasia of lymphoid tissue and a characteristic change in mononuclear cells of the blood
   2. Affects adolescents and young adults most commonly
   3. Caused by the Epstein-Barr virus, which is not highly contagious but is transmitted by saliva (the "kissing disease")
   4. Incubation period 2-6 weeks
   5. Pathophysiology: mononuclear infiltration of lymph nodes and other body tissue
B. Assessment findings
   1. Lethargy
   2. Sore throat/tonsilitis
   3. Lymphadenopathy; enlarged spleen, liver involvement
   4. Diagnostic tests
      a. Atypical WBCs increased
      b. Heterophil antibody and Monospot tests positive

REVIEW QUESTIONS

1. The mother of a child with classic hemophilia asks the nurse what her chances are of having another child with hemophilia. The nurse's best response is
   1. "All of your daughters will be carriers of the disease."
   2. "If you have another son, there is almost a 100% chance he will have hemophilia."
   3. "If you have a son, there is a 50% chance he will have hemophilia but none of your daughters are likely to have it."
   4. "There is a 25% chance of having another child with hemophilia."

2. A 4-year-old has been diagnosed as having iron deficiency anemia. A liquid iron preparation has been prescribed. When administering medication the nurse should
   1. ask the child if he wants to take his medicine.
   2. mix the medication in his milk bottle and give it to him at nap time.
   3. allow him to sip the medication through a straw.
   4. give the medication after lunch with a sweet dessert to disguise the taste.

3. A 10-year-old has hemophilia A and is admitted to the hospital for hemarthrosis of the right knee. He is in a great deal of pain. Which of the following interventions would aggravate his condition?
   1. Applying an ice bag to the affected knee.
   2. Administering children's aspirin for pain relief.
   3. Elevating the right leg above the level of his heart.
   4. Keeping the right leg immobilized.

4. The client with sickle cell trait
   1. has a chronic form of sickle cell anemia.
   2. has the most lethal form of the disease.
   3. will transmit the disease to all children.
   4. has some normal and some abnormal hemoglobin cells.

5. The mother of a child with sickle cell anemia tells the nurse that, when she was reading about sickle cell anemia, she learned that sickled blood cells do not have as long a life expectancy as normal red cells. The nurse knows the expectancy of a sickled blood cell is approximately
   1. 5 days.
   2. 15 days.

3. 30 days.

4. 60 days.

6. The child with sickle cell anemia may exhibit

1. vitiligo.

2. hyperactivity.

3. mild mental retardation.

4. delayed physical development.

7. A child who has sickle cell anemia has developed stasis ulcers on her lower extremities.This is due to

1. poor range of motion.

2. ruptured blood vessels.

3. impaired venous circulation.

4. hypertrophy of muscular tissue.

8. Which complication is associated with sickle cell anemia?

1. Constipation.

2. Hypothyroidism.

3. Addison's disease.

4. Cerebrovascular accidents.

9. Both parents carry the sickle cell anemia trait. Their 8-month-old child contracted chickenpox from his brother and now is very weak, febrile, and anorexic, and cries with pain when his wrists and elbows are moved. He is admitted to the hospital with a diagnosis of sickle cell crisis. The child's mother asks the nurse why he has not been symptomatic before now. The best response by the nurse would be

1. High fetal hemoglobin protected him against sickling.

2. His red blood cell levels remained normal.

3. Maternal antibodies protected him against sickling.

4. Sickle cell hemoglobin was not present until about 1 year of life.

10. In planning care for a child with newly diagnosed sickle cell anemia, his mother should be taught that vaso-occlusive crises may be prevented by

1. prophylactic administration of acetaminophen.

2. eating food with a high iron content.

3. exercising regularly.

4. promoting hydration.

11. How could the nurse best evaluate if parents are giving their child with iron deficiency anemia iron as prescribed?

   1. Parents state they offer orange juice when they give the medication.
   2. Parents state the child has greenish black stools.
   3. Parents state the child experiences nausea with the iron preparation.
   4. Parents state they are giving the iron as prescribed.

12. Parents of a child who has sickle-cell anemia want to know why their child did not have the first episode until he was approximately a year old. The best reply for the nurse to make is,

   1. "Are you sure your child has sickle-cell anemia and not sickle-cell trait?"
   2. "Affected children can be asymptomatic in infancy because of high levels of fetal hemoglobin that inhibit sickling."
   3. "Have you asked your doctor about this?"
   4. "Your child probably had a crisis and you did not realize it."

13. A 5-year-old is admitted to the nursing care unit in vaso-occlusive crisis from sickle cell anemia. What is the priority nursing intervention?

   1. Teaching the family about sickle cell anemia and home care needs.
   2. Managing the child's pain.
   3. Encouraging a high protein, high calorie diet.
   4. Administering oxygen via nasal cannula.

14. A 3-year-old with a recent history of chickenpox is admitted to the unit with idiopathic thrombocytopenic purpura. His platelet count is 15,000 mm^3/dl. His lesions are enlarging. Which of the following nursing actions best provides for the child's safety?

   1. Supervised outdoor play.
   2. Set times of rest periods.
   3. Only allowing him to have soft stuffed toys to play with.
   4. Keeping him on complete bed rest.

15. A child is admitted to the pediatric unit with hemarthrosis secondary to hemophilia. The most appropriate nursing intervention would be

   1. daily bleeding times.
   2. prophylactic antibiotic therapy.
   3. elevating and immobilizing the affected joint.
   4. encouraging active range of motion of affected joint.

ANSWERS AND RATIONALES

1. **3.** Classic hemophilia is inherited as an X-linked recessive trait. If this family has another son, there is a 50% chance that he will have the disease. If they have a daughter she is very unlikely to have the disease but there is a 50% chance she will be a carrier.

2. **3.** Iron is given with a straw to prevent staining the teeth.

3. **2.** Aspirin is an anticoagulant. The child has a clotting disorder and has been bleeding into his knee joint. He should not receive an anticoagulant.

4. **4.** Clients with sickle cell trait inherit only one defective gene. They can synthesize both normal and abnormal hemoglobin chains.

5. **2.** The life span of a sickled cell is 6 to 20 days as opposed to 120 days for a normal red blood cell.

6. **4.** Children with sickle cell disease usually manifest growth impairment.

7. **3.** The tissues of a client with sickle cell disease are constantly vulnerable to microcirculatory interruptions.

8. **4.** The sudden appearance of a stroke in sickle cell anemia is related to the microcirculatory interruptions that are caused by the sickled cell.

9. **1.** High levels of fetal hemoglobin inhibit sickling of red cells prior to the age of 6 months.

10. **4.** Promoting good hydration is a major factor in maintaining the blood viscosity needed to maximize the circulation of red blood cells. Dehydration causes sickling of red blood cells.

11. **2.** When an adequate dosage of iron is reached, the stools usually turn a greenish black. Absence of this color stool usually gives a clue to poor compliance.

12. **2.** Children with sickle-cell anemia are often asymptomatic until at least 4 to 6 months of age. A crisis is usually precipitated by an acute upper respiratory or gastrointestinal infection.

13. **4.** During a vaso-occlusive crisis, tissue hypoxia and ischemia cause pain. By delivering oxygen at the prescribed rate, further tissue hypoxia can be avoided.

14. **4.** Initially when his platelets are below 20,000 mm^3/dl and he is experiencing active bleeding or progression of lesions, activity is restricted.

15. **3.** During bleeding episodes, hemarthrosis is managed by elevating and immobilizing the joint and applying ice packs.

6

The Respiratory System

■ VARIATIONS FROM THE ADULT

A. Infants are obligatory nose breathers and diaphragmatic breathers.

B. Number and size of alveoli continue to increase until age 8 years.

C. Until age 5, structures of the respiratory tract have a narrower lumen and children are more susceptible to obstruction/distress from inflammation.

D. Normal respiratory rate in children is faster than in adults.
   1. Infants: 40–60/minute
   2. 1 year: 20–40/minute
   3. 2–4 years: 20–30/minute
   4. 5–10 years: 20–25/minute
   5. 10–15 years: 17–22/minute
   6. 15 and older: 15–20/minute

E. Most episodes of acute illness in young children involve the respiratory system due to frequent exposure to infection and a general lack of immunity.

■ ASSESSMENT

History

A. Presenting problem: symptoms may include cough, wheezing, dyspnea

B. Medical history: incidence of infections, respiratory allergies or asthma, prescribed and OTC medications, recent immunizations

C. Exposure to other children with respiratory infections or other communicable diseases

Physical Examination

A. Inspect shape of chest; note
   1. Barrel chest: occurs with chronic respiratory disease.

    2. Pectus carinatum (pigeon breast): sternum protrudes outward, producing increased A-P diameter; usually not significant.

    3. Pectus excavatum (funnel chest): lower part of sternum is depressed; usually does not produce symptoms; may impair cardiac function.

B. Note pattern of respirations.

    1. Rate

    2. Regularity

        a. Periodic respirations (periods of rapid respirations, separated by periods of slow breathing or short periods of no respirations) normal in young infants

        b. Apnea episodes (cessation of breathing for 20 seconds or more accompanied by color change or bradycardia) an abnormal finding

    3. Respiratory effort

        a. Nasal flaring: attempt to widen airway and decrease resistance

        b. Open-mouth breathing: chin drops with each inhalation

        c. Retractions: from use of accessory muscles

C. Observe skin color and temperature, particularly mucous membranes and peripheral extremities.

D. Note behavior: position of comfort, signs of irritability or lethargy, facial expression (anxiety).

E. Note speech abnormalities: hoarseness or muffled speech.

F. Observe presence and quality of cough: productive; paroxysmal, with inspiratory "whoop" characteristic of pertussis.

G. Auscultate for abnormal breath sounds (auscultation may be more difficult in infants and young children because of shallowness of respirations).

    1. Grunting on expiration

    2. Stridor: harsh inspiratory sound associated with obstruction or edema

    3. Wheezing: whistling noise during inspiration or expiration due to narrowed airways, common in asthma

    4. "Snoring": noisy breathing associated with nasal obstruction

Laboratory/Diagnostic Tests

A. Pulmonary function testing is usually not done under age 6 years since children have difficulty following directions.

B. Chest X-rays: avoid unnecessary exposure; protect gonads and thyroid.

■ ANALYSIS

Nursing diagnoses for the child with a disorder of the respiratory system may include

A. Activity intolerance

B. Altered respiratory functions: ineffective airway clearance, ineffective breathing pattern, impaired gas exchange

C. Anxiety

D. Fatigue

DELEGATION TIP

A ncillary personnel should be instructed to report any changes in the child's activity tolerance, dyspnea, increased secretions, or any abnormal sounds like grunting.

E. Impaired oral mucous membrane
F. Altered nutrition
G. Disturbed sleep pattern

■ PLANNING AND IMPLEMENTATION
Goals
A. Child will have patent airway and satisfactory oxygenation.
B. Child will be free from symptoms of respiratory distress.
C. Child will have improved ability to tolerate exercise, conserve energy.
D. Parents will participate in caring for child.

Interventions
Oxygen Tent (Croup Tent, Mist Tent, Oxygen Canopy)
A. General information
　　1. Used when desired oxygen concentration is 40% or less as oxygen concentration can be difficult to control
　　2. Primarily used for croup, when mist is to be delivered
B. Nursing care
　　1. Keep sides of plastic down and tucked in.
　　2. If tent has been opened for a while, increase oxygen flow to raise concentration quickly.
　　3. If child has been out of the tent, return oxygen concentration to ordered percent before returning child to tent.
　　4. If tent enclosure gets too warm, add ice to cooling chamber as needed.
　　5. Mist is usually prescribed in addition to oxygen
　　　　a. Keep reservoir for humidification filled.
　　　　b. Do not allow condensation on tent walls to obstruct view of child.
　　　　c. Keep clothes and bedding dry to avoid chilling.
　　6. Provide safety measures.
　　　　a. Keep plastic away from child's face.
　　　　b. Avoid toys that produce spark or friction, such as mechanical toys.
　　　　c. Avoid stuffed toys because of tendency to absorb moisture.
　　　　d. Encourage use of one or two favorite toys or transitional object in tent; other toys may be kept outside of tent in child's view.

Vaporizers

A. General information
   1. Same principle as oxygen tent
   2. Used at home; placed at bedside; mist directed into room around child
   3. Usually cool mist
B. Nursing responsibilities: teach parents to clean frequently because bacteria that grow in vaporizer can be dispersed into air.

Chest Physical Therapy

A. Postural drainage: infants and young children do not have enough rib cage for a lower front position
   1. Combine side and lower front positions
   2. 5 positions: upper front, upper back, lower back, right side and front, and left side and front
   3. 2–5 minutes per position
B. Percussion
   1. Do not use with clients with an acute attack of asthma or croup (dislodged mucus may cause plugging because of bronchial edema).
   2. Use percussion 30 minutes before meals to clear mucus before eating, thus enhancing intake.
   3. If aerosol medications are being used, administer immediately before percussion.
   4. Percussion is done with cupped hand, never on bare skin, over the rib cage only
      a. Use an undershirt, gown, or diaper over skin.
      b. If infant's chest is too small for nurse's hand, a small face mask can be substituted.
      c. Be careful to avoid spine and neck during percussion.
      d. Infants can be percussed while being held on nurse's lap.
      e. If child is unable to cough during and after percussion, suction as needed.
C. Vibration: performed on expiration.

Suctioning

A. Bulb syringes can be used to clear nasal stuffiness.
B. For nasotracheal and nasopharyngeal suction, use low pressure.
C. Assess response, and for improved respiratory status.

Deep Breathing Exercises

A. Encourage deep breathing by making exercises into games (e.g., touch toes, sit-ups, jumping jacks, blowing out "flashlight," ping-pong ball games using blowing).
B. Encourage use of toys that require blowing (harmonica, bubbles).
C. Laughing and crying also stimulate coughing and deep breathing.

Apnea Monitor

A. General information: monitors often use same three chest leads for simultaneous cardiac and respiratory rate monitoring
   1. Lead placement will differ from that usually prescribed for cardiac monitoring if apnea monitoring is also required.
   2. To monitor respiratory rate, chest leads will need to be where chest moves during inspiration.
   3. As chest wall movement rather than air entry is monitored, obstruction and dyspnea may not be recognized early.
   4. Most useful for early recognition of cessation of breathing.
B. Nursing care: when alarm sounds
   1. Note whether cardiac or respiratory rate has triggered alarm.
   2. Assess child's color, activity, and presence of respiratory effort.
   3. Auscultate cardiac and respiratory sounds.
   4. If no physical distress, check lead placement.
   5. If apneic, gently stimulate lower extremities. May need oxygen.
   6. If no improvement with stimulation and oxygen, assess need for CPR.

▮ EVALUATION

A. Child is satisfactorily oxygenated.
   1. Absence of respiratory distress
   2. Normal color and activity
   3. Decreased need for supplementary oxygen therapy
B. Parents are able to care for child at home.
   1. Identify symptoms of increased oxygen need
   2. Perform prescribed treatments
   3. Have obtained and demonstrated use of necessary equipment

▮ DISORDERS OF THE RESPIRATORY SYSTEM

Tonsillitis

A. General information
   1. Inflammation of tonsils often as a result of a viral or bacterial pharyngitis
   2. 10–15% caused by group A beta-hemolytic streptococci
B. Medical management
   1. Comfort measures and symptomatic relief
   2. Antibiotics for bacterial infection, usually penicillin or erythromycin
   3. Surgery: removal of tonsils/adenoids if necessary
C. Assessment findings
   1. Enlarged, red tonsils; fever
   2. Sore throat, difficulty swallowing, mouth breathing, snoring
   3. White patches of exudate on tonsillar pillars, enlarged cervical lymph nodes

D. Nursing interventions
1. Provide soft or liquid diet.
2. Use cool-mist vaporizer.
3. Administer salt water gargles, throat lozenges.
4. Administer analgesics (acetaminophen) as ordered.
5. Administer antibiotics as ordered; stress to parents importance of completing entire course of medication.

Tonsillectomy

A. General information
1. One of the most common operations performed on children
2. Indications for tonsillectomy include recurrent tonsillitis, peritonsillar abscess, airway or esophageal obstruction
3. Indications for adenoidectomy include nasal obstruction due to hypertrophy

B. Nursing interventions: preoperative
1. Make pre-op preparation age-appropriate; child enters the hospital feeling well and will leave with a very sore throat.
2. Obtain baseline bleeding and clotting times.
3. Check for any loose teeth.

C. Nursing interventions: postoperative
1. Position on side or abdomen to facilitate drainage of secretions.
2. Avoid suctioning if possible; if not, be especially careful to avoid trauma to surgical site.
3. Provide ice collar/analgesia for pain.
4. Observe for hemorrhage; signs may include frequent swallowing, increased pulse, vomiting bright red blood (vomiting old dried blood or pink-tinged emesis is normal).
5. Offer clear, cool, noncitrus, nonred fluids when awake and alert.
6. Provide client teaching and discharge planning concerning
   a. Need to maintain adequate fluid and food intake and to avoid spicy and irritating foods
   b. Quiet activity for a few days
   c. Need to avoid coughing, mouth gargles
   d. Chewing gum (but not Aspergum): can help relieve pain and difficulty swallowing and aids in diminishing bad breath
   e. Mild analgesics for pain
   f. Signs and symptoms of bleeding and need to report to physician

Acute Spasmodic Laryngitis (Croup)

A. General information
1. Respiratory distress characterized by paroxysmal attacks of laryngeal obstruction

2. Etiology unclear but familial predisposition, allergy, viruses, psychologic factors, and anxious temperament have been implicated
3. Common in children ages 1–3 years
4. Attacks occur mostly at night; onset sudden and usually preceded by a mild upper respiratory infection
5. Respiratory symptoms last several hours; may occur in a milder form on a few subsequent nights

B. Assessment findings
1. Inspiratory stridor, hoarseness, barking cough, anxiety, retractions
2. Afebrile, skin cool

C. Nursing interventions
1. Instruct parents to take the child into the bathroom, close the door, turn on the hot water, and sit on floor of the steamy bathroom with child.
2. If the laryngeal spasm does not subside the child should be taken to the emergency department.
3. After the spasm subsides, provide cool mist with a vaporizer.
4. Provide clear fluids.
5. Try to keep child calm and quiet.
6. Assure parents this is self-limiting.

Laryngotracheobronchitis

A. General information
1. Viral infection of the larynx that may extend into trachea and bronchi
2. Most common cause for stridor in febrile child
3. Parainfluenza viruses most common cause
4. Infection causes endothelial insult, increased mucus production, edema, low-grade fever
5. Affects children less than 5 years of age
6. Onset more gradual than with croup, takes longer to resolve; usually develops over several days with upper respiratory infection
7. Usually treated on outpatient basis; indications for admission include dehydration and respiratory compromise

B. Medical management
1. Drug therapy
   a. Aerosolized racemic epinephrine
   b. Antibiotics only if secondary bacterial infection present
   c. Steroids
2. Oxygen therapy: low concentrations to relieve mild hypoxia
3. Oral or nasotracheal intubation for moderate hypoxia
4. IV fluids to maintain hydration

C. Assessment findings
1. Fever, coryza, inspiratory stridor, barking cough, tachycardia, tachypnea, retractions

> **NURSING ALERT**
>
> K eep emergency ventilation equipment at the bedside, along with endo-tracheal tubes and suction equipment.

    2. May have difficulty taking fluids
    3. WBC normal
D. Nursing interventions
    1. Instruct parents to take child into steamy bathroom for acute distress.
    2. Keep child calm.
    3. After distress subsides, use cool mist vaporizer in bedroom.
    4. Child can vomit large amounts of mucus after the episode; reassure parents that this is normal.
    5. For hospitalized child
        a. Monitor vital signs, I&O, skin color, and respiratory effort.
        b. Maintain hydration.
        c. Provide care for the intubated child.
        d. Plan care to disturb the child as little as possible.

Epiglottitis

A. General information
    1. Life-threatening bacterial infection of epiglottis and surrounding structures
    2. Primary organism: *H. influenzae,* type B
    3. Often preceded by upper respiratory infection
    4. Rapid progression of swelling causes reduction in airway diameter; may lead to sudden respiratory arrest
    5. Affects children ages 3–7 years
B. Assessment findings
    1. Fever, tachycardia, inspiratory stridor (possibly), labored respirations with retractions, sore throat, dysphagia, drooling, muffled voice
    2. Irritability, restlessness, anxious-looking, quiet
    3. Position: sitting upright, head forward and jaw thrust out
    4. Diagnostic tests
        a. WBC increased
        b. Lateral neck X-ray reveals characteristic findings
C. Nursing interventions
    1. Provide mist tent with oxygen.
    2. Administer IV antibiotics as ordered.
    3. Provide tracheostomy or endotracheal tube care (page 294); note the following

      a. Restlessness, fatigue, dyspnea, cyanosis, pallor, tachycardia, tachypnea, diminished breath sounds, adventitious lung sounds.

      b. Need for suctioning to remove secretions; note amount, color, consistency.

    4. Reassure child through touch, sound, and physically being present.

    5. Involve parents in all aspects of care.

    6. Avoid direct examination of the epiglottis as it may precipitate spasm and obstruction.

    7. Remember this is extremely frightening experience for child and parents; explain procedures and findings; reinforce explanations of physician.

Bronchiolitis

A. General information

    1. Pulmonary viral infection characterized by wheezing

    2. Usually caused by respiratory syncytial virus

    3. Virus invades epithelial cells of nasopharynx and spreads to lower respiratory tract, causing increased mucus production, decreased diameter of bronchi, hyperinflation, and possible atelectasis

    4. Affects infants ages 2-8 months

    5. Increased incidence of asthma as child grows older

B. Medical management

    1. Nebulized bronchodilators (e.g., Albuterol)

    2. Steroids

    3. Ribavirin—antiviral, given by aerosol (SPAG) through hood, tent, mask, or ventilator—for severe symptoms

    4. Humidity, oxygen, fluids

    5. Prevention: RSV antibodies

      a. RSV-IG (immune globulin)—given IV monthly

      b. Palivizumab (Synagis)—given IM monthly

C. Assessment findings

    1. Difficulty feeding, fever

    2. Cough, coryza

    3. Wheezing, prolonged expiratory phase, tachypnea, nasal flaring, retractions (intercostal more pronounced than supraclavicular retractions)

    4. Diagnostic tests

      a. WBC normal

      b. X-ray reveals hyperaeration

D. Nursing interventions

    1. Provide high-humidity environment, with oxygen in some cases (instruct parents to take child into steamy bathroom if at home).

    2. Offer small, frequent feedings; clear fluids if trouble with secretions.

    3. Provide adequate rest.

    4. Administer antipyretics as ordered to control fever.

Asthma

A. General information
  1. Obstructive disease of the lower respiratory tract
  2. Most common chronic respiratory disease in children, in younger children affects twice as many boys as girls; incidence equal by adolescence
  3. Often caused by an allergic reaction to an environmental allergen, may be seasonal or year-round
  4. Immunologic/allergic reaction results in histamine release, which produces three main airway responses
    a. Edema of mucous membranes
    b. Spasm of the smooth muscle of bronchi and bronchioles
    c. Accumulation of tenacious secretions
  5. *Status asthmaticus* occurs when there is little response to treatment and symptoms persist
B. Medical management
  1. Drug therapy: Bronchodilators
    a. Beta-adrenergic agonists
      1) metered does inhaler (MDI)—most children will need spacers
      2) nebulizer—infants and toddlers
      3) rescue drugs for acute attacks
    b. Corticosteroids
      1) inhaled by MDI or nebulizer
      2) oral for persistent wheezing
      3) IV in hospital
    c. Nonsteroid anti-inflammatory agents
      1) cromolyn sodium
      2) nedocromil
      3) leukotriene inhibitors and receptor—antagonists
      4) used for maintenance, not rescue
    d. Xanthine—derivatives
      1) theophylline (oral)
      2) aminophylline (IV)
      3) used for status asthmaticus
    e. Procedure for use of oral inhaler. See Figure 6-1.
  2. Physical therapy
  3. Hyposensitization
  4. Exercise
C. Assessment findings
  1. Family history of allergies
  2. Client history of eczema
  3. Respiratory distress: shortness of breath, expiratory wheeze, prolonged expiratory phase, air trapping (barrel chest if chronic), use

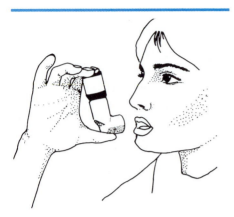

FIGURE 6-1 Instructions for use
of an oral inhaler

1. Remove the cap from the mouthpiece and shake the inhaler well.
2. Hold the inhaler so the metal canister containing the medication is upside down.
3. Breathe out as fully as possible.
4. Open your mouth and tilt your head back slightly. Hold the inhaler about 2 inches from your mouth.*
5. Firmly press the metal canister down into the mouthpiece. This releases the medication. At the same time, begin to inhale slowly through your mouth.
6. Hold your breath for about 10 seconds.
7. Slowly breathe out through your nose and pursed lips.
8. Wait about 5 minutes, shake the inhaler, and repeat if necessary. Cap and store the inhaler.
9. Rinse your mouth with water or gargle after the last inhalation.
10. Periodically clean the mouthpiece by removing the canister and rinsing the mouthpiece in warm water. Dry it and replace the canister.

*Note: This is a newer procedure. Many physicians and pharmacists will teach the client to place the mouthpiece in the mouth. The nurse should reinforce the procedure that has been taught.

of accessory muscles, irritability (from hypoxia), diaphoresis, change in sensorium if severe attack

    4. Diagnostic tests: ABGs indicate respiratory acidosis

D. Nursing interventions

    1. Place client in high-Fowler's position.

    2. Administer oxygen as ordered.

    3. Administer medications as ordered.

    4. Provide humidification/hydration to loosen secretions.

5. Provide chest percussion and postural drainage when bronchodilation improves.
6. Monitor for respiratory distress.
7. Provide client teaching and discharge planning concerning
   a. Modification of environment
      1) ensure room is well ventilated.
      2) stay indoors during grass cutting or when pollen count is high.
      3) use damp dusting.
      4) avoid rugs, draperies or curtains, stuffed animals.
      5) avoid natural fibers (wool and feathers).
   b. Importance of moderate exercise (swimming is excellent)
   c. Purpose of breathing exercises (to increase the end expiratory pressure of each respiration)

Aspiration of a Foreign Object

A. General information
   1. Relatively common airway problem.
   2. Severity depends on object (e.g., pins, coins, nuts, buttons, parts of toys) aspirated and the degree of obstruction.
   3. Depending on object aspirated, symptoms will increase over hours or weeks.
   4. The curious toddler is most frequently affected.
   5. If object does not pass trachea immediately, respiratory distress will be evident.
   6. If object moves beyond tracheal region, it will pass into one of the main stem bronchi; symptoms will be vague, insidious.
   7. Causes 400 deaths per year in children under age 4.
B. Medical management
   1. Objects in upper airway require immediate removal.
   2. Lower airway obstruction is less urgent (bronchoscopy or laryngoscopy).
C. Assessment findings
   1. Sudden onset of coughing, dyspnea, wheezing, stridor, apnea (upper airway)
   2. Persistent or recurrent pneumonia, persistent croupy cough or wheeze
   3. Object not always visible on X-ray
   4. Secondary infection
D. Nursing interventions
   1. Perform Heimlich maneuver if indicated.
   2. Reassure the scared toddler.
   3. After removal, place child in high-humidity environment and treat secondary infection if applicable.
   4. Counsel parents regarding age-appropriate behavior and safety precautions.

CLIENT TEACHING CHECKLIST

T each parents techniques to child proof their home against the aspiration of foreign objects by:

- Reviewing age-appropriate foods
- Raising awareness of food and objects children frequently aspirate, such as coins, nuts, hot dogs, and popcorn.
- Encouraging them to learn CPR and chest thrusts.

Cystic Fibrosis (CF)

A. General information
1. Disorder characterized by dysfunction of the exocrine glands (mucus-producing glands of the respiratory tract, GI tract, pancreas, sweat glands, salivary glands)
2. Transmitted as an autosomal recessive trait
3. Incidence: 1 in 1500–2000 live births
4. Most common lethal genetic disease among Caucasians in United States and Europe
5. Prenatal diagnosis of CF is not reliable
6. Secretions from mucous glands are thick, causing obstruction and fibrosis of tissue
7. Sweat and saliva have characteristic high levels of sodium chloride
8. Affected organs
   a. Pancreas: 85% of CF clients have pancreatic involvement
      1) obstruction of pancreatic ducts and eventual fibrosis and atrophy of the pancreas leads to little or no release of enzymes (lipase [fats], amylase [starch], and trypsin [protein])
      2) absence of enzymes causes malabsorption of fats and proteins
      3) unabsorbed food fractions excreted in the stool produce steatorrhea
      4) loss of nutrients and inability to absorb fat-soluble vitamins causes failure to thrive
   b. Respiratory tract: 99.9% of CF clients have respiratory involvement
      1) increased production of secretions causes increased obstruction of airway, air trapping, and atelectasis
      2) pulmonary congestion leads to cor pulmonale
      3) eventually death occurs by drowning in own secretions

    c. Reproductive system

        1) males are sterile

        2) females can conceive, but increased mucus in vaginal tract makes conception more difficult

        3) pregnancy causes increased stress on respiratory system of mother

    d. Liver: one-third of clients have cirrhosis/portal hypertension

  9. 95% of deaths are from abnormal mucus secretion and fibrosis in the lungs; shortened life span

B. Medical management

  1. Pancreatic involvement: aimed at promoting absorption of nutrients

    a. Diet modification

        1) infant: predigested formula

        2) older children: may require high-calorie, high-protein, or low/limited-fat diet, but many CF clients tolerate normal diet

    b. Pancreatic enzyme supplementation: enzyme capsules, tablets, or powders (Pancrease, Cotazym, Viokase) given with meals and snacks

  2. Respiratory involvement: goals are to maintain airway patency and to prevent lung infection

    a. Chest physiotherapy

    b. Antibiotics for infection

C. Assessment findings: symptoms vary greatly in severity and extent

  1. Pancreatic involvement

    a. Growth failure; failure to thrive

    b. Stools are foul smelling, large, frequent, foamy, fatty (steatorrhea), contain undigested food

    c. Meconium ileus (meconium gets stuck in bowel due to lack of enzymes) in newborns

    d. Rectal prolapse is possible

    e. Voracious appetite

    f. Characteristic protruding abdomen with atrophy of extremities and buttocks

    g. Symptoms associated with deficiencies in the fat-soluble vitamins

    h. Anemia

    i. Diagnostic tests

        1) trypsin decreased or absent in aspiration of duodenal contents

        2) fecal fat in stool specimen increased

  2. Respiratory involvement

    a. Signs of respiratory distress

    b. Barrel chest due to air trapping

    c. Clubbing of digits

    d. Decreased exercise tolerance due to distress

    e. Frequent productive cough

      f. Frequent pseudomonas infections

      g. Diagnostic tests

          1) chest X-ray reveals atelectasis, infiltrations, emphysemic changes

          2) pulmonary function studies abnormal

          3) ABGs show respiratory acidosis

  3. Electrolyte involvement

      a. Hyponatremia/heat exhaustion in hot weather

      b. Salty taste to sweat

      c. Diagnostic tests

          1) pilocarpine iontophoresis sweat test: indicates 2–5 times normal amount of sodium and chloride in the sweat

          2) fecal fat elevated

          3) fecal trypsin absent or decreased

D. Nursing interventions

  1. Pancreatic involvement

      a. Administer pancreatic enzymes with meals as ordered: do not mix enzymes until ready to use them; best to mix in applesauce.

      b. Provide a high-calorie, high-carbohydrate (no empty-calorie foods), high-protein, normal-fat diet.

      c. Provide a double dose of multivitamins per day, especially fat-soluble vitamins (A, D, E, K), in water-soluble form.

      d. If low-fat diet required, MCT (medium-chain triglycerides) oil may be used.

  2. Respiratory involvement

      a. Administer antibiotics as ordered (all antibiotics for pseudomonas are given IV; doses may be above recommended levels (for virulent organisms).

      b. Administer expectorants, mucolytics (rarely used) as ordered.

      c. Avoid cough suppressants and antihistamines.

      d. Encourage breathing exercises.

      e. Provide percussion and postural drainage 4 times a day.

      f. Provide aerosol treatments as needed; handheld nebulizers, mask, intermittent positive pressure breathing (IPPB), mist tent.

  3. Electrolyte involvement

      a. Add salt to all meals, especially in summer.

      b. Give salty snacks (pretzels).

  4. Provide appropriate long-term support to child and family.

  5. Provide client teaching and discharge planning concerning

      a. Genetic counseling

      b. Promotion of child's independence

      c. Avoidance of cigarette smoking in the house

      d. Availability of support groups/community agencies

      e. Alternative school education during extended hospitalization/ home recovery

REVIEW QUESTIONS

1. The nurse is caring for a child who had a tonsillectomy performed 4 hours ago. Which of the following is an abnormal finding and a cause for concern?

   1. An emesis of dried blood.
   2. Increased swallowing.
   3. Pink-tinged mucus.
   4. The child complains of a very sore throat.

2. A 7-year-old has been diagnosed as having cystic fibrosis. Chest physiotherapy has been ordered. Chest percussion should be performed

   1. before postural drainage.
   2. $1/2$ hour before meals.
   3. before an aerosol treatment.
   4. after suctioning.

3. The nurse is performing chest physiotherapy on a 6-year-old child who has congestion in his left lower lobe. The nurse should position the child on his

   1. left side in semi-Fowler's position.
   2. right side in semi-Fowler's position.
   3. left side in Trendelenburg position.
   4. right side in Trendelenburg position.

4. An infant is being evaluated for possible cystic fibrosis. The sweat test will show an elevation of which electrolyte?

   1. Chloride.
   2. Fluoride.
   3. Potassium.
   4. Calcium.

5. A 2-year-old is admitted to the hospital with cystic fibrosis. He is small for his age. What dietary suggestions can the nurse recommend to the child's mother to enhance his growth?

   1. Low-fat, low-residue, and high-potassium diet.
   2. Low-carbohydrate, soft diet with no sugar products.
   3. High-carbohydrate, high-fat diet with extra water between meals.
   4. High-protein, high-calorie meals with skim-milk milkshakes between meals.

6. The nurse is caring for a 2-year-old who has cystic fibrosis. His mother asks why the child developed cystic fibrosis. The nurse explains that cystic fibrosis

   1. develops due to meconium ileus at birth.
   2. is an autosomal recessive genetic defect.
   3. occurs during embryologic development.
   4. results from chromosomal nondysjunction that occurred at conception.

7. A 2-year-old is admitted to the hospital and will need to stay for several days. The child's mother is unable to stay overnight because there is no one to care for her other children. The nurse recommends that she

   1. leave something of hers with the child and tell him she'll be back in the morning.
   2. leave while he is in the playroom.
   3. leave after he has fallen asleep.
   4. tell him she'll be back in a few minutes after she has dinner.

8. The mother of a 2-year-old who has cystic fibrosis tells the nurse that the family is planning their first summer vacation. She wants to know if there are any special precautions needed because he has cystic fibrosis. The nurse should tell her that children with cystic fibrosis are particularly susceptible to

   1. severe sunburn.
   2. infectious diarrhea.
   3. heat prostration.
   4. respiratory allergies.

9. A 4-year-old is admitted to the hospital for the treatment of an acute asthma attack. Her health history reveals that she has been blind since birth and has had four asthma attacks in the past 6 months. She received nebulized albuterol (Proventil) in the emergency department and was transferred to the pediatric unit with an aminophylline infusion. When evaluating the child for positive effects of the aminophylline treatment, the most significant finding is

   1. a decrease in mucus production.
   2. a decrease in wheezing.
   3. an increase in blood pressure.
   4. a sleeping child.

10. A 12-month-old is hospitalized for a severe case of croup and has been placed in an oxygen tent. Today the oxygen order has been reduced from

35% to 25%. His blood gases are normal. The child refuses to stay in the oxygen tent. Attempts to placate him only cause him to become more upset. The most appropriate action for the nurse is to

1. restrain him in the tent and notify the physician.
2. take him out of the tent and notify the physician.
3. take him out of the tent and let him sit in the playroom.
4. tell him it will please his mother if he stays in the tent.

11. The nurse should recognize which of the following respiratory findings as normal in a 10-month-old infant?

1. Respiratory rate of 60 at rest.
2. Use of accessory muscles to assist in respiratory effort.
3. Respiratory rate of 32 at rest.
4. Diaphoresis with shallow respirations.

12. An 18-month-old presents with nasal flaring, intercostal and substernal retractions, and a respiratory rate of 50. What is the most appropriate nursing diagnosis?

1. Knowledge deficit.
2. Ineffective breathing pattern.
3. Ineffective individual coping.
4. High risk for altered body temperature: hyperthermia.

13. An 11-month-old is admitted to the hospital with bronchiolitis. He is currently in a croup tent with supplemental oxygen. Which toy is most appropriate for the nurse to recommend to the child's parents?

1. A stuffed animal made from a washable fabric.
2. A soft plastic stacking toy with multicolored rings.
3. A set of wooden blocks.
4. A pull toy.

14. Which of the following statements best assures the nurse that the parents understand the safety concerns related to use of a vaporizer at home?

1. "I have a high dresser in the bedroom on which to place the vaporizer. The cord will be concealed behind the dresser."
2. "I plan to put the vaporizer on a stool next to the bed so that my child will get the most benefit from the cool mist."
3. "I purchased a warm mist vaporizer because I don't want my child to get chilled from the mist in her face."
4. "I thought I could just set the vaporizer on the floor next to the bed."

15. A 4-year-old is experiencing an acute asthma attack. Why should the nurse avoid chest percussion with this child?

    1. Chest percussion may lead to increased bronchospasm and more respiratory distress.

    2. Chest percussion may cause mucous plugging of the alveoli.

    3. Chest percussion is useful in removing airway secretions and should be used.

    4. Chest percussion will produce increased coughing and thereby enhance respiratory distress.

16. A 5-month-old has severe nasal congestion. What is the best way for the nurse to clear his nasal passages?

    1. Administer saline nose drops and use a bulb syringe to clear passages.

    2. Ask him to blow his nose and keep tissues handy.

    3. Place him in a mist tent with 40% oxygen.

    4. Administer vasoconstrictive nose drops before meals and at bedtime.

17. A 30-week gestation infant who had apnea of prematurity is ready for discharge and will be going home on apnea monitoring. What should the nurse teach the parents for proper use of the monitor?

    1. The monitor is only used when the child is awake. It is not indicated at night or during naps.

    2. The alarms on the monitor should be turned off when an attendant is with the infant.

    3. The monitor should be kept on at all times except when the infant is being bathed. Careful attention to skin integrity and hygiene is important.

    4. It is best for the parents to have 24-hour home health supervision to watch the infant while monitoring is required.

18. A 3-year-old underwent a tonsillectomy this morning. As the nurse giving discharge instructions, which comment by the child's mother suggests that she understands the care requirements?

    1. "I plan to take her back to her play group tomorrow. I know she won't want to stay home."

    2. "I have bought fruit popsicles to give her later today."

    3. "I will give her aspirin if she gets irritable."

    4. "She is just waiting for the ice cream we promised her before she came to the hospital."

19. A 3-year-old boy presents in the ER with dysphagia, drooling, and respiratory difficulty that has increased significantly over the past 6 hours.

The nurse should know that these findings are suggestive of which of the following conditions?

1. Croup.
2. Pneumonia.
3. Bronchopulmonary dysplasia.
4. Epiglottitis.

20. A 2-year-old presents to an urgent care center with respiratory distress and cyanosis. Parents report an initial episode of choking. What is the best initial action for the nurse to take?

1. Call 911 and have parents wait for an ambulance to transport the child to a pediatric hospital.
2. Administer oxygen by face mask and call the child's pediatrician.
3. Perform abdominal thrusts as described in the Heimlich maneuver.
4. Start CPR after the child loses consciousness.

ANSWERS AND RATIONALES

1. **2.** Increased swallowing could be a sign of hemorrhage from the surgical site.

2. **2.** Chest percussion is done between meals to prevent vomiting, which might occur if done following meals.

3. **4.** The affected lobe must be uppermost to be drained by gravity.

4. **1.** There is increased excretion of chloride in the sweat of children with cystic fibrosis. A chloride level of over 60 mEq/liter is diagnostic for the disease.

5. **4.** A person with cystic fibrosis lacks pancreatic enzymes necessary for fat absorption. A diet high in protein and calories is necessary to meet the child's growth needs. Between-meal snacks milkshakes made with skim milk may be given to provide additional protein, vitamins, and calories.

6. **2.** Cystic fibrosis is an autosomal recessive genetic disease. If both parents have the cystic fibrosis trait, each child has a 25% chance of developing the disease, a 50% chance of being a carrier, and a 25% chance of not having the disease.

7. **1.** Leaving something of his mother's with the child and telling him that she will be back in the morning is the best approach in developing trust between the mother and her child.

8. **3.** Persons with cystic fibrosis are prone to electrolyte imbalances due to increased loss of sodium and potassium in their sweat. The mother should

avoid having her child become overheated and should frequently replenish body fluids with water or fruit juices.

9. **2.** Aminophylline is a bronchodilator. As it exerts its effects, wheezing will decrease.

10. **2.** The energy expended by the child in resisting the oxygen tent is causing increased respiratory effort. The child should be removed from the tent and closely monitored to be sure that he handles being in room air. The physician should be notified because the oxygen content of room air is only 20%, which is less than that ordered.

11. **3.** Rates of 20–40 breaths per minute are normal at this age.

12. **2.** The findings on assessment suggest respiratory distress. Ineffective breathing pattern is an appropriate diagnosis with the information now available.

13. **2.** Stacking toys with bright, large, colored plastic rings provide age-appropriate activity that is safe within the croup tent environment. The large rings can be held or stacked. They can be wiped down if damp. The size of the objects prevent them from creating any environmental hazards if the child is not continuously supervised.

14. **1.** It is best to keep the vaporizer out of the child's way. Concealing the cord and placing the appliance on a high surface is preferable.

15. **1.** During the course of an acute asthma attack, bronchospasm is a significant problem. Chest percussion can enhance the bronchospasm, leading to more pronounced respiratory distress.

16. **1.** Saline nose drops will help loosen secretions. The bulb syringe is necessary because the child is not old enough to effectively blow his nose.

17. **3.** Although apneic episodes are most common during sleep, they can occur at other times. Initially, it is particularly advisable to use the monitor continually except when bathing the infant.

18. **2.** Clear liquids are a good choice during the first 24 hours after surgery. Popsicles are appealing to children while providing fluids. They are less likely to irritate the surgical site than juices.

19. **4.** Epiglottitis is a medical emergency. The drooling and dysphagia are most often diagnostic of this condition.

20. **3.** The reported episode of choking and the child's condition suggest foreign body aspiration. The Heimlich maneuver should be attempted as an initial action to remove the object.

The Gastrointestinal System

■ VARIATIONS FROM THE ADULT

A. Mechanical functions of digestion are immature at birth.
1. No voluntary control over swallowing until 6 weeks
2. Stomach capacity decreased
3. Peristalsis increased, faster emptying time, more prone to diarrhea
4. Relaxed cardiac sphincter contributes to tendency to regurgitate food

B. Liver functions (glyconeogenesis and storage of vitamins) are immature throughout infancy.

C. Production of mucosal-lining antibodies is decreased.

D. Gastric acidity is low in infants, slowly rises until age 10, and then increases again during adolescence to reach adult levels.

E. Secretory cells are functional at birth, but efficiency of enzymes impaired by lower gastric pH.

F. Infant has decreased saliva, which causes decreased ability to digest starches.

G. Digestive processes are mature by toddlerhood.

H. Completion of myelinization of spinal cord allows voluntary control of elimination.

■ ASSESSMENT

History

A. Presenting problem: symptoms may include
1. Vomiting: type, color, amount, relationship to eating or other events
2. Abnormal bowel habits: diarrhea, constipation, bleeding
3. Weight loss or growth failure
4. Pain: location; relationship to meals or other events; effect on sleep, play, appetite
5. Any other parental concerns

B. Diet/nutrition history: appetite, daily caloric intake, food intolerances, feeding schedule, nutritional deficits

Physical Examination

A. General appearance
 1. Plot height and weight on growth chart.
 2. Measure midarm circumference and tricep skinfold thickness.
 3. Observe color: jaundiced or pale.
B. Mouth
 1. Note level of dentition, presence of dental caries.
 2. Observe mucosal integrity.
C. Abdomen
 1. Observe skin integrity.
 2. Note abdominal distention or visible peristaltic waves (seen in pyloric stenosis).
 3. Inspect for hernias (umbilical, inguinal).
 4. Auscultate for bowel sounds (a sound every 10-30 seconds is normal).
 5. Palpate for tenderness.
 6. Palpate for liver (inferior edge normally palpated 1-2 cm below right costal margin).
 7. Palpate for spleen (may be felt on inspiration 1-2 cm below left costal margin).
D. Vital signs: note presence of fever.

■ ANALYSIS

Nursing diagnoses for the child with a disorder of the gastrointestinal system may include
A. Constipation or diarrhea
B. Pain
C. Risk for deficient fluid volume
D. Imbalanced nutrition: less than body requirements
E. Impaired oral mucous membrane
F. Risk for impaired skin integrity
G. Ineffective tissue perfusion
H. Interrupted family processes

■ PLANNING AND IMPLEMENTATION
Goals

A. Child will maintain adequate nutritional intake.
B. Child will be free from complications of inadequate nutritional intake.
C. Pain will be relieved/controlled.
D. Child will reach optimal developmental level.
E. Parents will be able to care for child at home.

NURSING ALERT

U se specifically designed gastric feeding pump and bag to administer a liquid diet and to avoid confusion with parenteral infusions.

Interventions

Nasogastric Tube Feeding

A. Provide continuous NG tube feedings when child needs high-calorie intake.
B. Use infusion pump to ensure sustained intake.
C. Check tube placement every 4 hours.
D. Check residuals and refeed every 4 hours.

Gastrostomy

A. Used for clients at high risk for aspiration.
B. Regulate height of tube so feeding flows in over 20–30 minutes.

Parenteral Nutrition

A. Use central venous line for high dextrose solutions (greater than 10%).
B. Check infusion rate and amount every 30 minutes.
C. Monitor urine sugar and acetone every 4 hours for 24 hours after a solution change, then every 8 hours.
D. Monitor for signs of hyperglycemia (nausea, vomiting, dehydration).
E. Provide sterile care for insertion site.
  1. Change solution and tubing every 24 hours.
  2. Change dressing every 1–3 days.
  3. Apply restraints (if needed) to prevent dislodgment of central line.
F. Provide infants who are not receiving oral feedings with a pacifier to satisfy sucking needs.

■ EVALUATION

A. Child is receiving adequate nourishment as evidenced by normal growth and development.
B. Skin is intact, free from signs of redness or inflammation.
C. Child is free from infection, diarrhea, or vomiting.
D. Child is free from pain.
  1. Relaxed facial expression
  2. Level of activity
  3. No guarding of abdomen
E. Parents participate in care of child.
F. Child participates in normal daily activities with family and peers.

■ DISORDERS OF THE GASTROINTESTINAL SYSTEM
Congenital Disorders
Cleft Lip and Palate

A. General information
   1. Nonunion of the tissue and bone of the upper lip and hard/soft palate during embryologic development
   2. Familial disorder, often associated with other congenital abnormalities; incidence higher in Caucasians
      a. Cleft lip/palate: 1 in 1000 births
      b. Cleft palate: 1 in 2500 births
      c. Cleft lip with or without cleft palate affects more boys; cleft palate affects more girls
   3. With cleft palate, the failure of the bone and tissues to fuse results in a communication between the mouth and nose
B. Medical management: team approach for therapy
   1. Speech therapist
   2. Dentist and orthodontist
   3. Audiologist, otolaryngologist, pediatrician (these children are prone to otitis media and possible hearing loss)
   4. Surgical correction
      a. Timing varies with severity of defect; early correction helps to avoid speech defects.
      b. Cheiloplasty: correction of cleft lip
         1) goal is to unite edges to allow lips to be both functional and cosmetically attractive.
         2) usually performed approximately age 2 months (to prepare gums for eruption of teeth) when child is free from respiratory infection.
         3) Steri-Strips or Logan bar usually used to take tension off suture line.
      c. Cleft palate repair is usually not done until age 18 months in anticipation of speech development.
         1) between lip and palate repair child is maintained on normal nutritional and respiratory status; also maintains normal immunization schedule.
         2) child should be weaned and able to take liquids from a cup before palate repair.
C. Assessment findings
   1. Facial abnormality visible at birth: cleft lip or palate or both, unilateral or bilateral, partial or complete
   2. Difficulty sucking, inability to form airtight seal around nipple (size of defect may preclude breastfeeding)
   3. Formula/milk escapes through nose in infants with cleft palate
   4. Predisposition to infection because of free communication between mouth and nose

     5. Possible difficulty swallowing

     6. Abdominal distension due to swallowed air

D. Nursing interventions: pre-op cleft lip repair

     1. Feed in upright position to decrease chance of aspiration and decrease amount of air swallowed.

     2. Burp frequently; increased swallowed air causes abdominal distension and discomfort.

     3. Use a large-holed nipple; press cleft lip together with fingers to encourage sucking and to strengthen muscles needed later for speech.

     4. If infant unable to suck, use a rubber-tipped syringe and drip formula into side of mouth.

     5. Administer gavage feeding as ordered if necessary.

     6. Finish feeding with water to wash away formula in palate area.

     7. Provide small, frequent feedings.

     8. Provide emotional support for parents/family.

          a. Demonstrate benefits of surgery by showing before and after pictures.

          b. Reinforce that disorder is not their fault and that it will not affect child's life span or mental ability.

E. Nursing care: post-op cleft lip repair

     1. Maintain patent airway (child may appear to have respiratory distress because of closure of previously open space; adaptation occurs quickly).

     2. Assess color; monitor amount of swallowing to detect hemorrhage.

     3. Do not place in prone position or with pressure on cheeks; avoid any pressure or tension on suture line.

     4. Avoid straining on suture line by anticipating child's needs.

          a. Prevent crying.

          b. Keep child comfortable and content.

     5. Use elbow restraints or pin sleeves of shirt to diaper to keep child's hands away from suture line.

     6. Resume feedings as ordered.

     7. Keep suture line clean; clean after each feeding with saline, peroxide, or water to remove crusts and prevent scarring.

     8. Provide pain control/relief.

F. Nursing interventions: pre-op cleft palate repair

     1. Prepare parents to care for child after surgery.

     2. Instruct concerning feeding methods and positioning.

G. Nursing interventions: post-op cleft palate repair

     1. Position on side for drainage of blood/mucus.

     2. Have suction available but use only in emergency.

     3. Prevent injury or trauma to suture line.

          a. Use cups only for liquids; no bottles.

          b. Avoid straws, utensils, Popsicle sticks, chewing gum.

          c. Provide soft toys.

NURSING ALERT

Remove restraints at least every hour to encourage movement of extremities.

DELEGATION TIP

The application of restraints by ancillary personnel is acceptable if appropriate orders are in place and proper training has been provided.

---

    d. Use elbow restraints.
    e. Provide liquid diet initially, then progress to soft before returning to normal.
    f. Give water after each feeding to clean suture line.
    g. Hold and cuddle these babies to help distract them.

Altered Connections between Trachea, Esophagus, and Stomach

A. General information
    1. Types (Figure 7-1)
        a. *Esophageal atresia:* esophagus ends in a blind pouch; no entry route to stomach
        b. *Tracheoesophageal fistula* (*TEF*): open connection between trachea and esophagus
        c. *Esophageal atresia with TEF:* esophagus ends in a blind pouch; stomach end of esophagus connects with trachea
    2. These deformities are found more often in low-birth-weight or premature infants, and are associated with polyhydramnios in the mother and multiple congenital anomalies.
B. Medical management
    1. Drug therapy: antibiotics for respiratory infections
    2. Surgery
        a. Palliative
            1) gastrostomy for placement of a feeding tube
            2) esophagostomy to drain secretions
        b. Corrective
            1) end-to-end anastomosis to correct the defect and restore normal anatomy
            2) colon transplant for defects where there is insufficient tissue for an end-to-end anastomosis

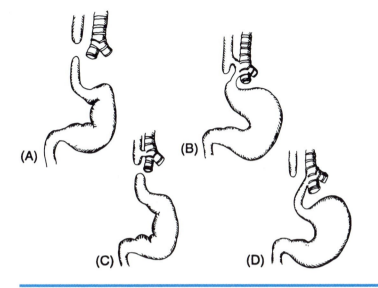

FIGURE 7-1 Esophageal defects: (A) Esophageal atresia; (B) (C) and (D) Esophageal atresia with tracheoesophageal fistula

C. Assessment findings
   1. Esophageal atresia
      a. History of polyhydramnios in mother (from infant's inability to swallow and excrete amniotic fluid)
      b. Inability to pass an NG tube
      c. Increased drooling and salivation
      d. Immediate regurgitation of undigested formula/milk when fed
      e. Intermittent cyanosis from choking on aspirated secretions
   2. TEF
      a. Normal swallowing but some food/mucus crosses fistula, causing choking and intermittent cyanosis
      b. Distended abdomen from inhaled air crossing fistula into stomach
      c. Aspiration pneumonia from reflux of gastric secretions into the trachea
   3. Esophageal atresia with TEF
      a. All findings for esophageal atresia
      b. Abdominal distension and aspiration pneumonia from gas and reflux of gastric acids into trachea
   4. Diagnostic tests: fluoroscopy with contrast material reveals type of defect
D. Nursing interventions: preoperative
   1. Maintain patent airway.
      a. Position according to type of defect (usually 30° head elevation).
      b. Provide continuous or prn nasal suctioning.

    2. Keep NPO.

    3. Administer IV fluids as ordered.

E. Nursing interventions: postoperative

    1. Provide nutrition.

        a. Provide gastrostomy tube feedings until the anastomosis site has healed.

        b. Start oral feedings when infant can swallow well.

        c. Progress from glucose water to small, frequent formula feedings.

    2. Promote respiratory function.

        a. Position properly.

        b. Suction as needed.

        c. Provide chest tube care.

    3. Provide client teaching and discharge planning concerning

        a. Alternative feeding methods

        b. Signs of respiratory distress and suctioning technique

Gastroesophageal Reflux (Chalasia)

A. General information

    1. Reversal of flow of stomach contents into lower portion of esophagus

    2. More common in premature infants due to hypotonia

    3. Caused by relaxed cardiac sphincter or overdistension of stomach by gas or overfeeding

    4. Results in local irritation of the lining of the esophagus from backflow of acidic gastric contents; sometimes causes aspiration pneumonia

B. Assessment findings

    1. Irritability

    2. "Spitting up" (versus vomiting or projectile vomiting); note relationship to feedings

    3. Diagnostic tests

        a. Muscle tone of cardiac sphincter reduced

        b. Esophageal pH: contents acidic

        c. Fluoroscopy: presence of refluxed contrast material not quickly cleared or repeated reflux

C. Nursing interventions

    1. Position with head elevated 30-45°.

    2. Give small, frequent feedings with adequate burping.

    3. Provide client teaching and discharge planning: teach parents how to position and feed infant.

Pyloric Stenosis

A. General information

    1. Hypertrophy (thickening) of the pyloric sphincter causing stenosis and obstruction

2. Incidence: 5 in 1000 births; more common in Caucasian, firstborn, full-term boys
3. Cause unknown; possibly familial
B. Medical management
   1. Correction of fluid electrolyte abnormalities
   2. Surgery: pyloromyotomy (Fredet-Ramstedt procedure)
C. Assessment findings
   1. Olive-size bulge under right rib cage
   2. Vomiting
      a. As obstruction increases, vomiting becomes more forceful and projectile.
      b. Vomitus does not contain bile (bile duct is distal to the pylorus).
   3. Peristaltic waves during and after feeding (look like rolling balls under abdominal wall)
   4. Failure to thrive, even though infant appears hungry after vomiting
   5. Dehydration: sunken fontanels, poor skin turgor, decreased urinary output
   6. Diagnostic tests
      a. Upper GI series reveals narrowing of the diameter of the pylorus
      b. Sodium, potassium, chloride decreased
      c. Hct increased
      d. Metabolic alkalosis
D. Nursing interventions: preoperative
   1. Administer replacement fluids and electrolytes as ordered.
   2. Prevent vomiting.
      a. May be NPO with NG tube to suction.
      b. Keep in high-Fowler's position.
      c. Place on right side after feedings.
      d. Minimize handling.
      e. Record strict I&O, daily weights, and urine specific gravity.
   3. Observe for symptoms of aspiration of vomitus.
E. Nursing interventions: postoperative
   1. Advance diet as tolerated.
   2. Place on right side after feeding. Elevate head.
   3. Monitor strict I&O, daily weights.
   4. Observe incision for signs of infection.
   5. Provide client teaching and discharge planning concerning feeding and positioning of infant.

Intussusception

A. General information
   1. Telescoping of bowel into itself (usually at the ileocecal valve) causing edema, obstruction, and possible necrosis of the bowel
   2. Most common at about age 6 months; occurs more often in boys than in girls; associated with cystic fibrosis and celiac disease
   3. Cause unknown

B. Medical management
   1. Barium or contrast medium enema to reduce telescoping by hydrostatic pressure
   2. Surgery if barium enema unsuccessful or if signs of peritonitis
C. Assessment findings
   1. Piercing cry
   2. Severe abdominal pain (pulls legs up)
   3. Vomiting of bile-stained fluid
   4. Bloody mucus in stool
   5. "Currant-jelly" stool
D. Nursing interventions
   1. Provide routine pre- and post-op care for abdominal surgery.
   2. Monitor for fluid and electrolyte imbalance and intervene as needed.
   3. Monitor for peritonitis and intervene as needed.
   4. Monitor stools. Report changes.

Hirschsprung's Disease (Aganglionic Megacolon)

A. General information
   1. Absence of autonomic parasympathetic ganglion cells in a portion of the large colon (usually occurs 4–25 cm proximally from anus), resulting in decreased motility in that portion of the colon and signs of functional obstruction
   2. Usually diagnosed in infancy
   3. Familial disease; more common in boys than girls; associated with Down syndrome
   4. When stool enters the affected part of the colon, lack of peristalsis causes it to remain there until additional stool pushes it through; colon dilates as stool is impacted.
B. Medical management
   1. Drug therapy: stool softeners
   2. Isotonic enemas
   3. Diet therapy: low residue
   4. Surgery
      a. Palliative: loop or double-barrel colostomy
      b. Corrective: abdominal-perineal pull through; bowel containing ganglia is pulled down and anastomosed to the rectum.
C. Assessment findings
   1. Failure or delay in passing meconium
   2. Abdominal distension; failure to pass stool
   3. Temporary relief following digital rectal exam
   4. Loose stools; only liquid can get around impaction (may also be a ribbonlike stool)
   5. Nausea, anorexia, lethargy

CLIENT TEACHING CHECKLIST

Provide the child and the family with instruction regarding:

- Colostomy care, rectal irritations, and skin management
- Dietary management
- Assessing complications such as infections and obstruction and when to notify changes in condition to the physician
- Techniques for coping with body image changes in the older child

---

6. Possibly bile-stained or fecal vomiting
7. Loss of weight, failure to grow
8. Volvulus (bowel twists upon itself, causing obstruction and necrosis) and enterocolitis due to fecal stagnation
9. Diagnostic tests: rectal biopsy confirms presence of aganglionic cells

D. Nursing interventions
   1. Administer enemas as ordered.
      a. Use mineral oil or isotonic saline.
      b. Do not use tap water or soap suds enemas in infants because of danger of water intoxication.
      c. Use volume appropriate to weight of child.
         1) infants: 150–200 ml
         2) children: 250–500 ml
   2. Do not treat the loose stools; the child actually is constipated.
   3. Administer TPN as ordered.
   4. Provide a low-residue diet.
   5. Provide client teaching and discharge planning concerning colostomy care and low-residue diet.

Imperforate Anus

A. General information
   1. Congenital malformation caused by abnormal fetal development
   2. Many variations; anal agenesis most frequent
   3. Often associated with fistula formation to rectum or vagina and other congenital anomalies
   4. Surgical correction performed in stages with completion at about age 1 year
   5. May need temporary colostomy

B. Medical management
  1. Manual dilatation
  2. Surgery: anoplasty (reconstruction of anus)
  3. Prophylactic antibiotics
C. Assessment findings
  1. No stool passage within 24 hours of birth
  2. Meconium stool from inappropriate orifice
  3. Inability to insert thermometer
D. Nursing interventions
  1. If suspected, do not take rectal temperature because of risk of perforating wall and causing peritonitis.
  2. Perform manual dilatation as ordered; instruct parents in proper technique.
  3. After surgery prevent infection; keep anal incisional area as clean as possible.
  4. After surgery use side-lying position, or have child lie prone with hips elevated.

Acquired Gastrointestinal Disorders

Celiac Disease

A. General information
  1. Malabsorption syndrome characterized by intolerance of gluten, found in rye, oats, wheat, and barley
  2. Familial disease, found more commonly in Caucasians
  3. Cause unknown; thought to be an inborn error of metabolism or an immunologic disorder
  4. Characterized by flat mucosal surface and atrophy of villi of the intestine; reduced absorptive surface causes marked malabsorption of fats
B. Medical management: diet therapy main intervention; gluten-free diet, TPN in children who are severely malnourished
C. Assessment findings
  1. Steatorrhea: frothy, pale, bulky, foul-smelling, greasy stools
  2. Chronic diarrhea during late infancy and throughout toddlerhood
  3. Failure to thrive
  4. Grossly distended abdomen; muscle wasting of limbs and buttocks
  5. Abdominal pain, irritability, listlessness, vomiting
  6. Symptoms of vitamin A, D, E, and K deficiency
  7. Diagnostic tests
      a. Pancreatic enzymes and sweat chloride test normal (performed to rule out the possibility of cystic fibrosis)
      b. Jejunal and duodenal biopsies show characteristic atrophy of the mucosa
D. Nursing interventions
  1. Monitor gluten-free diet (no wheat, barley, oats, and rye products)
  2. Provide supplemental fat-soluble vitamins in water-soluble form

3. Provide client teaching and discharge planning concerning
   a. Gluten-free diet; stress allowed foods and importance of reading labels carefully
   b. Avoidance of infection
   c. Assisting child to feel like a "normal" peer
   d. Importance of adhering to diet even though symptoms are controlled
   e. Importance of long-term follow-up management

Appendicitis

A. General information
   1. Inflammation of the appendix that prevents mucus from passing into the cecum; if untreated, ischemia, gangrene, rupture, and peritonitis occur
   2. Most common in school-age children
   3. May be caused by mechanical obstruction (fecaliths, intestinal parasites) or anatomic defect; may be related to decreased fiber in the diet
B. Assessment findings
   1. Diffuse pain, localizes in lower right quadrant
   2. Nausea/vomiting
   3. Guarding of abdomen, rebound tenderness, walks stooped over
   4. Decreased bowel sounds
   5. Fever
   6. Diagnostic tests
      a. WBC increased
      b. Elevated acetone in urine
C. Nursing interventions
   1. Administer antibiotics/antipyretics as ordered
   2. Prevent perforation of the appendix; do not give enemas or cathartics or use heating pad
   3. In addition to routine pre-op care for appendectomy
      a. Give support to parents if seeking treatment was delayed.
      b. Explain necessity of obtaining lab work prior to surgery.
   4. In addition to routine post-op care
      a. Monitor NG tube (usually with low suction).
      b. Monitor Penrose drains.
      c. Position in semi-Fowler's or lying on right side to facilitate drainage.
      d. Administer antibiotics as ordered.

Parasitic Worms

A. General information
   1. A parasite is an organism that lives in, on, or at the expense of the host.
   2. Common human GI parasites are pinworms and roundworms.
   3. Medication varies depending on type of parasite.

B. Assessment findings
1. Pinworms: anal irritation, itching, disturbed sleep
2. Roundworm: colic, abdominal pain, lack of appetite, weight loss
C. Nursing interventions
1. Obtain stool culture.
2. Observe for worms in all excreta (Scotch-tape test for stool).
3. Instuct parents to change clothing, bed linens, towels and launder in hot water.
4. Clean toilets with disinfectant.
5. Instruct all family members to scrub hands and fingernails prior to eating and after using toilet.
6. Follow specific medication and hygiene orders given by physician.

Giardiasis

A. General information
1. Common cause of diarrhea
2. Protozoan *Giardia lamblia*
3. Common in daycare centers
4. Cysts ingested, mature in GI tract, cysts excreted in stools, and complete maturation
5. Multiple stool cultures required as all stools don't contain cysts
6. Usually fecal–oral transmission, also contaminated water and animals
B. Assessment findings
1. Diarrhea
2. Vomiting, anorexia
3. Failure to thrive
4. Abdominal cramps
C. Medical management
1. Metronidazole (Flagyl)
2. Furazolidone (Furoxone)
D. Nursing interventions
1. Hygiene, especially with diaper changes
2. Handwashing
3. Instructions about drug therapy

Constipation

A. General information
1. Decrease in number of bowel movements with large, hard stools
2. May be caused by high fat and protein and low fluid in diet
3. May cause bowel obstruction if severe
B. Medical management
1. Drug therapy: stool softeners, suppositories, enemas
2. Diet therapy: increased fluids and fiber

C. Assessment findings
  1. Less frequent stools, difficulty eliminating stool, hard consistency compared to normal pattern (children do not have to stool every day)
  2. Bleeding with stooling
  3. Abdominal pain
D. Nursing interventions
  1. Assess for other pathologic causes of constipation.
  2. Dietary modification, increase fiber and fluids.
  3. Apply lubricant around anus.
  4. Remove stool digitally if possible.
  5. Provide prune juice (1 oz); add fruits to diet.
  6. Add small amount of Karo syrup to formula.
  7. Teach parents methods to prevent further episodes.

REVIEW QUESTIONS

1. A 9-year-old has celiac disease, which has been in good control since it was diagnosed 6 years ago. She has now been admitted to the hospital for an emergency appendectomy. Which preoperative procedure should the nurse withhold?

  1. A cleansing enema.

  2. Starting an IV.

  3. Keeping her NPO.

  4. Obtaining a blood sample for a CBC.

2. An 8-year-old has celiac disease. She had an emergency appendectomy. She is progressing well and is having her first real meal. Which food should the nurse remove from her tray?

  1. Chicken rice soup.

  2. Crackers.

  3. Hamburger patty.

  4. Fresh fruit cup.

3. A 10-month-old is brought to the clinic for a checkup and his MMR immunization. While talking to the nurse, the mother reports that her teenage babysitter has just come down with rubeola. The most appropriate plan of treatment for the child is to

  1. administer immune serum globulin.

  2. administer prophylactic penicillin.

3. vaccinate him now with MMR.

4. allow him to catch measles from the babysitter in order to develop active immunity.

4. The nurse is caring for a 12-month-old child who has a cleft palate. A cleft lip was repaired when he was 2 months old. His mother asks the nurse when he will be ready for a cleft palate repair. The most appropriate response is that cleft palate repair is usually done

   1. prior to development of speech.

   2. when the child is toilet trained.

   3. when the child is completely weaned from the bottle and pacifier.

   4. when a large-holed nipple is ineffective for his feedings.

5. A 2-year-old has had a cleft palate repair. A priority in the post-op plan of care for this child includes teaching his mother

   1. to resume toilet training after he is up and around.

   2. to use a cup or wide bowl spoon for feeding.

   3. that he will be more prone to respiratory infections now that his airway is smaller.

   4. that no further treatment will be needed until his adult teeth come in at age 6.

6. What is the appropriate feeding technique for the nurse to use with an infant who has a cleft palate?

   1. Suction client prior to feeding.

   2. Feed in sitting position.

   3. Have the nurse feed the client during hospitalization.

   4. Bubble client after feed to reduce risk of aspiration.

7. How would you evaluate that the new nurse is using appropriate technique to feed a 3-day-old with a cleft lip?

   1. NG tube is patent.

   2. Infant is seated in upright position.

   3. The nurse uses a Nuk nipple.

   4. The nurse adds rice to formula.

8. A baby girl is born prematurely to a mother with polyhydramnios. The baby is diagnosed with esophageal atresia with tracheoesophageal fistula. What assessment finding would the nurse be likely to note?

   1. Jaundice, high bilirubin.

   2. Seedy yellow stools.

3. Projectile emesis.

4. Frothy saliva, drooling.

9. A 5-month-old girl is admitted with gastroesophageal reflux. Her signs and symptoms include emesis, poor weight gain, hemepositive stools, irritability, and gagging with feeds. The nurse would include which intervention?

1. Urine dipstick each void.

2. Appropriate feeding positioning.

3. Biweekly weights.

4. Monitor white blood count as indicator for infection.

10. A 4-week-old is admitted for observation. Her assessment reveals projectile vomiting, visible gastric peristalsis, and an olive-shaped mass in the epigastrium. Which nursing diagnosis is of highest best priority?

1. Altered nutrition.

2. Self-care deficit.

3. Impaired gas exchange.

4. Fluid volume deficit.

11. The nurse would find which stool characteristic consistent with a diagnosis of intussusception?

1. Yellow seedy stools.

2. Currant jelly-like stools.

3. Mucous-like stools.

4. Hard black stools.

12. A 6-month-old boy is treated at home with saline enemas due to his Hirschsprung's disease. His mother asks if she can use tap water to reduce costs. The nurse responds,

1. "Yes, tap water is as effective as saline, just be sure to boil it first."

2. "No, saline enemas must be used to maintain his electrolyte balance."

3. "Yes; you can use tap water after letting it run for one minute to clear any lead from the pipes."

4. "No; tap water enemas are not allowed, but soap suds enemas are just as effective."

13. A 5-year-old boy has celiac disease. During a routine clinic visit, the nurse knows he is following his diet when he states,

1. "I had hot dogs and french fries for lunch."

2. "I ate chicken and vegetables for dinner."

    3. "I had macaroni and cheese for lunch."

    4. "I ate soup and crackers for dinner."

14. A 14-year-old is admitted to your unit following an emergency appendectomy. What is the nurse's goal for this client?

    1. Pain related to inflamed appendix.

    2. Patient will experience minimized risk of spread of infection.

    3. Maintain NG tube decompression until bowel motility returns.

    4. Child demonstrates resolution of peritonitis.

15. A 9-year-old girl comes into the clinic with a diagnosis of pinworms. What is it essential for the nurse to teach?

    1. Check for pinworms every morning for a week with a Scotch tape test.

    2. Save the girl's next bowel movement to check for pinworms.

    3. Follow-up with local doctor in 6 months to check for recurrence.

    4. Scrub hands and fingernails thoroughly before each meal and after each use of the toilet.

ANSWERS AND RATIONALES

1. 1. Enemas, cathartics, and heat to the abdomen should all be avoided in appendicitis because they may cause perforation of the appendix.

2. 2. The prescribed diet for children with celiac disease is gluten free. Crackers contain gluten.

3. 1. Administration of immune serum globulin will provide the child with passive immunity to prevent a full-blown case of measles or reduce the severity of symptoms.

4. 1. Cleft palate repair should be done before speech is well developed. This allows for the formation of a more normal speech pattern.

5. 2. Care must be taken not to put anything in the mouth that could damage the suture line.

6. 2. This position reduces the risk of aspiration.

7. 2. This position reduces the risk of aspiration.

8. 4. Infants with esophageal atresia (EA) with tracheoesophageal fistula (TEF) have difficulty handling their secretions.

9. 2. It may be a challenge to find the optimum position. Best positions include upright prone and 30° head of bed elevation.

10. 4. Infants with pyloric stenosis are at high risk for electrolyte imbalance and these need to be corrected prior to a pyloromyotomy.

11. 2. The obstruction causes bloody mucus known as currant jelly stools.

12. 2. Repeated water enemas cause electrolyte dilution.

13. 2. Chicken and vegetables do not contain gluten. Gluten is in barley, rye, oats, and wheat.

14. 2. This is an appropriate goal.

15. 4. Handwashing prevents reinfection and/or new infections in other people.

The Genitourinary System

■ VARIATIONS FROM THE ADULT

A. Nephrons continue to develop after birth.
B. Glomerular filtration rate is 30% below adult levels at birth; reaches normal level by age 2 years.
C. Tubular functions immature at birth; tubular absorption and secretion reach adult levels by age 2 years.
D. Urethra is shorter in children and more prone to ascending infection (particularly true in girls); the urethra is also closer to anus as source of contamination.
E. Many GU conditions in children become chronic.

■ ASSESSMENT

History

A. Presenting problem: symptoms may include
    1. Change in appearance, color, or smell of urine
    2. Change in amount, frequency, or pattern of urination
    3. Abdominal or back pain
    4. Anorexia, nausea, vomiting, weight loss
    5. Headaches, seizures
    6. Fatigue, lethargy
    7. Excessive thirst
    8. Drug use or accidental ingestions
B. Family history: kidney disease, hypertension

Physical Examination

A. General appearance: note presence of edema.
B. Abdomen and genitalia: note abdominal distension, presence of undescended testicle, tenderness to palpation, placement of urinary meatus, urinary stream during voiding

NURSING ALERT

Approximately 15–20 ml is needed for a urine analysis and culture.

C. Vital signs: note presence of fever; increased blood pressure (common in renal disease)

■ ANALYSIS

Nursing diagnoses for the child with a disorder of the genitourinary tract may include
A. Excess fluid volume
B. Impaired urinary elimination
C. Pain
D. Activity intolerance
E. Interrupted family process

■ PLANNING AND IMPLEMENTATION

Goals

A. Child will have normal urinary function.
B. Child's fluid and electrolyte and acid-base balances will be normal.
C. Child will be free from signs of infection.
D. Child's blood pressure will be within normal limits.
E. Parents will be able to care for child at home.

Intervention

Pediatric Urine Collector (PUC)

A. Used when child is not toilet trained
B. Nursing care
   1. Wash genitalia as for clean catch specimens.
   2. Apply bag directly to dry skin; do not use powder or creams.
   3. If child has not voided within 45 minutes, remove bag and repeat process.

■ EVALUATION

A. Child is adequately hydrated as evidenced by normal serum electrolyte levels and normal urine output.
B. Child is free from complications such as infection, skin breakdown, or hypertension.
C. Parents demonstrate ability to administer appropriate medications and treatments.

nform all ancillary staff regarding the need to collect a urine culture. However, the task of using the proper collection technique cannot be delegated.

■ DISORDERS OF THE GENITOURINARY SYSTEM
Urinary Tract Infection (UTI)

A. General information
   1. Bacterial invasion of the kidneys or bladder
   2. More common in girls, preschool, and school-age children
   3. Usually caused by *E. coli;* predisposing factors include poor hygiene, irritation from bubble baths, urinary reflux
   4. The invading organism ascends the urinary tract, irritating the mucosa and causing characteristic symptoms.

B. Assessment findings
   1. Low-grade fever
   2. Abdominal pain
   3. Enuresis, pain/burning on urination, frequency, hematuria

C. Nursing interventions
   1. Administer antibiotics as ordered; prevention of kidney infection/ glomerulonephritis important. (*Note:* obtain cultures before starting antibiotics.)
   2. Provide warm baths and allow child to void in water to alleviate painful voiding.
   3. Force fluids.
   4. Encourage measures to acidify urine (cranberry juice, acid-ash diet).
   5. Provide client teaching and discharge planning concerning
      a. Avoidance of tub baths (contamination from dirty water may allow microorganisms to travel up urethra)
      b. Avoidance of bubble baths that might irritate urethra
      c. Importance for girls to wipe perineum from front to back
      d. Increase in foods/fluids that acidify urine

Vesicoureteral Reflux

A. General information
   1. Regurgitation of urine from the bladder into the ureters due to faulty valve mechanism at the vesicoureteral junction
   2. Predisposes child to
      a. UTIs from urine stasis
      b. Pyelonephritis from chronic UTIs
      c. Hydronephrosis from increased pressure on renal pelvis

---

CLIENT TEACHING CHECKLIST

Suggest the following to the client with a UTI:

- Wear cotton undergarments that are comfortable and not restrictive.
- Take showers instead of tub baths.
- For a sexually active client, encourage voiding after sexual activity.

B. Assessment findings: same as for urinary tract infections
C. Nursing interventions for surgical reimplantation of ureters
    1. Assist with preoperative studies as needed (IVP, voiding cystourethrogram, cystoscopy).
    2. Provide postoperative care.
        a. Monitor drains; may have one from bladder and one from each ureter (ureteral stents).
        b. Check output from all drains (expect bloody drainage initially) and record carefully.
        c. Observe drainage from abdominal dressing; note color, amount, frequency.
        d. Administer medication for bladder spasms as ordered.

Exstrophy of the Bladder

A. General information
    1. Congenital malformation in which nonfusion of abdominal and anterior walls of the bladder during embryologic development causes anterior surface of bladder to lie open on abdominal wall
    2. Varying degrees of defect
B. Assessment findings
    1. Associated structural changes
        a. Prolapsed rectum
        b. Inguinal hernia
        c. Widely split symphysis
        d. Rotated hips
    2. Associated anomalies
        a. Epispadias
        b. Cleft scrotum or clitoris
        c. Undescended testicles
        d. Chordee (downward deflection of the penis)
C. Medical management: two-stage reconstructive surgery, possibly with urinary diversion; usually delayed until age 3–6 months

D. Nursing interventions: preoperative
  1. Provide bladder care; prevent infection.
      a. Keep area as clean as possible; urine on skin will cause irritation and ulceration.
      b. Change diaper frequently; keep diaper loose fitting.
      c. Wash with mild soap and water.
      d. Cover exposed bladder with Vaseline gauze.
E. Nursing interventions: postoperative
  1. Design play activities to foster toddler's need for autonomy (e.g., Play-Doh, talking toys, books); child will be immobilized for extended period of time.
  2. Prevent trauma; as child gets older and more mobile, trauma more likely; teach parents to avoid areas such as sandboxes.

Undescended Testicles (Cryptorchidism)

A. General information
  1. Unilateral or bilateral absence of testes in scrotal sac
  2. Testes normally descend at 8 months of gestation, will therefore be absent in premature infants
  3. Incidence increased in children having genetically transmitted diseases
  4. Unilateral cryptorchidism most common
  5. 75% will descend spontaneously by age 1 year
B. Medical management
  1. Whether or not to treat is still controversial; if testes remain in abdomen, damage to the testes (sterility) is possible because of increased body temperature.
  2. If not descended by age 8 or 9, chorionic gonadotropin can be given.
  3. Orchipexy: surgical procedure to retrieve and secure testes placement; performed between ages 1–3 years.
C. Assessment findings: unable to palpate testes in scrotal sac (when palpating testes be careful not to elicit cremasteric reflex, which pulls testes higher in pelvic cavity)
D. Nursing interventions
  1. Advise parents of absence of testes and provide information about treatment options.
  2. Support parents if surgery is to be performed.
  3. Post-op, avoid disturbing the tension mechanism (will be in place for about 1 week).
  4. Avoid contamination of incision.

Hypospadias

A. General information
  1. Urethral opening located anywhere along the ventral surface of penis
  2. Chordee (ventral curvature of the penis) often associated, causing constriction
  3. In extreme cases, child's sex may be uncertain

NURSING ALERT

D ouble diaper the child if a stent is in place. The inner diaper collects stool and the outer diaper collects urine and protects the stent.

B. Medical management
  1. Minimal defects need no intervention
  2. Neonatal circumcision delayed, tissue may be needed for corrective repair
  3. Surgery performed at age 3–9 months; 2 years of age for complex repairs
C. Assessment findings
  1. Urinary meatus misplaced
  2. Inability to make straight stream of urine
D. Nursing interventions
  1. Diaper normally.
  2. Provide support for parents.
  3. Provide support for child at time of surgery.
  4. Postoperatively check pressure dressing, monitor catheter drainage, assess pain.

Enuresis

A. General information
  1. Involuntary passage of urine after the age of control is expected (about 4 years)
  2. Types
    a. Primary: in children who have never achieved control
    b. Secondary: in children who have developed complete control and lose it
  3. May occur at any time of day but is most frequent at night
  4. More common in boys
  5. No organic cause can be identified; familial tendency
  6. Etiologic possibilities
    a. Sleep disturbances
    b. Delayed neurologic development
    c. Immature development of bladder leading to decreased capacity
    d. Psychologic problems
B. Medical management
  1. Bladder retention exercises
  2. Behavior modification, e.g., bed alarm devices
  3. Drug therapy: results are temporary; side effects may be unpleasant or even dangerous
    a. Tricyclic antidepressants: imipramine HCI (Tofranil)

  b. Anticholinergics

  c. DDAVP

C. Assessment findings

 1. Physical exam normal

 2. History of repeated involuntary urination

D. Nursing interventions

 1. Provide information/counseling to family as needed.

  a. Confirm that this is not conscious behavior and that child is not purposely misbehaving.

  b. Assure parents that they are not responsible and that this is a relatively common problem.

 2. Involve child in care; give praise and support with small accomplishments.

  a. Age 5-6 years: can strip bed of wet sheets.

  b. Age 10-12 years: can do laundry and change bed.

 3. Avoid scolding and belittling child.

Nephrosis (Nephrotic Syndrome)

A. General information

 1. Autoimmune process leading to structural alteration of glomerular membrane that results in increased permeability to plasma proteins, particularly albumin

 2. Course of the disease consists of exacerbations and remissions over a period of months to years

 3. Commonly affects preschoolers, boys more often than girls

 4. Pathophysiology

  a. Plasma proteins enter the renal tubule and are excreted in the urine, causing proteinuria.

  b. Protein shift causes altered oncotic pressure and lowered plasma volume.

  c. Hypovolemia triggers release of renin and angiotensin, which stimulates increased secretion of aldosterone; aldosterone increases reabsorption of water and sodium in distal tubule.

  d. Lowered blood pressure also stimulates release of ADH, further increasing reabsorption of water; together with a general shift of plasma into interstitial spaces, results in edema.

 5. Prognosis is good unless edema does not respond to steroids.

B. Medical management

 1. Drug therapy

  a. Corticosteroids to resolve edema

  b. Antibiotics for bacterial infections

  c. Thiazide diuretics in edematous stage

 2. Bed rest

 3. Diet modification: high protein, low sodium

C. Assessment findings
 1. Proteinuria, hypoproteinemia, hyperlipidemia
 2. Dependent body edema
  a. Puffiness around eyes in morning
  b. Ascites
  c. Scrotal edema
  d. Ankle edema
 3. Anorexia, vomiting and diarrhea, malnutrition
 4. Pallor, lethargy
 5. Hepatomegaly
D. Nursing interventions
 1. Provide bed rest.
  a. Conserve energy.
  b. Find activities for quiet play.
 2. Provide high-protein, low-sodium diet during edema phase only.
 3. Maintain skin integrity.
  a. Do not use Band-Aids.
  b. Avoid IM injections (medication is not absorbed into edematous tissue).
  c. Turn frequently.
 4. Obtain morning urine for protein studies.
 5. Provide scrotal support.
 6. Monitor I&O, vital signs and weigh daily.
 7. Administer steroids to suppress autoimmune response as ordered.
 8. Protect from known sources of infection.

Acute Glomerulonephritis

A. General information
 1. Immune complex disease resulting from an antigen-antibody reaction
 2. Secondary to a beta-hemolytic streptococcal infection occurring elsewhere in the body
 3. Occurs more frequently in boys, usually between ages 6–7 years
 4. Usually resolves in about 14 days, self-limiting
B. Medical management
 1. Antibiotics for streptococcal infection
 2. Antihypertensives if blood pressure severely elevated
 3. Digitalis if circulatory overload
 4. Fluid restriction if renal insufficiency
 5. Peritoneal dialysis if severe renal or cardiopulmonary problems develop
C. Assessment findings
 1. History of a precipitating streptococcal infection, usually upper respiratory infection or impetigo
 2. Edema, anorexia, lethargy
 3. Hematuria or dark-colored urine, fever

4. Hypertension
5. Diagnostic tests
   a. Urinalysis reveals RBCs, WBCs, protein, cellular casts
   b. Urine specific gravity increased
   c. BUN and serum creatinine increased
   d. ESR elevated
   e. Hgb and hct decreased
D. Nursing interventions
   1. Monitor I&O, blood pressure, urine; weigh daily.
   2. Provide diversional therapy.
   3. Provide client teaching and discharge planning concerning
      a. Medication administration
      b. Prevention of infection
      c. Signs of renal complications
      d. Importance of long-term follow-up

Hydronephrosis

A. General information
   1. Collection of urine in the renal pelvis due to obstruction to outflow
   2. Obstruction most common at ureteral-pelvic junction but may also be caused by adhesions, ureterocele, calculi, or congenital malformation
   3. Obstruction causes increased intrarenal pressure, decreased circulation, and atrophy of the kidney, leading to renal insufficiency
   4. May be unilateral or bilateral; occurs more often in left kidney
   5. Prognosis good when treated early
B. Medical management: surgery to correct or remove obstruction
C. Assessment findings
   1. Repeated UTIs
   2. Failure to thrive
   3. Abdominal pain, fever
   4. Fluctuating mass in region of kidney
D. Nursing interventions: prepare child for multiple urologic studies.

REVIEW QUESTIONS

1. A 4-year-old has just been diagnosed as having nephrotic syndrome. His potential for impairment of skin integrity is related to
   1. joint inflammation.
   2. drug therapy.

   3. edema.

   4. generalized body rash.

2. A 20-month-old is admitted to the hospital with a diagnosis of cryptorchidism. Surgical correction is performed at this time to prevent

   1. difficulty in urinating.

   2. sterility.

   3. herniation.

   4. peritonitis.

3. A 3-day-old is diagnosed with hypospadias. His parents are very upset and have been willing listeners as the nurse has explained this problem to them. The nurse explained that in hypospadias, the physical problem is primarily

   1. ambiguous genitalia.

   2. urinary incontinence.

   3. ventral curvature of the penis.

   4. altered location of the urethral meatus.

4. The parents of a newborn who has hypospadias ask about surgical repair. They are told that the preferred time to schedule surgical repair of hypospadias is when the boy is

   1. 9 months old.

   2. 5 years old.

   3. 12 years old.

   4. 17 years old.

5. The parents of a baby boy who was born with hypospadias want to know about the surgical repair. The nurse tells them that they will be able to evaluate the success of hypospadias surgery by

   1. the cosmetic appearance of the penis.

   2. maintaining stable blood pressure in the child.

   3. observing a straight stream when he voids.

   4. his ability to void without discomfort.

6. The nurse is teaching parents about post-op care of their child who has had an orchiopexy. The nurse states,

   1. "You must tighten the rubber band around the scrotum every 4 hours to maintain the testicle."

   2. "You must increase tension on the rubber band every 4 hours."

   3. "You must check the rubber band every 4 hours to check for disconnection."

   4. "Cut the rubber band after 24 hours."

7. A baby boy is born with a hypospadias. The parents decide to wait until the child is 6 months old for the repair. The father asks the nurse why the doctor said not to have the baby circumcised. The nurse's best response is,

   1. ''It is best to wait until the baby is older and understands the surgery.''

   2. ''Circumcision carries a high infection rate and that may delay his hypospadias repair.''

   3. ''The foreskin may be used during the hypospadias repair.''

   4. ''He will need the foreskin to help anchor the Foley catheter after the repair.''

8. The nurse is planning care for a 2-year-old who has nephrotic syndrome and is in remission. What type of diet would the nurse plan to feed this child?

   1. High protein, low calorie.

   2. High calorie, low protein.

   3. Low sodium, low fat.

   4. Regular diet, no added salt.

9. A 5-year-old girl recovered from a strep infection 2 weeks ago. She now presents with loss of appetite, dark colored urine, and orbital edema. What is the nurse's assessment?

   1. Nephrotic syndrome.

   2. Glomerulonephritis.

   3. Renal tubular acidosis.

   4. Hemolytic uremic syndrome.

10. A 4-year-old boy is admitted with glomerulonephritis. His mother asks why his eyes are so puffy. The nurse responds,

   1. ''This is a common finding due to circulatory congestion in the kidneys.''

   2. ''Children cry a lot with glomerulonephritis and the puffiness should subside when he feels better.''

   3. ''Has he been rubbing his eyes excessively?''

   4. ''Periorbital edema is associated with hypertension.''

ANSWERS AND RATIONALES

1. **3.** A child with nephritic syndrome will have massive edema. A child with edema is prone to skin breakdown.

2. **2.** If the testes remain in the abdomen beyond the age of 5, damage resulting from exposure to internal body temperature can cause sterility.

3. 4. In hypospadias, the urethral opening may be anywhere along the underside of the penis.

4. 1. Most surgical repairs are scheduled for the child between 6 and 18 months of age.

5. 3. Observing the child void in a straight stream while standing is the expected successful outcome of hypospadias repair.

6. 3. The Torek procedure attaches a rubber band from the testicle to the scrotal sac to the thigh to maintain the testicle in the pouch. The family must check the rubber band every 4 hours and call the doctor if the rubber band breaks or becomes disconnected.

7. 3. The foreskin is frequently used as a flap during the repair.

8. 4. The child who is in remission is allowed a regular diet; salt is restricted in the form of no added salt at the table and excluding foods with very high salt content.

9. 2. Acute poststreptococcal glomerulonephritis is the most common of the noninfectious renal diseases in children.

10. 1. Periorbital edema is often associated with circulatory congestion in the kidneys.

9

The Musculoskeletal System

■ VARIATIONS FROM THE ADULT

Bones

A. Linear growth results from skeletal development
1. Centers of ossification
    a. Primary centers in diaphyses
    b. Secondary centers in epiphyses
    c. Used in assessment of bone age; number of ossification centers in wrist equals age in years plus 1
    d. Centers appear earlier in girls than in boys
2. Metaphysis
    a. Cartilaginous plate between diaphysis and epiphysis
    b. The site of active growth in long bones
    c. Disappears over time with bony fusion of diaphysis and epiphysis
    d. Linear growth ends with epiphyseal fusion
    e. Assessment of bone age includes the advancing bone edges
B. Bone circumference growth occurs as new bone tissue is formed beneath the periosteum.
C. Skeletal maturity is reached by age 17 in boys and 2 years after menarche in girls.
D. Certain characteristics of bone in children affect injury and healing, bones are more prone to injury, and injury results from relatively minor accidents.
1. Metaphysis
    a. Absorbs shock, protects joints from injury.
    b. Traumatic injury or infection to this growth plate can cause deformity.
    c. If not injured, this growth plate participates in healing and straightening of limbs by process of remodeling.
2. Porous bone
    a. Increases flexibility; absorbs force on impact.
    b. Allows bones to bend, buckle, and break in "greenstick" or incomplete fracture.

   3. Thicker periosteum
      a. More active osteogenic potential
      b. Healing more rapid
         1) neonatal period: may take 2-3 weeks
         2) early childhood: may take 4 weeks
         3) later childhood: may take 6 weeks
         4) adolescence: 8-10 weeks
      c. Stiffness after immobilization is rare unless joint has been injured.
E. Bone growth is affected by Wolff's law: bone will grow in the direction in which stress is placed on it.

Muscles

A. Muscle growth is responsible for a large part of increase in body weight.
B. The number of muscle fibers is constant throughout life; growth results from an increase in the size of the muscle fibers and by an increased number of nuclei per fiber.
C. Muscle growth most apparent in adolescence, influenced by growth hormone, adrenal androgens, and in boys by testosterone.

■ ASSESSMENT

History

A. Presenting problem: symptoms may include
   1. Delayed motor development
   2. Injury
   3. Pain, loss of sensation, tingling
   4. Muscle weakness, loss of function of an extremity
   5. Interference with normal activity or play
   6. Other parental concerns
B. Family history: genetic disorders, skeletal deformities
C. Inadequate nutrition (e.g., vitamin A deficiency causes rickets)

Physical Examination

A. General appearance: note any asymmetry, visible deformities, swelling (of joints or over bones), quality of movement (ROM, gait, guarding).
B. Measure muscle strength.
C. Identify warmth or tenderness over bones and joints.
D. Assess pain: note type, location, onset, relationship to activity.
E. Perform examination in standing, lying, and sitting positions.

■ ANALYSIS

Nursing diagnoses for the child with a disorder of the musculoskeletal system may include

NURSING ALERT

A spiral fracture in a child may indicate child abuse.

A. Risk for activity intolerance
B. Pain
C. Deficient diversional activity
D. Risk for injury
E. Impaired physical mobility
F. Self-care deficit
G. Disturbed body image
H. Risk for impaired skin integrity
I. Ineffective tissue perfusion

■ PLANNING AND IMPLEMENTATION

Goals

A. Injury or deformity will be identified and treated early.
B. Child will achieve maximum level of mobility.
C. Pain will be relieved/controlled.
D. Child will be free from injury.
E. Parents will be able to care for child at home.

Interventions

Care of the Child with a Cast

A. General information
   1. Initial chemical hardening reaction may cause a change in an infant's body temperature; monitor and intervene as needed.
   2. Choose toys too big to fit down cast.
   3. Do not use baby powder near cast since it clumps and provides a medium for bacterial growth.
   4. Prepare for anticipated casting by having child help apply a cast to a doll the day before.
   5. Demonstrate the use of a cast cutter on a doll before using on child to show it does not cut skin.
B. Care of child in hip spica cast (cast encases child from nipples to knees; legs are abducted with a bar between the thighs)
   1. Use firm mattress to allow for increased weight of plaster cast.
   2. Do not lift cast by crossbar.
   3. Protect cast from water and urine.

NURSING ALERT

Observations of pain, unusual odor, swelling, discoloration, or inability to move toes should be reported immediately to the health care provider.

---

     a. Put waterproof material over petaling (Chux®, plastic diapers).
     b. Elevate head of bed slightly to prevent urine and stool from seeping under cast; confirm that entire body is on a slant, not just the head.
     c. Use Bradford frame (canvas board with opening near genitalia) and place a bedpan under opening.
  4. Use pillows to support all parts of the cast.
  5. Drape towel across top of chest part of cast during feedings to prevent crumbs from entering cast.
  6. Monitor for pain/pressure points due to growth if cast is on for a long time.

Care of the Child in Traction

A. General information
  1. Infants and young toddlers do not have enough body weight to use traditional tractions effectively.
  2. Children do not understand the necessity of maintaining proper body alignment and will need frequent repositioning.
B. Bryant's traction: used primarily in children
  1. Child is own counterweight.
  2. Both legs are at 90° angle to bed.
  3. Buttocks must be slightly off mattress in order to ensure sufficient traction on legs.
  4. Used with children under age 2 years whose weight is too low (under 30 lb [14 kg]) to counterbalance without additional gravitational force.
  5. Used for fractured femur and dislocated hip.
  6. Monitor for vascular injury to feet with frequent neurovascular checks.

Care of the Child with a Brace

A. General information
  1. Orthopedic device made of metal or leather applied to the body, particularly the trunk and lower extremities, to support the weight of the body, to correct or prevent deformities, and to prevent involuntary movements in spastic conditions
  2. Types
     a. Milwaukee brace
       1) steel and leather brace fitted and adapted to child individually
       2) extends from chin cup and neck pad to pelvis

    3) used in scoliosis to correct curvature

    4) worn 23 hours/day, removed once daily for bathing

    5) causes little interference with activity

  b. Rotowalker

    1) used to provide upright mobility in children with lower limb paralysis

    2) child shifts weight to achieve mobility

  c. Leg brace

    1) designed to stabilize extremity and offer support during ambulation

    2) special hinges permit hip, knee, and ankle to flex during sitting

B. Nursing care: provide client teaching and discharge planning concerning

  1. Importance of meticulous skin care

  2. Need to wear protective clothing under brace

  3. Potential problems of ill-fitting braces

    a. Difficulty in balancing

    b. Muscle stress and skin breakdown

  4. Need for frequent checking and adjustment of braces with growth

■ EVALUATION

A. Child's musculoskeletal development is normal as evidenced by normal growth and activity.

B. Child experiences minimal discomfort.

C. Injuries are prevented.

D. Parents demonstrate ability to identify complications and administer treatments correctly.

■ DISORDERS OF THE MUSCULOSKELETAL SYSTEM
Congenital Dislocation of the Hip (Developmental Dysplasia of the Hip)

A. General information

  1. Displacement of the head of the femur from the acetabulum; present at birth, although not always diagnosed immediately

  2. One of the most common congenital malformations; incidence is 1 in 500–1000 live births

  3. Familial disorder, more common in girls; may be associated with spina bifida

  4. Cause unknown; may be fetal position in utero (breech delivery), genetic predisposition, or laxity of ligaments

  5. The acetabulum is shallow and the head of the femur cartilaginous at birth, contributing to the dislodgment.

B. Medical management

  1. Goal is to enlarge and deepen socket by pressure.

  2. The earlier treatment is initiated, the shorter and less traumatic it will be.

3. Early treatment consists of positioning the hip in abduction with the head of the femur in the acetabulum and maintaining it in position for several months.
4. If these measures are unsuccessful, traction and casting (hip spica) or surgery may be successful.

C. Assessment findings
1. May be unilateral or bilateral, partial or complete
2. Limitation of abduction (cannot spread legs to change diaper)
3. Ortolani's click (should only be performed by an experienced practitioner)
    a. With infant in supine position (on the back), bend knees and place thumbs on bent knees, fingers at hip joint.
    b. Bring femurs 90° to hip, then abduct.
    c. With dislocation there is a palpable click where the head of the femur snaps over edge of acetabulum.
4. Barlow's test
    a. With infant on back, bend knees.
    b. Affected knee will be lower because the head of the femur dislocates towards bed by gravity (referred to as telescoping of limb).
5. Additional skin folds with knees bent, from telescoping
6. When lying on abdomen, buttocks of affected side will be flatter because head of femur falls toward bed from gravity
7. Trendelenburg test (used if child is old enough to walk)
    a. Have child stand on affected leg only.
    b. Pelvis will dip on normal side as child attempts to stay erect.

D. Nursing interventions
1. Maintain proper positioning: keep legs abducted.
    a. Pavlik harness (place undershirt under harness and socks on legs)
    b. Frejka pillow splint (jumperlike suit to keep legs abducted)
    c. Place infant on abdomen with legs in "frog" position
    d. Other immobilization devices (splints, casts, braces)
2. Provide adequate nutrition; adapt feeding position as needed for immobilization device.
3. Provide sensory stimulation; adapt to immobilization device and positioning.

4. Provide client teaching and discharge planning concerning
   a. Application and care of immobilization devices
   b. Modification of child care using immobilization devices

Clubfoot (Talipes)

A. General information
   1. Abnormal rotation of foot at ankle
      a. Varus (inward rotation): would walk on ankles, bottoms of feet face each other
      b. Valgus (outward rotation): would walk on inner ankles
      c. Calcaneous (upward rotation): would walk on heels
      d. Equinas (downward rotation): would walk on toes
   2. Most common deformity (95%) is talipes equinovarus.
   3. Deformity almost always congenital; usually unilateral
   4. Occurs more frequently in boys than in girls; may be associated with other congenital disorders but cause unknown
   5. General incidence: 1 in 700–1000
B. Medical management
   1. Exercises
   2. Casting (cast is changed periodically to change angle of foot)
   3. Denis Browne splint (bar shoe): metal bar with shoes attached to the bar at specific angle
   4. Surgery and casting for several months
C. Assessment findings: foot cannot be manipulated by passive exercises into correct position (differentiate from normal clubbing of newborn's feet)
D. Nursing interventions
   1. Perform exercises as ordered.
   2. Provide cast care or care for child in a brace.
   3. Child who is learning to walk must be prevented from trying to stand; apply restraints if necessary.
   4. Provide diversional activities.
   5. Adapt care routines as needed for cast or brace.
   6. Assess toes to be sure cast it not too tight.
   7. Provide skin care.
   8. Provide client teaching and discharge planning concerning
      a. Application/care of immobilization device
      b. Preparation for surgery if indicated
      c. Need to monitor special shoes for continued fit throughout treatment.

Tibial Torsion

A. General information
   1. Rotational deformity of tibia (greater than that normally found in newborn)
   2. Types
      a. Internal: knee forward and foot inward

    b. External: knee forward and foot outward (rare, associated with muscle paralysis)

  3. Majority of cases resolve without treatment

B. Medical management

  1. Splinting: use of Denis Browne splint at night

  2. Surgical correction if still evident by age 3 years

C. Assessment findings: with child lying supine, assess for straight line between tibial tuberosity and 2nd toe; in tibial torsion, the line intersects the 4th or 5th toe.

D. Nursing interventions

  1. If no treatment needed, encourage parents to be patient and emphasize that condition usually resolves by itself

  2. If stretching exercises are recommended, teach parents normal ROM exercises and how to carry them out.

  3. Instruct parents on use of Denis Browne splint if needed.

Legg-Calvé-Perthes Disease

A. General information

  1. Aseptic necrosis of femoral head due to disturbance of circulation to the area

  2. Primarily affects boys ages 4–10 years

  3. Stages: lasting from 18 months to a few years

    a. Initial stage: may not be distinguishable from transient synovitis

    b. Avascular stage: often the first stage noticed

    c. Revascularization stage: regeneration of vascular and connective tissue

    d. Regeneration stage: formation of new bone

B. Medical management: goal is to minimize deformity until healing process is completed

  1. Initial bed rest with traction and then an abduction brace

  2. Possible surgery

C. Assessment findings

  1. Limp, limitation of movement

  2. Pain in groin, hip, and referred to knee; often difficult for child to localize pain

  3. Diagnostic test: X-ray reveals opaque ossification center of head of the femur (softened in avascular stage)

D. Nursing interventions

  1. Provide care for a child with a cast or brace.

  2. Provide diversional activities.

Slipped Femoral Capital Epiphysis

A. General information

  1. Spontaneous displacement of proximal femoral epiphysis in a posterior and inferior direction

---

CLIENT TEACHING CHECKLIST

- Reinforce ambulation and weight bearing instructions, such as avoiding contact sports, as ordered by the health care provider.
- Assist the family in developing a strategy for returning to school.
- Review clinical manifestations and discuss monitoring the unaffected hip for the same problem.

---

    2. Onset insidious; usually occurs during fast growth period of adolescence (growth hormones weaken epiphyseal plate)

    3. Occurs most often in very tall and very obese adolescents; boys affected more frequently

B. Medical management

    1. Skeletal traction

    2. Surgical stabilization with pinning

C. Assessment findings

    1. Limp and referred pain to groin, hip, or knee

    2. Limited internal rotation and abduction of hip

D. Nursing interventions

    1. Suggest weight reduction program for obese children to decrease stress on bones.

    2. Provide care for the child with a cast or traction.

Osteogenesis Imperfecta

A. General information

    1. An inherited disorder affecting collagen formation and resulting in pathologic fractures

    2. Types

        a. Osteogenesis imperfecta congenita: autosomal recessive, prognosis poor

        b. Osteogenesis imperfecta tarda: autosomal dominant, less severe form, involvement of varying degrees

    3. Classic picture includes soft, fragile bones; blue sclera; otosclerosis

    4. Severity of symptoms decreases at puberty due to hormone production and child's ability to prevent injury

B. Medical management

    1. Magnesium oxide supplements

    2. Reduction and immobilization of fractures

C. Assessment findings

    1. Osteogenesis imperfecta congenita

        a. Multiple fractures at birth

        b. Possible skeletal deformity due to intrauterine fracture

      c. Bones of skull are soft

      d. Occasional intracranial hemorrhage

  2. Osteogenesis imperfecta tarda

      a. Delayed walking, fractures, structural scoliosis as child grows

      b. Lower limbs more frequently affected

      c. Hypermobility of joints

      d. Prone to dental caries

D. Nursing interventions

  1. Support limbs, do not stretch.

  2. Position with care; use blankets to aid in mobility and provide support.

  3. Instruct parents in bathing, dressing, diapering.

  4. Support parents; encourage expression of feelings of anger or guilt (parents may have been unjustly suspected of child abuse).

Scoliosis

A. General information

  1. Lateral curvature of the spine

  2. Most commonly occurs in adolescent girls

  3. Disorder has a familial pattern; associated with other neuromuscular disorders

  4. Majority of the time (75% of cases) disorder is idiopathic; others causes include congenital abnormality of vertebrae, neuromuscular disorders, and trauma

  5. May be functional or structural

      a. Nonstructural/functional: "C" curve of spine

         1) due to posture, can be corrected voluntarily and disappears when child lies down

         2) not progressive

         3) treated with posture exercises

      b. Structural/progressive: "S" curve of spine

         1) usually idiopathic

         2) structural change in spine, does not disappear with position changes

         3) more aggressive intervention needed

B. Medical management

  1. Stretching exercises of the spine for nonstructural changes

  2. Bracing

      a. Milwaukee brace

      b. TSLO-custom molded plastic orthotic brace

      c. Braces worn 16–23 hours/day; off only for hygiene

  3. Surgical correction

      a. Spinal alignment

      b. Fusion with bone chips

      c. Instrumentation to stabilize position

      1) Harrington rod

      2) Luque instrumentation: wires and hooks

C. Assessment findings (structural scoliosis)

  1. Failure of curve to straighten when child bends forward with knees straight and arms hanging down to feet (curve disappears with functional scoliosis)

  2. Uneven bra strap marks

  3. Uneven hips

  4. Uneven shoulders

  5. Asymmetry of rib cage

  6. Diagnostic test: X-ray reveals curvature

D. Nursing interventions

  1. Teach/encourage exercises as ordered.

  2. Provide care for child with Milwaukee brace

    a. Child wears brace 23 hours/day; is removed once a day for bathing.

    b. Monitor pressure points, adjustments may be needed to accommodate increase in height or weight.

    c. Promote positive body image with brace.

  3. Provide cast/traction care.

  4. Assist with modifying clothing for immobilization devices.

  5. Adjust diet for decreased activity.

  6. Provide diversional activities.

  7. Provide care for child with Harrington rod insertion (see below).

  8. Provide client teaching and discharge planning concerning

    a. Exercises

    b. Brace/traction/cast care

    c. Correct body mechanics

    d. Alternative education for long-term hospitalization/home care

    e. Availability of community agencies

Surgical Correction for Scoliosis

A. General information

  1. Spinal fusion and installation of supports along spine

  2. Used for moderate to severe curvatures

  3. Usually results in increase in height; positive body image changes

B. Nursing interventions

  1. Provide general pre-op teaching and care.

  2. In addition to routine post-op care.

    a. Log roll.

    b. Do not raise head of bed.

    c. Usually out of bed to chair after 48 hours with Luque procedure.

    d. Discuss adapting home environment to allow for privacy yet interaction with family during recovery.

    e. Discuss alternate methods of education during recovery period.

Muscular Dystrophy

A. General information
   1. A group of muscular diseases in children characterized by progressive muscle weakness and deformity
   2. Genetic in origin; biochemical defect is suspected
   3. Types
      a. *Pseudohypertrophic* (*Duchenne type*): most frequent type
         1) X-linked recessive
         2) affects only boys
         3) usually manifests in first 4 years
      b. *Facioscapulohumeral*
         1) autosomal dominant
         2) mild form, with weakness of facial and shoulder girdle muscles
         3) onset usually in adolescence
      c. *Limb girdle*
         1) autosomal recessive
         2) affects boys and girls
         3) onset usually in adolescence
      d. *Congenital*
         1) autosomal recessive
         2) onset in utero
      e. *Myotonic*
         1) autosomal dominant
         2) more common in boys
         3) onset in infancy or childhood, or adult onset
         4) prognosis in childhood form is guarded
   4. Disease causes progressive disability throughout childhood; most children with Duchenne's muscular dystrophy are confined to a wheelchair by age 8–10 years.
   5. Death occurs by age 20 in 75% of clients with Duchenne's muscular dystrophy.
B. Assessment findings (Duchenne type)
   1. Pelvic girdle weakness is early sign (child waddles and falls)
   2. Gower's sign (child uses hands to push up from the floor)
   3. Scoliosis (from weakness of shoulder girdle)
   4. Contractures and hypertrophy of muscles
   5. Diagnostic tests
      a. Muscle biopsy reveals histologic changes: degeneration of muscle fibers and replacement of fibers with fat.
      b. EMG shows decrease in amplitude and duration of potentials.
   6. Serum enzymes increased, especially CPK
C. Nursing interventions
   1. Prepare child for EMG and muscle biopsy.
   2. Maintain function at optimal level; keep child as active and independent as possible.

3. Plan diet to prevent obesity.
4. Continually evaluate capabilities.
5. Support child and parents and provide information about availability of community agencies and support groups.

Juvenile Rheumatoid Arthritis

A. General information
   1. Systemic, chronic disorder of connective tissue, resulting from an autoimmune reaction
   2. Results in eventual joint destruction
   3. Affected by stress, climate, and genetics
   4. More common in girls; peak ages 2–5 and 9–12 years
   5. Types
      a. *Mono/pauciarticular JRA*
         1) fewer than four joints involved (usually in legs)
         2) asymmetric; rarely systemic
         3) generally mild signs of arthritis
         4) symptoms may decrease as child enters adulthood
         5) prognosis good
      b. *Polyarticular JRA*
         1) multiple joints affected
         2) symmetrical symptoms of arthritis, disability may be mild to severe
         3) involvement of temporomandibular joint may cause earaches
         4) characterized by periods of remissions and exacerbations
         5) prognosis poorer
         6) treatment symptomatic for arthritis: physical therapy, ROM exercises, aspirin
      c. *Systemic disease with polyarthritis (Still's disease)*
         1) explosive course with remissions and exacerbations lasting for months
         2) begins with fever, rash, lymphadenopathy, anorexia, and weight loss
B. Medical management, assessment findings, and nursing interventions: see Rheumatoid Arthritis.

REVIEW QUESTIONS

1. An 18-month-old has a fractured femur and is in Bryant's traction. To evaluate correct application of the traction the nurse should note that
   1. the child is being continuously and gradually pulled toward bottom of bed.
   2. the child's buttocks are raised slightly.

3. the child's leg is at a 45° angle to the bed.

4. the child can move the unaffected leg freely.

2. A 14-year-old is in a hip spica cast. To turn her correctly, the nurse should

   1. use the cross bar.

   2. turn her upper body first, then turn the lower body.

   3. log-roll her.

   4. tell her to pull on the trapeze and sit up to help in turning.

3. A routine physical examination on a 2-day-old uncovered evidence of congenital dislocation, or dysplasia, of the right hip. When assessing the infant, a sign of one-sided hip displacement is

   1. an unusually narrow perineum

   2. pain where her leg is abducted.

   3. symmetrical skin folds near her buttocks and thigh.

   4. asymmetrical skin folds over the buttocks and thigh.

4. An infant is being treated for congenital hip dysplasia with a Pavlik harness. The baby's mother asks if she can remove the harness if it becomes soiled. The best response for the nurse to make is

   1. No, the harness may not be removed.

   2. No, she will only be wearing it a few days.

   3. Yes, just long enough to clean the area.

   4. Yes, just overnight while she is sleeping.

5. A 10-year-old takes aspirin QID for Still's disease (juvenile rheumatoid arthritis). What symptoms would her mother observe that would be indicative of aspirin toxicity?

   1. Hypothermia.

   2. Hypoventilation.

   3. Decreased hearing acuity.

   4. Increased urinary output.

6. Which of the following would the nurse include in a plan of care for a toddler with a newly applied hip spica cast?

   1. Petal the cast around the perineum area with waterproof tape.

   2. Teach the parents care of the child just before discharge.

   3. Give the child small blocks and beads to promote eye-hand coordination.

   4. Check neurovascular status every shift.

7. The mother of a 6-year-old asks why she was told not to use powder under her child's long leg cast. Which of the following is the most accurate basis for the nurse's response?

   1. Promoting adequate circulation is a top priority.
   2. Drying the cast is very important.
   3. Assessing the smell of a cast is a top priority.
   4. Preserving skin integrity is of the utmost importance.

8. In examining a newborn, the nurse notes the following: asymmetric gluteal folds, shortened right leg, and limited abduction of the right thigh. The nurse would correctly interpret these observations as which of the following?

   1. Right congenital dislocated hip.
   2. Spastic cerebral palsy.
   3. Left hip dysplasia.
   4. Myelodysplasia.

9. An infant with congenital hip dysplasia is placed in a Pavlik harness. In the nurse's teaching plan for the mother, which of the following would be important to include?

   1. Adjustment of daily care routines as the harness is worn 24 hours a day.
   2. Clothing should not be worn under the harness.
   3. The harness should be removed for bathing and diapering only.
   4. The infant should be confined to the crib.

10. In assessing a newborn for talipes equinovarus, the nurse would note which of the following?

    1. The feet turn inward when the infant lies still, but they are flexible.
    2. The feet are rigid and cannot be manipulated to a neutral position.
    3. Uneven knee length occurs when both knees are flexed.
    4. Limited abduction is observed when performing the Ortolani maneuver.

11. The nurse would evaluate that the parents correctly understand the care of their infant being treated for talipes equinovarus if the parents said which of the following?

    1. "We will unwrap the cast every night and massage his feet with lotion to prevent skin breakdown."
    2. "We'll petal the cast around the baby's groin to protect it from urine and bowel movements."

3. "Every day we'll check the baby's toes for movement and color after we squeeze them."

4. "We're so glad that the casts will cure his club feet."

12. Which of the following comments by the school nurse would be most appropriate in screening for scoliosis of a 13-year-old?

1. "You may leave your shirt on, but stand erect and turn to the side."

2. "Do you have any back pain?"

3. "Remove your clothes from the waist up and bend over at your waist."

4. "Have you noticed that your skirts don't hang evenly?"

13. A child is admitted to the hospital for a spinal fusion and Harrington rod insertion. A nursing priority in the first 8 hours postoperatively will be to

1. give fluids and fiber to promote bowel elimination.

2. check neurovascular function in extremities.

3. log roll every 4 hours.

4. monitor hourly urine output.

14. The nurse would evaluate that a child understood the effective use of her Milwaukee brace for her scoliosis if she said which of the following?

1. "I'm so glad that I don't have to sleep in this brace."

2. "I've toughened my skin so I can wear the brace right next to my skin."

3. "I can't believe that I'm not allowed to chew gum anymore."

4. "I'm going to look forward to my bath time each day without this brace."

15. A 4-year-old has recently been diagnosed with Duchenne's muscular dystrophy. His parents ask if their 2-year-old daughter will get the disease. The nurse's best response would be which of the following?

1. "Every child you have has a 25% chance of developing the disease and a 50% chance of being a carrier."

2. "Sons are affected 50% of the time, whereas 50% of the time daughters will become carriers who have no symptoms."

3. "Only your sons have a 25% chance of developing the disease."

4. "Every child has a 50% chance of developing the disease."

ANSWERS AND RATIONALES

1. 2. In Bryant's traction both legs are in traction at a 90° angle and the buttocks are raised slightly off the bed.

2. 3. The client in a hip spica cast should be turned as a unit.

3. **4.** Displacement of the hip on one side causes asymmetry of skin folds.

4. **1.** The harness is not to be removed until the hip is stable with 90° of flexion and X-ray confirmation. This usually occurs after about 3 weeks in a Pavlik harness.

5. **3.** Tinnitus or ringing in the ears is a side effect of aspirin therapy. In salicylate poisoning the child will have hypothermia, hyperventilation to compensate for metabolic acidosis, and may develop renal failure.

6. **1.** It is important to protect the cast from urine and stool to prevent skin and cast breakdown.

7. **4.** Powder may irritate the skin, leading to skin breakdown and infection.

8. **1.** These are all signs of right congenital dislocated hip in a newborn.

9. **1.** The harness is worn 24 hours a day so that parents must learn how to manage daily care (sponging and dressing the baby) with the harness on.

10. **2.** Talipes equinovarus is a rigid deformity with forefoot adduction, inversion of the heel, and plantar flexion of the feet.

11. **3.** Parents should be taught to assess neurovascular status of the toes because babies grow quickly and may outgrow the casts.

12. **3.** This is part of the screening process for scoliosis. The nurse is checking for rib hump and flank asymmetry. Also included is visual inspection of frontal and dorsal posture, observation for uneven hip and shoulder levels as well as for muscular disproportion.

13. **2.** One of the greatest risks of spinal surgery is of paralysis if the spinal cord is injured or compressed by swelling. Monitoring for sensation and movement is the top priority.

14. **4.** For best results in correction, the brace should be worn for 20–23 hours a day and only removed for hygiene and skin care.

15. **2.** Duchenne's muscular dystrophy is an X-linked recessive disorder. The defective gene is transmitted through carrier females to affected sons 50% of the time depending on which X is transmitted. Daughters have a 50% chance of becoming carriers.

The Endocrine System

■ VARIATIONS FROM THE ADULT

A. Adenohypophysis (anterior lobe of pituitary gland)
   1. Growth hormone
      a. Does not affect prenatal growth.
      b. Main effect on linear growth is through increase of cells in skeletal bones.

   c. Maintains rate of synthesis of body protein.
   2. Thyroid-stimulating hormone (TSH)
      a. Important for normal development of bones, teeth, and brain.
      b. Secretion decreases throughout childhood, then increases at puberty.
   3. Adrenocorticotropic hormone (ACTH)
      a. Little is produced throughout childhood.
      b. Becomes active in adolescence.
      c. Stimulates adrenals to secrete sex hormones.
      d. Influences production of gonadotropic hormone by hypothalamus.
         1) gonadotropic hormones activate gonads.
         2) gonads secrete estrogen or testosterone, which stimulate development of secondary sex characteristics.
   4. Estrogen has an inhibitory effect on epiphyseal growth.

■ ANALYSIS

Nursing diagnoses for the child with a disorder of the endocrine system may include

A. Ineffective health maintenance
B. Impaired home maintenance
C. Noncompliance
D. Disturbed body image
E. Low self-esteem

■ PLANNING AND IMPLEMENTATION
Goals

A. Any endocrine imbalance in childhood will be identified and treated.
B. Child will achieve a normal metabolic state.
C. Child will develop successful coping mechanisms for manifestations of disease.
D. Child will have no signs of complications of the disease.

■ EVALUATION

A. Child receives appropriate medication, and nutritional requirements are met; symptoms of endocrine disease are controlled.
B. Child is free from complications of disease.
C. Child is achieving growth and developmental tasks on as normal a timetable as possible.
D. Child discusses feelings about body image and uses coping mechanisms that promote a positive self-image.

■ DISORDERS OF THE ENDOCRINE SYSTEM
Diabetes Mellitus

A. General information
  1. Most common endocrine disease of children; onset may be at any age
  2. Children typically develop Type I: insulin dependent diabetes mellitus
  3. Possible genetic predisposition to disease
  4. Treatments vary based on rapid growth rate in children, increased incidence of infections, and dietary fads of peers; all include insulin administration.
  5. Risk of complications is high; most commonly retinopathy, neuropathy, nephropathy, skin changes, predisposition to infection
  6. Children sometimes have one honeymoon period that occurs shortly after a child is regulated on insulin for the first time
     a. Lasts from 1 month to 1 year.
     b. Represents final effort of pancreas to provide insulin until beta cells are completely destroyed.
     c. Parents may distrust the diagnosis of diabetes and need to be reminded that symptoms will reappear and child will need insulin for life.
B. Medical management
  1. Insulin
  2. Diet therapy
  3. Exercise
  4. Prevention of complications
C. Assessment findings
  1. Rapid onset
  2. Polyuria, polydipsia, polyphagia, fatigue

NURSING ALERT

D o not use candy bars or cake frosting to treat hypoglycemia. The fat decreases the rapid absorption of the glucose in the candy.

DELEGATION TIP

B lood glucose testing may be performed by ancillary personnel and also the child and parents. Proper recording of results and prompt reporting to the nurse is essential if findings are abnormal.

3. Weight loss
4. Ketoacidosis
5. Dry, flushed skin with hyperglycemia
D. Nursing interventions
1. Administer insulin (regular and NPH) as ordered.
2. Force fluids without sugar.
3. Monitor blood glucose levels daily.
4. Observe for hypoglycemia (insulin shock): behavior changes, sweating.
5. Provide client teaching and discharge planning concerning
    a. Daily regimen for home care
    b. Urine and blood glucose monitoring
    c. Nutrition management
    d. Effects of infection and exercise on carbohydrate metabolism
    e. Prevention of acute and chronic complications

Congenital Hypothyroidism (Cretinism)
A. General information
1. Disorder related to absent or nonfunctioning thyroid
2. Newborns are supplied with maternal thyroid hormones that last up to 3 months
B. Medical management
1. Prevention: neonatal screening blood test (mandatory in many states)
2. Drug therapy: thyroid hormone replacement
3. Without treatment mental retardation and developmental delay will occur after age 3 months
C. Assessment findings
1. Altered body proportions; short stature with legs shorter than they should be in proportion to trunk

CLIENT TEACHING CHECKLIST

- Medication may be crushed and added to a small amount of formula because it is tasteless.
- Instruct parents regarding the signs of overdose such as rapid pulse, sweating, and fever.
- Teach parents to count infant's pulse and withhold dose if pulse is too rapid.

NURSING ALERT

Medications should never be added to infant formula. Incomplete ingestion will result in under-medicating the client.

    2. Tongue is enlarged and protrudes from mouth; may result in breathing and feeding difficulties
    3. Hypothermia with cool extremities
    4. Short, thick neck; delayed dentition
    5. Hypotonia
    6. Low levels of T_3 and T_4
D. Nursing interventions
    1. Administer oral thyroxine and vitamin D as ordered to prevent mental retardation.
    2. Provide client teaching and discharge planning concerning
        a. Medication administration and side effects
        b. Importance of continued therapy

■ HYPOPITUITARISM (PITUITARY DWARFISM)

A. General information
    1. Hyposecretion of growth hormone by the anterior lobe of the pituitary gland
    2. Cause may be unknown or it may be due to craniopharyngioma
B. Medical management: administration of growth hormone (limited in supply since it is rendered from human cadavers)
C. Assessment findings
    1. Newborn is of normal size, but child falls below the third percentile by age 1.
    2. Child is well proportioned, but may be overweight for height.
    3. Underdeveloped jaw, abnormal position of teeth, high voice, delayed puberty

4. Diagnostic tests
a. X-rays reveal delayed closing of epiphyseal plates of long bones
   b. Normal IQ
D. Nursing interventions
   1. Interact with child according to chronologic age/developmental level, and not according to physical appearance.
   2. Administer growth hormone as ordered (because of delay in bone development, these children can still grow even when their peers have stopped).
   3. Monitor for signs and symptoms of additional neurologic disorders.
   4. Keep careful records of height and weight.
   5. Encourage child/parents to express feelings.
   6. Assist child in learning to interact normally with peers.

■ HYPERPITUITARISM (GIGANTISM)

A. General information
   1. Hypersecretion of growth hormone (usually related to a tumor of the anterior pituitary) resulting in enlargement of bones of head, hands, and feet, and overgrowth of long bones
   2. Especially noticeable at puberty
B. Medical management
   1. Surgery to remove tumor
   2. Radiation therapy if there is no tumor
C. Assessment findings
   1. Height beyond maximum upper percentile
   2. Proportional weight and muscle growth
   3. Coarse facial features
   4. Signs of increased ICP if caused by a tumor
D. Nursing interventions
   1. Record height and head circumference.
   2. Provide nursing care for a client receiving radiation therapy.
   3. Provide care for the child with a brain tumor.
   4. Assist child in interacting normally with peers.

REVIEW QUESTIONS

1. An 8-year-old is newly diagnosed with diabetes mellitus. Which of the following symptoms is different from what you would expect to find in maturity-onset (Type II) diabetes?
    1. Increased appetite.
    2. Increased thirst.
    3. Increased urination.
    4. Weight loss.

2. A 7-year-old is newly diagnosed with diabetes mellitus. She had an injection of regular and NPH insulin at 7:30 A.M. At 3:10 P.M. she complains that she does not feel well. She is pale, perspiring, and trembling. The nurse should
    1. tell her to lie down and wait for the dinner trays to arrive.
    2. ask her to give a urine specimen and test it for sugar and acetone.
    3. give her a carbohydrate snack.
    4. administer the afternoon dose of regular insulin.

3. A 10-year-old with diabetes mellitus is learning how to administer her insulin. She asks the nurse why she cannot take pills like her grandmother who also has diabetes. The best response for the nurse to make is
    1. How long has your grandmother been taking oral medication?
    2. You'll be able to stop taking insulin once you stop growing.
    3. You have a different kind of diabetes and you will need to take insulin throughout your life.
    4. You'll be able to switch to pills when you reach your grandmother's age.

ANSWERS AND RATIONALES

1. 4. Weight loss is associated with juvenile diabetes, whereas weight gain develops in maturity-onset diabetes.

2. 3. The symptoms suggest she is having a hypoglycemic reaction from the NPH insulin and needs an afternoon snack.

3. 3. Juvenile or Type I diabetics need lifetime insulin since they no longer produce their own.

The Integumentary System

■ VARIATIONS FROM THE ADULT

A. Skin is only 1 mm thick at birth; approximately twice as thick at maturity.
B. Evaporative water loss is greater in infants and small children.
C. Skin is more susceptible to bacterial infection in children.
D. Children are more prone to toxic erythema as a result of drug reactions and skin eruptions.
E. Children's skin is more susceptible to sweat retention and maceration.

■ ASSESSMENT

History

A. Medical history: previous skin disease, allergic conditions
B. History of present condition: onset, relationship to eating or other activities, medication usage

Physical Examination

A. Lesion type: note petechiae, erythema, ecchymosis; note secondary symptoms from rubbing, scratching, or healing.
B. Observe distribution pattern.
C. Note presence of pain or altered sensation.
D. Check scalp for signs of lice or nits.

■ ANALYSIS

Nursing diagnoses for the child with a disorder of the integumentary system may include
A. Pain
B. Disturbed body image
C. Disturbed sensory perception
D. Risk for impaired skin integrity
E. Low self-esteem

■ PLANNING AND IMPLEMENTATION
Goals

A. Child will be free from discomfort.
B. Skin integrity will be restored.
C. Spread of infection and secondary infection will be prevented.

■ EVALUATION

A. Child is free from discomfort.
   1. Minimal scratching or rubbing
   2. Relaxed facial expression
   3. Minimal restlessness
B. Child's skin is clean, dry, and free from redness or signs of irritation.
C. Child is free from complications such as spread of infection.
D. Parents demonstrate satisfactory hygiene measures when caring for child with disorder of skin or scalp.

■ DISORDERS OF THE INTEGUMENTARY SYSTEM
Burns

A. For children, the rule of nines is modified; the head of a small child is 18–19%, the trunk 32%, each leg 15%, each arm 9½%.
B. Burns in infants and toddlers are frequently due to spills (pulling hot fluids on them or falling into hot baths); for older children, flame burns are more frequent.

Impetigo

A. General information
   1. Superficial bacterial infection of the outer layers of skin (usually staphylococcus or streptococcus)
   2. Common in toddlers and preschoolers
   3. Related to poor sanitation
   4. Very contagious
B. Medical management: topical and systemic antibiotics
C. Assessment findings
   1. Well-demarcated lesions
   2. Macules, papules, vesicles that rupture, causing a superficial moist erosion
   3. Moist area dries, leaving a honey-colored crust
   4. Spreads peripherally
   5. Most commonly found on face, axillae, and extremities
   6. Pruritus
D. Nursing interventions
   1. Implement skin isolation techniques.
   2. Soften the skin and crusts with Burrow's solution compresses.

3. Remove crusts gently.
4. Cover draining lesions to prevent spread of infection.
5. Administer antibiotics as ordered, both orally and as bacteriocidal ointments.
6. Prevent secondary infection.
7. Provide client teaching and discharge planning concerning
   a. Medication administration
   b. Proper hygiene techniques

Ringworm

A. General information
   1. Dermatomycosis due to various species of fungus
   2. Infected sites include
      a. Scalp (tinea capitis)
      b. Body (tinea corporis)
      c. Feet (tinea pedis or athlete's foot)
   3. May be transmitted from person to person or acquired from animals or soil
B. Assessment findings
   1. Scalp
      a. Scaly circumscribed patches on the scalp
      b. Base of hair shafts are invaded by spores of the fungus; causes hair to break off, resulting in alopecia
      c. Spreads in a circular pattern
      d. Detected by Wood's lamp (fluoresces green at base of the affected hair shafts)
   2. Skin: red-ringed patches of vesicles; pain, scaling, itching
C. Nursing interventions
   1. Prevention: isolate from known infected persons.
   2. Apply antifungal ointment as ordered.
   3. Administer oral griseofulvin as ordered.

Pediculosis (Head Lice)

A. General information
   1. Parasitic infestation
   2. Adult lice are spread by close physical contact (sharing combs, hats, etc.)
   3. Occurs in school-age children, particularly those with long hair
B. Medical management: special shampoos followed by use of fine-tooth comb to remove nits
C. Assessment findings
   1. White eggs (nits) firmly attached to base of hair shafts
   2. Pruritus of scalp

NURSING ALERT

Apply pediculicidal agent to scalp and then add water to lather.

D. Nursing interventions
    1. Institute skin isolation precautions (especially head coverings and gloves to prevent spread to self, other staff, and clients)
    2. Use special shampoo and comb the hair
    3. Provide client teaching and discharge planning concerning
        a. How to check self and other family members and how to treat them
        b. Washing of clothes, bed linens, etc.; discouraging sharing of brushes, combs, and hats

Allergies

Diaper Rash

A. General information
    1. Contact dermatitis
    2. Plastic/rubber pants and linings of disposable diapers exacerbate the condition by prolonging contact with moist, warm environment; skin is further irritated by acidic urine
    3. May also be caused by sensitivity to laundry soaps used
B. Medical management: exposure of skin to air/heat lamp
C. Assessment findings
    1. Erythema/excoriation in the perineal area
    2. Irritability
D. Nursing interventions
    1. Keep area clean and dry; clean with mild soap and water after each stool and as soon as child urinates.
    2. Take off diaper and expose area to air during the day.
    3. Use heat lamp as ordered.
    4. Provide client teaching and discharge planning concerning
        a. Proper hygiene/infant care
        b. Diaper laundering methods
        c. Avoiding use of plastic pants or disposable diapers with a plastic lining
        d. Avoiding use of cornstarch (a good medium for bacteria once it becomes wet)
        e. Need to avoid use of commercially prepared diaper wipes since they contain chemicals and alcohol, which may be irritating

---

CLIENT TEACHING CHECKLIST

Instruct the client with poison ivy to:

- Not rub fingers against skin or eyes
- Not burn the poison ivy plants to remove them from the environment

---

NURSING ALERT

Wet occlusive dressings increase the penetration of corticosteroid ointments.

Poison Ivy

A. General information
   1. Contact dermatitis; mediated by T-cell response so rash is not seen for 24–48 hours after contact.
   2. Poison ivy is not spread by the fluid in the vesicles; can be spread by clothes and animals that retain the plant resin.

B. Assessment findings: very pruritic impetigo-like lesions

C. Nursing interventions
   1. Administer antihistamines and cortisone as ordered.
   2. Provide client teaching and discharge planning concerning
      a. Plant identification
      b. Need to wash with soap and water after contact with plant
      c. Importance of washing clothes to get the resin out

Eczema

A. General information
   1. Atopic dermatitis, often the first sign of an allergic predisposition in a child; many later develop respiratory allergies
   2. Usually manifests during infancy

B. Medical management
   1. Drug therapy
      a. Topical steroids
      b. Antihistamines
      c. Emollients
      d. Cautious administration of immunizations
      e. Medicated or colloid baths
   2. Diet therapy: elimination diet to detect offending foods

C. Assessment findings
1. Erythema, weeping vesicles that rupture and crust over
2. Usually evident on cheeks, scalp, behind ears, and on flexor surfaces of extremities (rarely on diaper area)
3. Severe pruritus; scratching causes thickening and darkening of skin
4. Dry skin, sometimes urticaria
D. Nursing interventions
1. Avoid heat and prevent sweating; keep skin dry (moisture aggravates condition).
2. Monitor elimination diet to detect food cause.
   a. Remove all solid foods from diet (formula only).
   b. If symptoms disappear after 3 days, start 1 new food group every 3 days to see if symptoms reappear.
   c. The food that is suspected of causing the rash is withdrawn again to make sure symptoms go away in 3 days and is then introduced a second time (challenge test).
3. Check materials in contact with child's skin (sheets, lotions, soaps).
4. Tepid baths, mild soaps.
   a. Provide lubricant immediately after bath.
   b. Pat dry gently with soft towel (do not rub) and pat in lubricant.
   c. Avoid the use of harsh soaps (dry skin).
5. Administer topical steroids as ordered (penetrate better if applied within 3 minutes after bath). Thin layer of topical steroid.
6. Use cotton instead of wool clothing.
7. Keep child's nails short to prevent scratching and secondary infection; use gloves or elbow restraints if needed.
8. Apply wet saline or Burrow's solution compresses.
9. Double-rinse laundry.
10. Assess skin for infection.

Acne

A. General information
1. Skin condition associated with increased production of sebum from sebaceous glands at puberty.
2. Lesions include pustules, papules, and comedones.
3. Majority of adolescents experience some degree of acne, mild to severe.
4. Lesions occur most frequently on face, neck, shoulders, and back.
5. Caused by a variety of interrelated factors including increased activity of sebaceous glands, emotional stress, certain medications, menstrual cycle.
6. Secondary infection can complicate healing of lesions.
7. There is no evidence to support the value of eliminating any foods from the diet; if cause and effect can be established, however, a particular food should be eliminated.

B. Assessment findings
   1. Appearance of lesions is variable and fluctuating
   2. Systemic symptoms absent
   3. Psychologic problems such as social withdrawal, low self-esteem, feelings of being "ugly"
C. Nursing interventions
   1. Discuss OTC products and their effects.
   2. Instruct child in proper hygiene (handwashing, care of face, not to pick or squeeze any lesions).
   3. Demonstrate proper administration of topical ointments and antibiotics if indicated.

REVIEW QUESTIONS

1. A 2-year-old was recently found to have impetigo. What measures should be given the highest priority to prevent its spread while in the hospital?
   1. Keeping it covered.
   2. Good handwashing.
   3. Applying A&D ointment.
   4. Placing the child in isolation.

2. A 7-year-old boy has a loss of scalp hair and is diagnosed with ringworm. What question will the nurse most likely ask?
   1. Whether the family owns any pets.
   2. From what economic background is the family.
   3. Whether other children in his classroom have ringworm.
   4. Whether the child can read the medicine directions.

3. Three school children have pediculosis capitus. The school nurse has been instructing the parents of all three students on prevention. Which statement made by one mother indicates an understanding of prevention?
   1. "I will put all of the stuffed animals in plastic bags for 2 weeks."
   2. "Since the sheets are now clean, the kids can share beds, too."
   3. "Once I cut her hair, all the nits should be gone."
   4. "I will now bathe my child every day to prevent reinfection."

4. Prior to discharge home with their new baby, the nurse knows that the parents understand diaper rash prevention when
   1. they articulate that the baby should be checked for wet diapers every half an hour.
   2. they are observed wiping with soap and water at diaper changes.

3. the mother discusses needs to use tight rubber pants to keep diapers from leaking.

4. the father wipes carefully and uses a mild ointment to protect the skin.

5. A 3-year-old girl has had eczema since 4 months of age. Which statement made by her father indicates to the nurse that he understands the management of eczema?

    1. "Benadryl should be given every night before bedtime."

    2. "It's beneficial to keep her in the bubble bath for as long as possible each day."

    3. "Typical eruption areas that need to be treated include flexor surfaces of joints."

    4. "Hot water is better in which to bathe."

ANSWERS AND RATIONALES

1. 2. Good handwashing is of paramount importance in preventing its spread.

2. 1. Pets are known to be carriers of ringworm.

3. 1. Stuffed animals can harbor eggs and cause reinfection.

4. 4. Careful cleansing on delicate skin and use of ointments helps to preserve the skin's integrity.

5. 3. These are the joint areas typically affected in the childhood years.

12

Pediatric Oncology

■ OVERVIEW

A. Cancer is the leading cause of death from disease in children from 1–14 years.

B. Incidence
   1. 6000 children develop cancer per year.
   2. 2500 children die from cancer annually.
   3. Boys are affected more frequently.

C. Leukemia is the most frequent type of childhood cancer, followed by tumors of the CNS.

D. Etiologic factors include environmental agents, viruses, familial/genetic factors, and host factors.

Major Stressful Events

Five events have been identified as major stressors:

A. *Diagnosis:* child is initially hospitalized to determine extent of disease, plan course of treatment, and to educate child and family.

B. *Treatment:* multimodal
   1. May include surgery, radiation, chemotherapy
   2. Side effects are serious and unpleasant; child/family may complain that the "treatment is worse than the disease."

C. *Remission:* child is without evidence of disease, treatment continues; goals for this period include
   1. Maintenance of normal family patterns: discipline and usual household chores
   2. Maintenance of relationships among family and friends
      a. Parents' marriage may be strained
      b. Siblings may feel neglected or jealous
   3. Attendance at school
      a. Child may fear rejection by peers due to change in appearance or not being able to keep up
      b. Teacher may be unsure as to what to say or how to treat the child

    c. Classmates need to be prepared for child's return; may have fears/concerns about whether the disease is catching and whether their friend will die
D. *Recurrence*
    1. An event of enormous magnitude and a cause of severe disappointment
    2. May occur while still on treatment or after treatment has been completed
E. *Death*

■ ASSESSMENT
History

A. Family history: some cancers suggest patterns of inheritance
B. Prenatal exposure
C. Children with chromosomal disorders have a higher-than-average incidence of cancer
D. History may elicit symptoms that have been present for a period of time
E. Presenting problems: symptoms may include
    1. Fever, pain, bleeding
    2. Abdominal mass
    3. Night sweats, weight loss
    4. Hematuria, hypertension

Physical Examination

A. General appearance
    1. Skin: note color, bruises, or petechiae
    2. Neurologic status: note fatigue, activity level, behavior, headache, dizziness, gait disturbances
    3. Pain: guarding of any body part, changes in range of motion
B. Measure vital signs including BP
C. Plot height and weight on growth chart
D. Inspect and palpate abdomen; note enlargement of liver and spleen
E. Palpate for enlarged lymph nodes
F. Inspect eyes for nystagmus

Laboratory/Diagnostic Test

A. Blood studies, e.g., CBC
B. X-rays, bone scans, CT scans, MRI, ultrasound
C. Lumbar puncture
D. Bone marrow aspiration

Analysis

Nursing diagnoses for the child with cancer may include
A. Risk for infection
B. Risk for injury

NURSING ALERT

The American Academy of Pediatrics recommends that the child be sedated prior to a lumbar puncture.

C. Fear/anxiety
D. Disturbed body image
E. Deficient knowledge

Planning and Implementation

Goals

A. Child will be free from infection
B. Child will be free from pain
C. Optimum developmental level will be achieved
D. Family will develop effective coping strategies

■ INTERVENTIONS

Surgery

A. May be performed for tumor removal, to obtain a biopsy, to determine extent of disease, or for palliation
B. Often used in conjunction with radiation or chemotherapy

Radiation Therapy

A. Primarily used in children to improve prognosis
B. Goal is to achieve maximum effect on tumor while sparing normal tissue
   1. May be used for palliative relief from pain, disfigurement
   2. May be curative, destroys cancer cells/reduces size of tumor
   3. Frequently used as an adjunct to chemotherapy and surgery
   4. Must weigh gain versus risks of permanent damage to normal tissue
   5. Infants particularly susceptible to developing skeletal deformities in later years as a result of radiation
   6. Complications to growing child include scoliosis, arrested skeletal development, and pulmonary fibrosis (depends on site radiated)
   7. Dosage range varies; may be as low as 1000 rad to relieve bone pain in a specific area, to as high as 7000 rad to achieve a cure in Ewing's sarcoma
   8. Usually performed 5 days a week for 2-6 weeks

NURSING ALERT

N urses who care for children receiving radiation therapy must wear a dosi-meter film badge at all times.

Chemotherapy

Almost all pediatric cancer clients receive some form of drug therapy.

A. Childhood cancers are more sensitive and responsive to drugs than are adult cancers.
B. Childhood cancers tend to metastasize early and systemic treatment is needed in addition to localized treatment.

Bone Marrow Transplant

A. General information
  1. Treatment alternative for a variety of childhood diseases including
     a. Definite: acute lymphoblastic leukemia, acute nonlymphocytic leukemia, severe aplastic anemia, immunodeficiencies, and malignant infantile osteopetrosis
     b. Possible: chronic myelogenous leukemia, solid tumors, some hematologic disorders, and some inherited metabolic disorders
  2. Types
     a. Autologous: client transplanted with own harvested marrow
     b. Syngeneic: transplant between identical twins
     c. Allogeneic: transplant from a genetically nonidentical donor
        1) most common transplant type
        2) sibling most common donor
  3. Procedure
     a. Donor suitability determined through tissue antigen typing; includes human leukocyte antigen (HLA) and mixed leukocyte culture (MLC) typing.
     b. Donor bone marrow is aspirated from multiple sites along the iliac crests under general anesthesia.
     c. Donor marrow is infused IV into the recipient.
  4. Early evidence of engraftment seen during the second week posttransplant; hematologic reconstitution takes 4–6 weeks; immunologic reconstitution takes months.
  5. Hospitalization of 2 or 3 months required.
  6. Prognosis is highly variable depending on indication for use.
B. Complications
  1. Failure of engraftment
  2. Infection: highest risk in first 3–4 weeks

3. Pneumonia: nonbacterial or interstitial pneumonias are principal cause of death during first 3 months posttransplant

4. *Graft vs host disease* (*GVHD*): principal complication; caused by an immunologic reaction of engrafted lymphoid cells against the tissues of the recipient

   a. Acute GVHD: develops within first 100 days posttransplant and affects skin, gut, liver, marrow, and lymphoid tissue

   b. Chronic GVHD: develops 100–400 days posttransplant; manifested by multiorgan involvement

5. Recurrent malignancy

6. Late complications such as cataracts, endocrine abnormalities

C. Nursing care: pretransplant

   1. Extensive time must be spent with child/parents in preparing for this procedure.

   2. Recipient immunosuppression attained with total body irradiation (TBI) and chemotherapy to eradicate existing disease and create space in host marrow to allow transplanted cells to grow.

   3. Provide protected environment.

      a. Child should be in a laminar air flow room or on strict reverse isolation; surveillance cultures done twice a week.

      b. Encourage use of toys and familiar objects; they must be sterilized before being brought into the room.

      c. Encourage frequent contact with schoolteacher/play therapist.

      d. Introduce new people where they can be seen, but outside child's room so child can see what they look like without isolation garb.

   4. Monitor central lines frequently; check patency and observe for signs of infection (fever, redness around site).

   5. Provide care for the child receiving chemotherapy and radiation therapy to induce immunosuppression.

      a. Administer chemotherapy as ordered, assist with radiation therapy if required.

      b. Monitor side effects and keep child as comfortable as possible.

      c. Monitor carefully for potential infection.

      d. Child will become very ill; prepare parents.

D. Nursing care: posttransplant

   1. Prevent infection.

      a. Maintain protective environment.

      b. Administer antibiotics as ordered.

      c. Assess all mucous membranes, wounds, catheter sites for swelling, redness, tenderness, pain.

      d. Monitor vital signs frequently (every 1–4 hours as needed).

      e. Collect specimens for cultures as needed and twice a week.

      f. Change IV set-ups every 24 hours.

   2. Provide mouth care for stomatitis and mucositis (severe mucositis develops about 5 days after irradiation).

    a. Note tissue sloughing, bleeding, changes in color.

    b. Provide mouth rinses, viscous lidocaine, and antibiotic rinses.

    c. Do not use lemon and glycerin swabs.

    d. Administer parenteral narcotics as ordered if necessary to control pain.

    e. Provide care every 2 hours or as needed.

3. Provide skin care: skin breakdown may result from profuse diarrhea from the TBI.

4. Monitor carefully for bleeding.

    a. Check for occult blood in emesis and stools.

    b. Observe for easy bruising, petechiae on skin, mucous membranes.

    c. Monitor changes in vital signs.

    d. Check platelet count daily.

    e. Replace blood products as ordered (all blood products should be irradiated).

5. Maintain fluid and electrolyte balance and promote nutrition.

    a. Measure I&O carefully.

    b. Provide adequate fluid, protein, and caloric intake.

    c. Weigh daily.

    d. Administer fluid replacement as ordered.

    e. Monitor hydration status: check skin turgor, moisture of mucous membranes, urine output.

    f. Check electrolytes daily.

    g. Check urine for glucose, ketones, protein.

    h. Administer antidiarrheal agents as needed.

6. Provide client teaching and discharge planning concerning

    a. Home environment (e.g., cleaning, pets, visitors)

    b. Diet modifications

    c. Medication regimen: schedule, dosages, effects, and side effects

    d. Communicable diseases and immunizations

    e. Daily hygiene and skin care

    f. Fever

    g. Activity

■ STAGES OF CANCER TREATMENT

A. Induction

    1. Goal: to remove bulk of tumor

    2. Methods: surgery, radiation/chemotherapy, bone marrow transplant

    3. Effects: often the most intensive phase; side effects of treatment are potentially life threatening

B. Consolidation

    1. Goal: to eliminate any remaining malignant cells

    2. Methods: often chemotherapy/radiation therapy

    3. Effects: side effects will still be evident

CLIENT TEACHING CHECKLIST

- Instruct the parents and family members to provide adequate rest periods for the child receiving treatment for cancer because they will fatigue easily.
- Report any changes in the child's condition to the health care provider.

C. Maintenance
  1. Goal: to keep child disease free
  2. Method: chemotherapy (this phase may last for several years)
D. Observation
  1. Goal: to monitor the child at intervals for evidence of recurrent disease and complications of treatment
  2. Method: treatment is complete; child may continue in this stage indefinitely
E. Late effects of treatment
  1. Impaired growth and development, usually related to radiation of growth centers
  2. CNS damage resulting in intellectual, psychologic, or neurologic sequelae
  3. Impaired pubertal development including hormonal or reproductive problems
  4. Development of secondary malignancy
  5. Psychologic problems (poor self-esteem, depression, anxiety) related to living with a life-threatening disease and complex treatment regimen

Side Effects

A. From combined effects of treatment: nausea, vomiting, diarrhea, alopecia, anemia (low RBCs), increased susceptibility to infection (low WBCs), bleeding (low platelets), stomatitis, mucositis, pain, learning problems
B. From radiation (findings differ according to site radiated): sleepiness, reddened skin
C. From chemotherapy: drug toxicity specific to agents used
D. Developmental: behavior problems, avoidance of school and friends, low self-esteem or self-image

Nursing Interventions

A. Help child cope with intrusive procedures.
  1. Provide information geared to developmental level and emotional readiness.
  2. Explain what is going to happen, why it is necessary, and how it will feel.
  3. Allow child to handle and manipulate equipment.
  4. Use needle play as indicated.

    5. Allow child some control in situations (e.g., positioning, selecting injection site).

B. Support child and parents.

    1. Maintain frequent clinical conferences to keep all informed.

    2. Always tell the truth.

    3. Acknowledge feelings and encourage child/family to express them, assure them that feelings are normal.

    4. Provide contact with another parent or an organized support group such as Candlelighters.

    5. Try to keep daily life as normal as possible.

C. Minimize side effects of treatment.

    1. Skin breakdown

        a. Keep clean and dry; wash with warm water, no soaps or creams.

        b. Do not wash off radiation markings.

        c. Avoid exposure to sunlight.

        d. Avoid all topical agents with alcohol (perfumes and powders).

        e. Do not use electric heating pads or hot water bottles.

    2. Bone marrow suppression

        a. Decreased RBCs

            1) allow child to determine activities.

            2) provide frequent rest periods.

        b. Decreased WBCs

            1) avoid crowds, isolate from children with known communicable disease.

            2) evaluate any potential site of infection.

            3) monitor temperature elevations.

        c. Decreased platelets

            1) make environment safe.

            2) select activities that are physically safe.

            3) avoid use of salicylates.

        d. Administer transfusions as ordered.

        e. Interpret peripheral blood counts to guide specific interventions and precautions.

    3. Nausea and vomiting

        a. Administer antiemetic at least half an hour before chemotherapy; repeat as necessary.

        b. Encourage relaxation techniques.

        c. Eat light meal prior to administration of therapy.

        d. Ensure adequate oral intake or administer IV fluids as necessary.

    4. Alopecia

        a. Reduce trauma of hair loss (especially in children over age 5 years).

        b. Buy wig before hair falls out.

        c. Discuss various head coverings with boys and girls.

        d. Avoid exposing head to sunlight.

        e. Discuss feelings.

5. Stomatitis, mucositis.
6. Nutrition deficits
   a. Establish baseline prior to start of treatment.
   b. Measure height and weight regularly.
   c. Provide small, frequent meals.
   d. Consult dietitian as needed.
   e. Provide high-calorie, high-protein supplements.
7. Developmental delays
   a. Discuss limit setting, discipline.
   b. Some behavior problems might be side effects of drug therapy.
   c. Facilitate return to school as soon as able.
   d. Realize changing needs of child.

■ CANCERS

Leukemia

A. General information
   1. Most common form of childhood cancer
   2. Peak incidence is 3 to 5 years of age
   3. Proliferation of abnormal white blood cells that do not mature beyond the blast phase
   4. In the bone marrow, blast cells crowd out healthy white blood cells, red blood cells, and platelets, leading to bone marrow depression
   5. Blast cells also infiltrate other organs, most commonly the liver, spleen, kidneys, and lymph tissue
   6. Symptoms reflect bone marrow failure and associated involvement of other organs
   7. Types of leukemia, based on course of disease and cell morphology
      a. Acute lymphocytic leukemia (ALL)
         1) 80–85% of childhood leukemia
         2) malignant change in the lymphocyte or its precursors
         3) acute onset
         4) 95% chance of obtaining remission with treatment
         5) 75% chance of surviving 5 years or more
         6) prognostic indicators include: initial white blood count (less than 10,000/mm^3), child's age (2–9 years), histologic type, sex
      b. Acute nonlymphocytic leukemia (ANLL)
         1) includes granulocytic and monocytic types
         2) 60–80% will obtain remission with treatment
         3) 30–40% cure rate
         4) prognostic indicators less clearly defined
B. Medical management
   1. Diagnosis: blood studies, bone marrow biopsy
   2. Treatment stages

  a. Induction: intense and potentially life threatening

  b. CNS prophylaxis: to prevent central nervous system disease. Combination of radiation and intrathecal chemotherapy.

  c. Maintenance: chemotherapy for 2 to 3 years.

C. Assessment findings

 1. Anemia (due to decreased production of RBCs), weakness, pallor, dyspnea

 2. Bleeding (due to decreased platelet production), petechiae, spontaneous bleeding, ecchymoses

 3. Infection (due to decreased WBC production), fever, malaise

 4. Enlarged lymph nodes

 5. Enlarged spleen and liver

 6. Abdominal pain with weight loss and anorexia

 7. Bone pain due to expansion of marrow

D. Nursing interventions

 1. Provide care for the child receiving chemotherapy and radiation therapy.

 2. Provide support for child/family; needs will change as treatment progresses.

 3. Support child during painful procedures (frequent bone marrow aspirations, lumbar punctures, venipunctures needed).

  a. Use distraction, guided imagery.

  b. Allow child to retain as much control as possible.

  c. Administer sedation prior to procedure as ordered.

Brain Tumors

A. General information

 1. A space-occupying mass in the brain tissue; may be benign or malignant

 2. Males affected more often; peak age 3–7 years

 3. Second most prevalent type of cancer in children

 4. Cause unknown; genetic and environmental factors may play a role; familial tendency for brain tumors, which are found with preexisting neurocutaneous disorders.

 5. Two-thirds of all pediatric brain tumors are beneath the tentorium cerebelli (in the posterior fossa), often involving the cerebellum or brain stem.

 6. Three-fourths of brain tumors in children are gliomas (medulloblastoma and astrocytoma).

B. Types

 1. *Medulloblastoma:* highly malignant tumor usually found in cerebellum; runs a rapid course

  a. Findings include increased ICP plus unsteady walk, ataxia, anorexia, early morning vomiting

  b. Treated with radiation since complete removal is impossible

 2. *Astrocytoma:* a benign, cystic, slow-growing tumor usually found in cerebellum

      a. Onset of symptoms is insidious.

      b. Findings include focal disturbances, papilledema, optic nerve atrophy, blindness.

  3. *Ependymoma:* a usually benign tumor that arises in the ventricles of the brain, causing noncommunicating hydrocephalus and damage (by pressure) to other vital tissues of the brain

  4. *Craniopharyngioma:* tumor that arises from remnants of embryonic tissue near the pituitary gland in the sella turcica, causes pressure on the third ventricle

      a. Decreased secretion of ADH causes diabetes insipidus (these children may need Pitressin).

      b. Additional symptoms include altered growth pattern, visual difficulties, difficulty regulating body temperature.

  5. *Brain stem glioma:* slow-growing tumor, indicated by cranial nerve palsies, ataxia

C. Medical management

  1. Surgery: some tumors entirely or partially resected; others are not amenable to surgery because of proximity to vital brain parts

  2. Radiation therapy: often used to shrink tumors

  3. Chemotherapy: vincristine, lomustine, procarbazine, intrathecal methotrexate; not as effective with brain tumors as with other childhood cancers

D. Assessment findings

  1. Symptoms dependent on location and type of tumor.

  2. A definite diagnosis is difficult in children because of the elasticity of child's skull and generally poor coordination of the young child.

  3. A decrease in school performance may be the first sign.

  4. Increased ICP

      a. Morning headache

      b. Morning vomiting without nausea; vomiting without relation to feeding schedule; projectile vomiting

      c. Personality changes

      d. Diplopia

         1) difficult to assess in young children

         2) observe child for tilting of head, closing or covering one eye, rubbing the eyes, or impaired eye-hand coordination

      e. Papilledema: a late sign

      f. Increased blood pressure with decreased pulse: also a late sign

      g. Cranial enlargement

         1) more readily noticeable prior to 18 months when suture lines are still open

         2) bulging, tense, pulsating fontanels

         3) widened suture lines

         4) 90% or more on head circumference chart

5. Focal signs and symptoms
   a. Ataxia
      1) in cerebellar tumors
      2) may not be readily identified because of uncoordinated movements of young children
   b. Muscle strength
      1) weakness with cerebellar tumors
      2) weakness, spasticity, and paralysis of lower extremities with cerebral or brain stem tumors
      3) change in handedness, posture, or manual coordination: may be early signs
   c. Head tilt
      1) in posterior fossa tumors
      2) early sign of visual impairment
      3) associated with nuchal rigidity
      4) due to traction on the dura
   d. Ocular signs
      1) nystagmus: corresponds to the same side as the infratentorial lesion
      2) diplopia/strabismus: from palsy of cranial nerve VI with brain stem glioma or increased ICP
      3) visual field deficit (child does not react to activity on periphery of vision): with craniopharyngiomas
   e. Seizures: with cerebral tumors
6. Diagnostic tests
   a. Skull X-ray reveals presence and location of tumor
   b. CT scan (with or without contrast dye) reveals position, consistency, size of tumor, and effect on surrounding tissue
   c. EEG may show seizure activity
E. Nursing interventions
   1. Obtain baseline vital signs and perform thorough neurologic assessment; monitor vital signs and neurologic status frequently.
   2. Prevent injury/complications.
      a. Institute seizure precautions.
      b. Monitor for fluid and electrolyte imbalance from vomiting.
      c. Observe for increased ICP.
      d. Provide safety measures (bed rails up).
   3. Promote comfort/relief of headache.
      a. Decrease environmental stimuli.
      b. Administer analgesics as ordered.
   4. Prevent constipation (straining increases ICP).
      a. Provide appropriate foods and fluids as ordered.
      b. Provide stool softeners as ordered.
      c. Avoid enemas, which increase ICP.

5. Provide care for the child undergoing brain surgery.
6. Provide care for the child undergoing radiation or chemotherapy.
7. Provide client teaching and discharge planning concerning
   a. Diagnostic tests (instruction needs to be appropriate to the child's developmental level)
      1) machines will make clicking sounds
      2) wires attached to the head for an EEG will not electrocute child
      3) head is immobilized for a CT scan
      4) the use of contrast dye and expected sensations if used
      5) need to lie still with the technician out of the room for most tests (younger children will be sedated for fuller cooperation)
   b. Importance of family discussion of fears/anxiety about surgery and prognosis
   c. Need to assist in implementing child's interaction with peers
   d. Available support groups and community agencies

Brain Surgery

A. General information
   1. Indications
      a. Removal of a tumor
      b. Evacuation of a hematoma
      c. Removal of a foreign body or skull fragments resulting from trauma
      d. Aspiration of an abscess
      e. Insertion of a shunt
B. Nursing interventions: preoperative
   1. Assess the child's understanding of the procedure; have the child draw a picture, tell a story; observe doll play.
   2. Explain the procedure in terms according to the child's developmental level.
   3. Allow the child to visit the operating room/intensive care unit, if permitted, depending on the child's emotional and developmental levels.
   4. Explain that pre-op symptoms such as headache and ataxia may be temporarily aggravated.
   5. Advise child/parents that blindness may result, depending on the location of the tumor.
   6. Inform the child/parents that the head will be shaved; long hair may be saved; hats or scarves may be used to cover the head once the dressings are removed.
   7. Support the child/family if a tumor cannot be totally removed.
   8. Provide instruction about radiation and chemotherapy (may need to be delayed since detail may be overwhelming).
   9. Explain to the child/parents about the post-op dressing, monitoring devices, and possibility of facial edema.

C. Nursing interventions: postoperative
  1. Prevent injury/complications.
    a. Monitor vital signs and neuro status frequently until stable.
    b. Apply hypothermia blanket as ordered.
    c. Assess respiratory status/signs of infection.
    d. Observe the dressing for discharge/hemorrhage.
    e. Close or cover eyes, apply ice, instill saline drops or artificial tears.
    f. Position as ordered according to the location of the tumor and type of surgery.
    g. Assess for increased ICP.
    h. Institute seizure precautions.
  2. Promote comfort.
    a. Decrease environmental stimuli.
    b. Administer analgesics as ordered, first assessing LOC.
  3. Promote adequate nutrition.
    a. Administer fluids as ordered.
    b. Monitor I&O.
    c. Provide diet as ordered.
  4. Provide emotional support and encourage child/family to discuss prognosis.
  5. Provide client teaching and discharge planning concerning
    a. Wound care
    b. Signs of increased ICP
    c. Activity level
    d. Sensation and time period of hair growth
    e. Peer acceptance
    f. Radiation/chemotherapy, if indicated
    g. Availability of support groups/community agencies

Hodgkin's Lymphoma

A. General information
  1. Malignant neoplasm of lymphoid tissue, usually originating in localized group of lymph nodes; a proliferation of lymphocytes
  2. Metastasizes first to adjacent lymph nodes
  3. Cause unknown
  4. Most prevalent in adolescents; accounts for 5% of all malignancies
  5. Prognosis now greatly improved for these children; influenced by stage of disease and histologic type
  6. Long-term treatment effects include increased incidence of second malignancies, especially leukemia and infertility
B. Medical management
  1. Diagnosis: extensive testing to determine stage, which dictates treatment modality

     a. Lymphangiogram determines involvement of all lymph nodes (reliable in 90% of clients); is helpful in determining radiation fields

     b. Staging via laparotomy and biopsy

        1) stage I: single lymph node involved; usually in neck; 90–98% survival

        2) stage II: involvement of 2 or more lymph nodes on same side of diaphragm; 70–80% survival

        3) stage III: involvement of nodes on both sides of diaphragm; 50% survival

        4) stage IV: metastasis to other organs

     c. Laparotomy and splenectomy

     d. Lymph node biopsy to identify presence of Reed-Sternberg cells and for histologic classification

  2. Radiation: used alone for localized disease

  3. Chemotherapy: used in conjunction with radiation therapy for advanced disease

C. Assessment findings

  1. Major presenting symptom is enlarged nodes in lower cervical region; nodes are nontender, firm, and movable

  2. Recurrent, intermittent fever

  3. Night sweats

  4. Weight loss, malaise, lethargy

  5. Pruritus

  6. Diagnostic test: presence of Reed-Sternberg cells

D. Nursing interventions

  1. Provide care for child receiving radiation therapy.

  2. Administer chemotherapy as ordered and monitor/alleviate side effects.

  3. Protect client from infection, especially if splenectomy performed.

  4. Provide support for child/parents; specific needs of adolescent client must be considered.

Non-Hodgkin's Lymphoma

A. General information

  1. Tumor originating in lymphatic tissue

  2. Significantly different from Hodgkin's lymphoma

     a. Control of primary tumor is difficult

     b. Disease is diffuse, cell type undifferentiated

     c. Tumor disseminates early

     d. Includes wide range of disease entities: lymphosarcoma, reticulum cell sarcoma, Burkitt's lymphoma

  3. Primary sites include GI tract, ovaries, testes, bone, CNS, liver, breast, subcutaneous tissues

  4. Affects all age groups.

B. Medical management
1. Chemotherapy: multiagent regimens including cyclophosphamide (Cytoxan), vincristine, prednisone, procarbazine, doxorubicin, bleomycin
2. Radiation therapy: primary treatment in localized disease
3. Surgery for diagnosis and clinical staging

C. Assessment findings
1. Depend on anatomic site and extent of involvement
2. Rapid onset and progression
3. Many have advanced disease at diagnosis

D. Nursing interventions: provide care for child receiving chemotherapy, radiation therapy, and surgery.

Wilms' Tumor (Nephroblastoma)

A. General information
1. Large, encapsulated tumor that develops in the renal parenchyma, more frequently in left kidney (usually unilateral)
2. Originates during fetal life from undifferentiated embryonic tissues
3. Peak age of occurrence: 1–3 years
4. Prognosis good if there are no metastases.

B. Medical management
1. Nephrectomy, with total removal of tumor
2. Postsurgical radiation in treatment of stages II, III, and IV; stage I disease does not usually require radiation, but it may be used if the tumor histology is unfavorable.
3. Postsurgical chemotherapy: vincristine and daunorubicin, doxorubicin

C. Assessment findings
1. Staging
   a. Stage I: limited to kidney
   b. Stage II: tumor extends beyond kidney, but is completely encapsulated
   c. Stage III: tumor confined to abdomen
   d. Stage IV: tumor has metastasized to lung, liver, bone, or brain
   e. Stage V: bilateral renal involvement at diagnosis
2. Usually mother notices mass while bathing or dressing child; nontender, usually midline near liver
3. Hypertension and possible hematuria, anemia, and signs of metastasis
4. Diagnostic test: IVP reveals mass

D. Nursing interventions
1. Do not palpate abdomen to avoid possible dissemination of cancer cells.
2. Handle child carefully when bathing and giving care.
3. Provide care for the client with a nephrectomy; usually performed within 24–48 hours of diagnosis.
4. Provide care for the child receiving chemotherapy and radiation therapy.

Neuroblastoma

A. General information
   1. A highly malignant tumor that develops from embryonic neural crest tissue; arises anywhere along the craniospinal axis, usually from the adrenal gland
   2. Incidence
      a. One in 10,000
      b. Males slightly more affected
      c. From infancy to age 4
   3. Staging
      a. Stage I: tumor confined to the organ of origin
      b. Stage II: tumor extends beyond primary site but not across midline
      c. Stage III: tumor extends beyond midline
      d. Stage IV: tumor metastasizes to skeleton (bone marrow), soft tissue (liver), and lymph nodes
B. Medical management: depends on the staging of tumor and age of child; includes surgery, radiation therapy, chemotherapy
C. Assessment findings vary, depending on the tumor site and stage
   1. If in the abdomen, may initially resemble Wilms' tumor
   2. Local signs and symptoms caused by pressure of the tumor on surrounding tissue
   3. Metastatic manifestations
      a. Ocular: supraorbital ecchymosis, periorbital edema, exophthalmos
      b. Cervical or supraclavicular lymphadenopathy
      c. Bone pain: may or may not occur with bone metastasis
      d. Nonspecific complaints; pallor, anorexia, weight loss, irritability, weakness
   4. Diagnosis usually made after metastasis has occurred
   5. Diagnostic tests
      a. X-rays of the head, chest, or abdomen reveal presence of primary tumor or metastases
      b. IVP: if tumor is adrenal, shows a downward displacement of the kidney on the affected side
      c. Bone marrow aspiration: to rule out metastasis; neuroblasts have a clumping pattern
      d. CBC: RBCs and platelets decreased
      e. Coagulation studies: abnormal due to thrombocytopenia
      f. Catecholamine excretion: VMA levels in urine increased
         1) child must not ingest vanilla, chocolate, bananas, or nuts for 3 days prior to the test
         2) 24-hour urine specimen needed
D. Nursing interventions: same as for leukemia and brain tumors.

Bone Tumors

Osteogenic Sarcoma

A. General information
   1. Primary bone tumor arising from the mesenchymal cells and characterized by formation of osteoid (immature bone)
   2. Invades ends of long bones, most frequently distal end of femur or proximal end of tibia
   3. Occurs more often in boys, usually between ages 10 and 20 years
   4. Lungs most frequent site of metastasis
   5. 5-year survival rate is 10-20%
B. Medical management
   1. Surgery: treatment of choice
      a. Amputation: temporary prosthesis used immediately after surgery; permanent one usually fitted a few weeks later
      b. Limb salvage procedures
      c. Lung surgery if there are metastases
   2. Radiation: only in areas where tumor is not accessible to surgery
   3. Chemotherapy: adjuvant therapy being studied
C. Assessment findings
   1. Insidious pain, increasing with activity, gradually becoming more severe
   2. Tender mass, warm to touch; limitation of movement
   3. Pathologic fractures
D. Nursing interventions
   1. Prepare child for amputation: discuss fears, concerns, and facts of procedure; answer questions regarding prosthetic devices, limited activity
   2. Assure child that phantom limb pain will subside

Ewing's Sarcoma

A. General information
   1. Primary tumor arising from cells in bone marrow
   2. Invades bone longitudinally, destroying bone tissue; no new bone formation
   3. Femur most frequently affected site
   4. More common in males, between ages 5 and 15 years
   5. Lungs most frequent site of metastasis
B. Medical management
   1. High-dose radiation is primary treatment
   2. Chemotherapy
   3. Value of surgery presently being reassessed
C. Assessment findings
   1. Pain and swelling
   2. Palpable mass, may be tender, warm to touch
   3. 15-35% of clients have metastatic disease at time of diagnosis

D. Nursing interventions
1. Promote exercise of affected limb to maintain function.
2. Avoid activities that may cause added stress to affected limb.

REVIEW QUESTIONS

1. A 10-year-old is being prepared for a bone marrow transplant. The nurse can assess how well he understands this treatment when he says

    1. "I'll be much better after this blood goes to my bones."

    2. "I won't feel too good until my body makes healthy cells."

    3. "This will help all of the medicine they give me to work better."

    4. "You won't have to wear a mask and gown after my transplant."

2. A 4-year-old has leukemia. Her mother understands the white count involvement in this disease but doesn't understand why her child has bruises and anemia. The nurse explains that

    1. all blood cells are made in the bone marrow and therefore all types will be affected.

    2. the anemia is because her child hasn't been eating well; the bruises are from the multiple needle sticks.

    3. they are related to inactivity.

    4. this is indicative that the end is near.

3. A 14-year-old has had an exacerbation of acute lymphocytic leukemia. The primary effect of leukemia on the bone marrow is

    1. crowding out of normal bone marrow cells.

    2. proliferation of cells producing blood components.

    3. a selective reduction in the number of neutrophils.

    4. leukopenia, thrombocytopenia, and anemia.

4. A 14-year-old girl has acute lymphocytic leukemia and is admitted. She is terminally ill. An appropriate nursing action would be to

    1. leave her alone as much as possible and whisper when in her room in order not to disturb her.

    2. assist her in giving away her possessions to friends and family.

    3. encourage her parents to explain to her 5-year-old sister that she will be asleep for a long time.

    4. reduce emotional stress by not having the child's parents/family participate in her care.

5. A 10-year-old is receiving cranial irradiation for a brain tumor. He has developed alopecia. Which of the following is an appropriate nursing intervention?

   1. Have the child identify famous movie stars and sports heroes who are bald.

   2. Assure the child that his hair will grow in before he leaves the hospital.

   3. Wrap a bandage around his head.

   4. Help him select a variety of hats.

6. A 6-year-old girl is newly diagnosed with acute lymphoid leukemia (ALL). During your assessment, which of the following signs and symptoms would you expect?

   1. Fever, pallor, bone and joint pain.

   2. Fever, ruddy complexion, petechiae.

   3. Abdominal pain, cystitis, swollen joints.

   4. Enlarged lymph nodes, low grade fever, night sweats.

7. A 12-year-old girl with ALL is receiving induction therapy with vincristine, prednisone, and L-asparaginase. She presents with paresthesia, alopecia, and moon face. Which of the following nursing diagnoses would be most appropriate for this child?

   1. High risk for injury.

   2. Impaired physical mobility.

   3. Body image disturbance.

   4. Altered nutrition: less than body requirements.

8. You are caring for a 10-year-old with ALL who underwent a bone marrow transplant. To provide a safe, effective care environment, what would be included in a plan of care?

   1. Rectal temperature every 4 hours to monitor for infection.

   2. Encouraging the child to go to the playroom to limit isolation.

   3. Use of egg crate or other pressure reducing mattress.

   4. Inserting a Foley catheter to monitor output.

9. A 15-year-old girl with ALL has been on maintenance therapy for 6 months. She is receiving chemotherapy of L-asparaginase, methotrexate, and cytarabine. Her absolute neutrophil count is 500/mm^3. In planning for her care, which of the following would be included in a nursing care plan?

   1. Good handwashing by visitors and staff.

   2. Daily CBCs drawn.

   3. Daily physical therapy.

   4. Restriction of activity.

10. A 5-year-old boy is newly diagnosed with an astrocytoma brain tumor. His symptoms include headache, nausea, and seizures. Based on this information, which nursing diagnosis would be most appropriate for him?

   1. High risk for infection.
   2. High risk for injury.
   3. Anticipated grief.
   4. Impaired physical mobility.

11. Which of the following statements made by parents of an 8-year-old boy who just had surgery for a brain tumor reflect understanding of safety needs?

   1. "We will obtain a tutor to teach him at home."
   2. "We will not allow him to participate in sports anymore."
   3. "We will tell our other children to let him have his way and not upset him."
   4. "He will wear a helmet for sports."

12. A 16-year-old boy is admitted with Hodgkin's lymphoma. Which assessment finding would you expect?

   1. Small, tender lymph nodes in the groin.
   2. Enlarged, firm nontender nodes in the supraclavicular area.
   3. Enlarged, tender nodes all over the body.
   4. Small, nontender, nonmoveable nodes in the cervical area.

13. A 3-year-old with a Wilms' tumor is returning to the unit after surgery to remove the tumor. Which of the following actions have the highest priority in caring for this child?

   1. Maintaining NPO.
   2. Frequent blood pressure.
   3. Turning every 4 hours.
   4. Administering pain medication every 4 hours.

14. A child is to receive radiation therapy following surgery for Wilms' tumor. Which of the following measures would be important to include in the care plan prior to radiation therapy?

   1. Give compazine every 6 hours for nausea.
   2. Place a sign over the bed that reads "no needle punctures."
   3. Practice lying in the required position.
   4. Encourage play appropriate to age.

15. A 6-year-old boy with Ewing's sarcoma has just finished his course of chemotherapy. Which of the following statements by his parents indicate they understand the signs of complications from the chemotherapy?

1. "He will be playing football next week."

2. "We will keep him on a liquid diet until he feels better."

3. "We understand he is more susceptible to infections; we will keep him away from any sick family members."

4. "He will wear a baseball hat to bed."

ANSWERS AND RATIONALES

1. **2.** The goal of a bone marrow transplant is to have the donor cells produce functioning blood cells for the client.

2. **1.** In leukemia, bone marrow is replaced by blast cells, resulting in decreased white cells, red cells, and platelets. The bruises are due to the child's decreased platelet count.

3. **1.** Leukemia cells are capable of an increased rate of production and a long cell life, causing crowding out of the normal bone marrow cells. Cells producing normal blood components are then unable to reproduce.

4. **2.** Adolescents who know they are dying frequently want to give away their belongings.

5. **4.** Selecting hats to cover his head will help the child deal with the change in body image.

6. **1.** The signs and symptoms of leukemia are a result of infiltration of the bone marrow. These include fever, pallor, fatigue, anorexia, petechiae, and bone and joint pain.

7. **3.** This may be especially true for this child as she is entering adolescence. Her loss of hair and "fat face" will make her different from her friends. Adolescents need to belong and be accepted by a group of peers.

8. **3.** Skin breakdown and impaired healing are common with bone marrow transplant. This is a preventive measure for the integrity of the skin.

9. **1.** Because of the maintenance therapy and neutrophil count, this client may have bone marrow suppression, which increases her risk for infection. Good handwashing is essential to help prevent infection.

10. **2.** Seizure precautions should be instituted to prevent an injury.

11. **4.** To protect the skull while it is healing, a child may need to wear a padded helmet for active sports.

12. **2.** The most common symptom of Hodgkin's disease is enlarged, firm, nontender moveable nodes in the supraclavicular area.

13. **2.** Frequent blood pressure measurements are needed to watch for signs of shock and as an indication of the functioning of the remaining kidney.

14. 3. The child may stay in a fixed position during each therapy session, which may last 10-20 minutes. Having the child practice the required position prior to beginning radiation therapy can be helpful.

15. 3. This client is likely to have bone marrow suppression, which increases his risk for infection and bleeding.

Appendices Table of Contents

Appendix A

Recommended Childhood and Adolescent Immunization Schedule **UNITED STATES · 2005**

Vaccine ▼ / Age ▶	Birth	1 month	2 months	4 months	6 months	12 months	15 months	18 months	24 months	4-6 years	11-12 years	13-18 years
Hepatitis B	HepB #1	HepB #2			HepB #3						HepB Series	
Diphtheria, Tetanus, Pertussis			DTaP	DTaP	DTaP			DTaP		DTaP	Td	Td
Haemophilus influenzae type b			Hib	Hib	Hib	Hib						
Inactivated Poliovirus			IPV	IPV		IPV				IPV		
Measles, Mumps, Rubella						MMR #1				MMR #2	MMR #2	
Varicella						Varicella					Varicella	
Pneumococcal Conjugate			PCV	PCV	PCV	PCV			PCV	PPV		
Influenza						Influenza (Yearly)				Influenza (Yearly)		
Hepatitis A										Hepatitis A Series		

Vaccines below red line are for selected populations

This schedule indicates the recommended ages for routine administration of currently licensed childhood vaccines, as of December 1, 2004, for children through age 18 years. Any dose not administered at the recommended age should be administered at any subsequent visit when indicated and feasible. ▒ Indicates age groups that warrant special effort to administer those vaccines not previously administered. Additional vaccines may be licensed and recommended during the year. Licensed combination vaccines may be used whenever any components of the combination are indicated and other components of the vaccine

are not contraindicated. Providers should consult the manufacturers' package inserts for detailed recommendations. Clinically significant adverse events that follow immunization should be reported to the Vaccine Adverse Event Reporting System (VAERS). Guidance about how to obtain and complete a VAERS form is available at www.vaers.org or by telephone, 800-822-7967.

▒ Range of recommended ages	▒ Only if mother HBsAg(−)
▒ Preadolescent assessment	▓ Catch-up immunization

The Childhood and Adolescent Immunization Schedule is approved by:
Advisory Committee on Immunization Practices www.cdc.gov/nip/acip
American Academy of Pediatrics www.aap.org
American Academy of Family Physicians www.aafp.org

DEPARTMENT OF HEALTH AND HUMAN SERVICES
CENTERS FOR DISEASE CONTROL AND PREVENTION

FIGURE A-1 Recommended Childhood and Adolescent Immunization Schedule, 2005 (Courtesy of U.S. Centers for Disease Control and Prevention. Retrieved June 1, 2005, from http://www.cdc.gov/nip/recs/child-schedule.pdf)

Appendix B: Physical Growth Charts

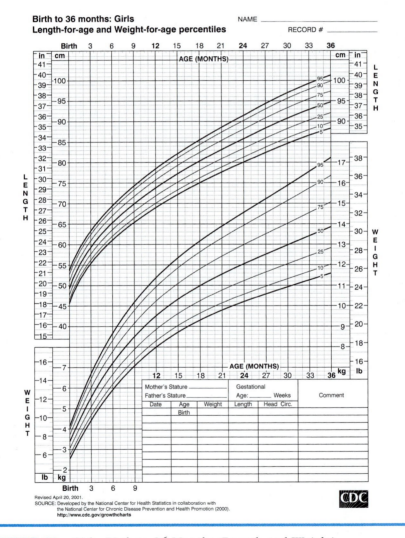

Birth to 36 months: Girls
Length-for-age and Weight-for-age percentiles

NAME _____

RECORD # _____

Revised April 20, 2001.
SOURCE: Developed by the National Center for Health Statistics in collaboration with
the National Center for Chronic Disease Prevention and Health Promotion (2000).
http://www.cdc.gov/growthcharts

FIGURE B-1A Girls: Birth to 36 Months (Length and Weight)

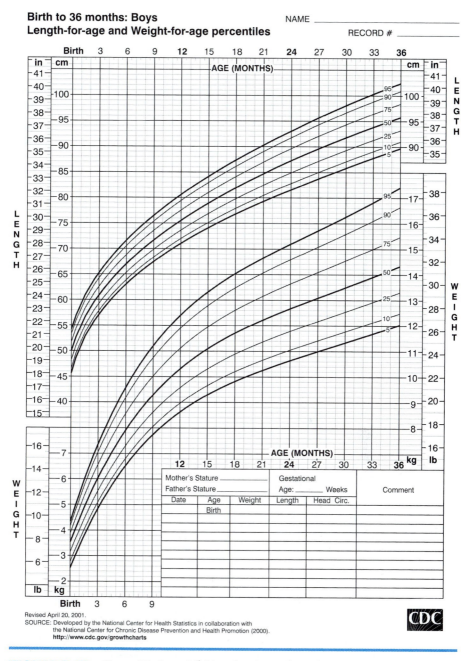

Birth to 36 months: Boys
Length-for-age and Weight-for-age percentiles

NAME _____

RECORD # _____

Revised April 20, 2001.
SOURCE: Developed by the National Center for Health Statistics in collaboration with
the National Center for Chronic Disease Prevention and Health Promotion (2000).
http://www.cdc.gov/growthcharts

FIGURE B-1B   Boys: Birth to 36 Months (Length and Weight)

Birth to 36 months: Girls
Head circumference-for-age and
Weight-for-length percentiles

NAME _____

RECORD # _____

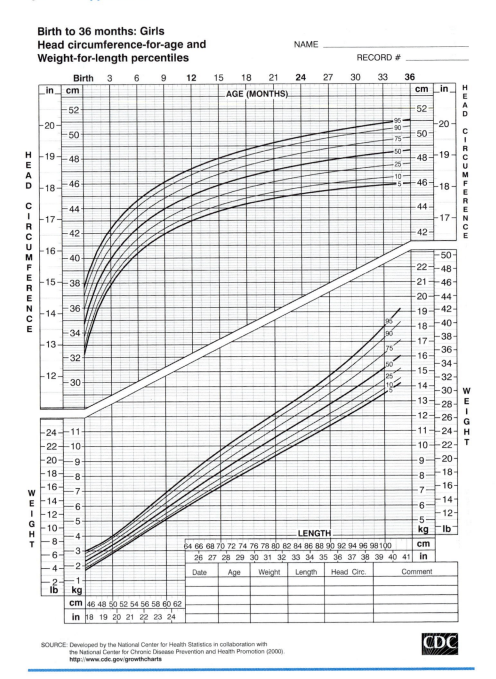

SOURCE: Developed by the National Center for Health Statistics in collaboration with
the National Center for Chronic Disease Prevention and Health Promotion (2000).
http://www.cdc.gov/growthcharts

FIGURE B-1C   Girls: Birth to 36 Months (Head Circumference)

Birth to 36 months: Boys
Head circumference-for-age and
Weight-for-length percentiles

NAME _____

RECORD # _____

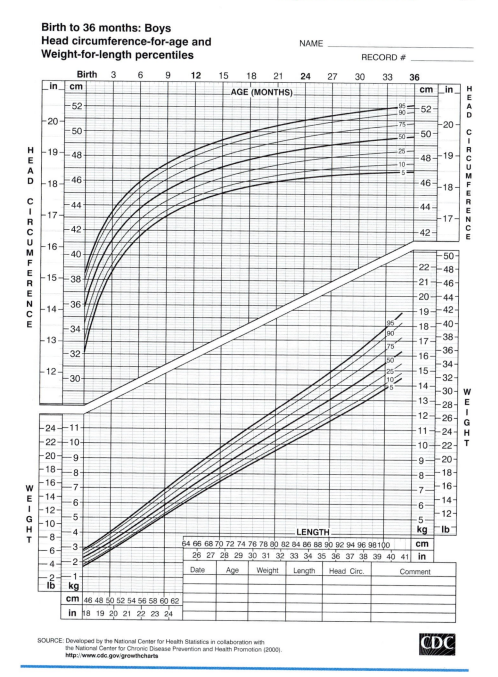

SOURCE: Developed by the National Center for Health Statistics in collaboration with
the National Center for Chronic Disease Prevention and Health Promotion (2000).
http://www.cdc.gov/growthcharts

FIGURE B-1D   Boys: Birth to 36 Months (Head Circumference)

2 to 20 years: Girls
Stature-for-age and Weight-for-age percentiles

NAME _____

RECORD # _____

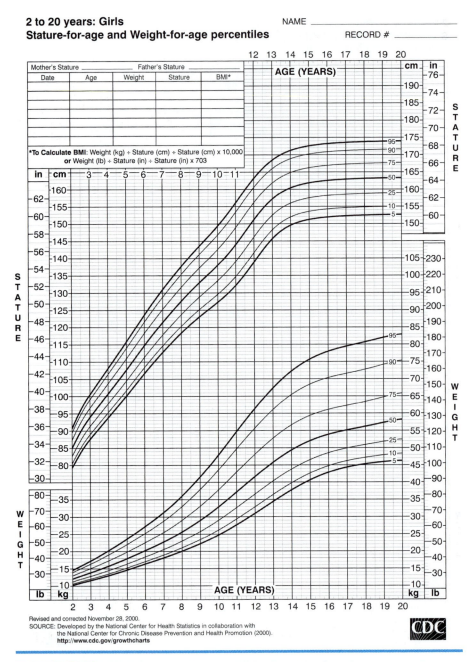

Revised and corrected November 28, 2000.
SOURCE: Developed by the National Center for Health Statistics in collaboration with
the National Center for Chronic Disease Prevention and Health Promotion (2000).
http://www.cdc.gov/growthcharts

FIGURE B-1E Girls: 2 to 20 Years (Stature and Weight)

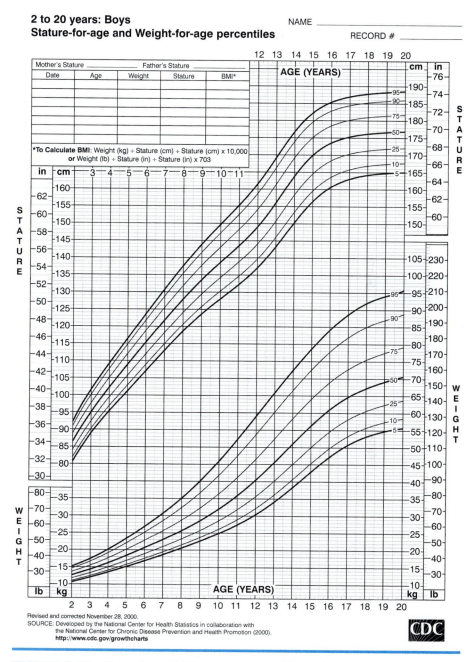

FIGURE B-1F Boys: 2 to 20 Years (Stature and Weight)

Appendix C: Common Laboratory Tests and Normal Values

Acetaminophen (serum or plasma)

Therapeutic concentration	10–30 µg/ml
Toxic concentration	>200 µg/ml

Albumin (plasma)

Newborn	2.5–3.4 g/dl
<5 yr	3.4–5.0 g/dl
5–19 yr	4.0–5.6 g/dl

Alkaline phosphatase (ALP) (serum)

1–9 yr	145–420 U/L
2–10 yr	100–320 U/L
11–18 yr male	100–390 U/L
11–18 yr female	100–320 U/L

Ammonia nitrogen (serum or plasma)

Newborn	90–150 mg/dl
Child	40–80 mg/dl

Amylase (serum)

1–19 yr	35–127 U/L

Antistreptolysin O titer (ASO titer) (serum)

2-4 yr	<166 Todd units
School-aged	170-330 Todd units

Bicarbonate (HCO$_3$) (serum)

Infant (venous)	20-24 mEq/L
>2 years (venous)	22-29 mEq/L
>2 years (arterial)	21-28 mEq/L

Bilirubin (total) (serum)

Premature Infant	
Cord blood	<2 mg/dl
0-1 day	<8 mg/dl
1-2 days	<12 mg/dl
2-5 days	<16 mg/dl
>5 days	<20 mg/dl
Full-term Infant	
Cord	<2.8 mg/dl
0-1day	<2-6 mg/dl
1-2 days	<6-8 mg/dl
2-5 days	<4-6 mg/dl
>5 days	<10 mg/dl

Bilirubin (conjugated) (serum)

	0.0-0.2 mEq/L

Blood volume (whole blood)

Female	50-75 ml/Kg
Male	52-83 ml/Kg

C-reactive protein (CRP) (serum)

2-12 yr	67-1800 ng/ml

Calcium (Ca)—Total (serum)

Newborn	9.0-10.6 mg/dl
Child	8.8-10.8 mg/dl

Continued

Carbon dioxide
Partial pressure (PCO$_2$) (whole blood, arterial)

Newborn	27–40 mm Hg
Infant	27–41 mm Hg
Thereafter: Male	35–48 mm Hg
Female	32–45 mm Hg

Total (tCO$_2$) (serum or plasma)

Newborn	13–22 mmol/L
Infant	20–28 mmol/L
Child	20–28 mmol/L
Thereafter	23–30 mmol/L

Chloride (Cl) (serum)

Newborn	97–110 mmol/L
Thereafter	98–106 mmol/L

Chloride (sweat)

Normal	<40 mmol/L
Borderline	45–60 mmol/L
Cystic Fibrosis	>60 mmol/L

Cholesterol (total)

Newborn	53–135 mg/dl
Infant	70–175 mg/dl
Child	120–200 mg/dl
Adolescent	<200 mg/dl

Creatine kinase (CK, CPK) (serum)

Newborn	87–725 U/L

Creatine (serum)

Newborn	0.3–1.0 mg/dl
Infant	0.2–0.4 mg/dl
Child	0.3–0.7 mg/dl
Adolescent	0.5–1.0 mg/dl

Digoxin (serum or plasma)

Therapeutic concentration

Congestive heart failure (CHF)	0.8–1.5 ng/ml
Arrhythmias	1.5–2.0 ng/ml
Toxic concentration	>2.5 ng/mt

Erythrocyte (RBC) count (whole blood)

Newborn	4.8–7.1 million/mm^3
3–6 mo	3.1–4.5 million/mm^3
0.5–2 yr	3.7–5.3 million/mm^3
2–6 yr	3.9–5.3 million/mm^3
6–12 yr	4.0–5.2 million/mm^3
12–18 yr: Male	4.5–5.3 million/mm^3
Female	4.1–5.1 million/mm^3

Erythrocyte sedimentation rate (ESR) (whole blood)

Westergren (modified)	
Child	0–10 mm/hr
Wintrobe	
Child	0–13 mm/hr

Fibroginogen (plasma)

Newborn	125–300 mg/dl
Thereafter	200–400 mg/dl

Glucose (serum)

Newborn	50–90 mg/dl
Child	60–100 mg/dl
Thereafter	70–105 mg/dl

Growth hormone (hGH, somatotropin) (plasma, fasting)

Newborn	5–40 ng/ml
Child	0–10 ng/ml

Hematocrit (HCT, Hct) (whole blood)

Newborn	44–72%
2 mo	28–42%

Continued

6-12 yr	35-45%
12-18 yr: Male	37-49%
Female	36-46%

Hemoglobin (Hb) (whole blood)

Newborn	14-27 g/dl
2 mo	9-14 g/dl
6-12 yr	11.5-15.5 g/dl
12-18 yr: Male	13-16 g/dl
Female	12-16 g/dl

Iron (serum)

Newborn	100-250 µg/dl
Infant	40-100 µg/dl
Child	50-120 µg/dl
Thereafter: Male	50-160 µg/dl
Female	40-150 µg/dl

Lead (whole blood)

Child	<10 µg/dl

Leukocyte (WBC) Count (whole blood)

Newborn	$9\text{-}30 \times 1000$ cells/mm^3
1-3 yr	$6.0\text{-}17.5 \times 1000$ cells/mm^3
4-7 yr	$5.5\text{-}15.5 \times 1000$ cells/mm^3
8-13 yr	$4.5\text{-}13.5 \times 1000$ cells/mm^3
Adult	$4.5\text{-}11.0 \times 1000$ cells/mm^3

Leukocyte differential count (whole blood)

Myelocytes	0%
Neutrophils—"bands"	3-5%
Neutrophils—"segs"	54-62%
Lymphocytes	25-33%
Monocytes	3-7%
Eosinophils	1-3%
Basophils	0-0.75%

Osmolality (serum)

Child, adult	275-295 mOsmol/kg H_2O

Oxygen, partial pressure (PO_2) (whole blood, arterial)

Birth	8-24 mm Hg
1 d	54-95 mm Hg
Thereafter (decreased with age)	83-108 mm Hg

Oxygen saturation (SaO_2) (whole blood, arterial)

Newborn	85-90%
Thereafter	95-99%

Partial thromboplastin time (PTT) (whole blood) (Na citrate)

Nonactivated	60-85 seconds (Platelin)
Activated	25-35 seconds (differs with methods)

Phenylalanine (serum)

Premature	2.0-7.5 mg/dl
Newborn	1.2-3.4 mg/dl
Thereafter	0.8-1.8 mg/dl

Plasma volume (plasma)

Male	25-43 ml/kg
Female	28-45 ml/kg

Platelet count (thrombocyte count) (whole blood)

Newborn (After 1 wk. same as adult)	$84-478 \times 10^3$ mm^3 (μl)
Adult	$150-400 \times 10^3$ mm^3 (μl)

Potassium (serum)

<2 yr	3.0-6.0 mmol/L
2-12 yr	3.5-7.0 mmol/L
>12 yr	3.5-5.0 mmol/L

Protein (serum, total)

Premature	4.3-7.5 g/dl
Newborn	4.6-7.4 g/dl
1-7 yr	6.1-7.9 g/dl

Continued

8–12 yr	6.4–8.1 g/dl
13–19 yr	6.6–8.2 g/dl

Prothrombin time (PT)

One-stage (Quick) (whole blood)

In general	11–15 seconds (varies with type of thromboplastin)
Newborn	Prolonged by 2–3 sec

Sodium (serum or plasma)

Newborn	136–146 mmol/L
Infant	139–146 mmol/L
Child	138–145 mmol/L
Thereafter	136–146 mmol/L

Specific gravity (urine)

Newborn	1.016–1.030
Infants	1.002–1.006
Thereafter	1.016–1.030

Thyroxine (T_4, T_4 total, T_4 RIA) (serum)

Newborn	9–18 µg/dl
Infant	7–15 µg/dl
1–5 yr	7.3–15 µg/dl
5–10 yr	6.4–13.3 µg/dl
Thereafter	5–12 µg/dl

Thyrotropin (thyroid stimulating hormone [TSH])

Newborn	3–18 µIU/L by day 3 of life
Thereafter	2–10 mU/L

Triglycerides (TG) (serum) (after ≥12 hr fast)

	M	F
0–5 yr	30–86 mg/dl	32–99 mg/dl
6–11 yr	31–108 mg/dl	35–114 mg/dl
12–15 yr	36–138 mg/dl	41–138 mg/dl
16–19 yr	40–163 mg/dl	40–128 mg/dl

Triiodothyronine (T_3, T_3 total, T_3 RIA) (serum)

Newborn	72–260 ng/dl
1–5 yr	100–260 ng/dl
5–10 yr	90–240 ng/dl
10–15 yr	80–210 ng/dl
Thereafter	115–190 ng/dl

Urea nitrogen (serum or plasma)

Newborn	3–12 mg/dl
Infant/child	5–18 mg/dl
Thereafter	7–18 mg/dl

Urine volume (urine, 24 hr)

Newborn	50–300 ml/d
Infant	350–550 ml/d
Child	500–1000 ml/d
Adolescent	700–1400 ml/d
Thereafter: Male	800–1800 ml/d
Female	600–1600 ml/d (varies with intake and other factors)

Note: Normal lab values differ depending on lab used. Verify your facility's normal values.
SOURCE: Modified from *Delmar's Guide to Laboratory and Diagnostic Tests* by R. Daniels. (2001). Albany, NY: Delmar; *Nelson Textbook of Pediatrics* (16th ed.), by R. Behrman, R. Kliegman, and H. Jenson. (2000). Philadelphia, PA: W. B. Saunders; *A Manual of Laboratory and Diagnostic Tests* (6th ed.) by F. Fischbach. (1999). Philadelphia PA: Lippincott.

Appendix D: Temperature Equivalents and Pediatric Weight Conversion

Celsius and Fahrenheit
Temperature Equivalents

Celsius	Fahrenheit
34.0	93.2
34.2	93.6
34.4	93.9
34.6	94.3
34.8	94.6
35.0	95.0
35.2	95.4
35.4	95.7
35.6	96.1
35.8	96.4

36.0	96.8
36.2	97.1
36.4	97.5
36.6	97.8
36.8	98.2
37.0	98.6
37.2	98.9
37.4	99.3
37.6	99.6
37.8	100.0
38.0	100.4
38.2	100.7
38.4	101.1
38.6	101.4
38.8	101.8
39.0	102.2
39.2	102.5
39.4	102.9
39.6	103.2
39.8	103.6
40.0	104.0

Continued

40.2	104.3
40.4	104.7
40.6	105.1
40.8	105.4
41.0	105.8
41.2	106.1
41.4	106.5
41.6	106.8
41.8	107.2
42.0	107.6
42.2	108.0
42.4	108.3
42.6	108.7
42.8	109.0

Conversion formulas:
Fahrenheit to Celsius ($°F - 32$) $\times$ (5/9) = $°C$
Celsius to Fahrenheit ($°C$) $\times$ (9/5) + 32 = $°F$

PEDIATRIC WEIGHT CONVERSION (POUNDS TO KILOGRAMS)

Pounds	0	1	2	3	4	5	6	7	8	9
0	0.00	0.45	0.90	1.36	1.81	2.26	2.72	3.17	3.62	4.08
10	4.53	4.98	5.44	5.89	6.35	6.80	7.35	7.71	8.16	8.61
20	9.07	9.52	9.97	10.43	10.88	11.34	11.79	12.24	12.70	13.15
30	13.60	14.06	14.51	14.96	15.42	15.87	16.32	16.78	17.23	17.69
40	18.14	18.59	19.05	19.50	19.95	20.41	20.86	21.31	21.77	22.22
50	22.68	23.13	23.58	24.04	24.49	24.94	25.40	25.85	26.30	26.76
60	27.21	27.66	28.22	28.57	29.03	29.48	29.93	30.39	30.84	31.29
70	31.75	32.20	32.65	33.11	33.56	34.02	34.47	34.92	35.38	35.83
80	36.28	36.74	37.19	37.64	38.10	38.55	39.00	39.46	39.93	40.37
90	40.82	41.27	41.73	42.18	42.63	43.09	43.54	43.99	44.45	44.90
100	45.36	45.81	46.26	46.72	47.17	47.62	48.08	48.53	48.98	49.44

Continued

Pounds	0	1	2	3	4	5	6	7	8	9
110	49.89	50.34	50.80	51.25	51.71	52.16	52.61	53.07	53.52	53.97
120	54.43	54.88	55.33	55.79	56.24	56.70	57.15	57.60	58.06	58.51
130	58.96	59.42	59.87	60.32	60.78	61.23	61.68	62.14	62.59	63.05
140	63.50	63.95	64.41	64.86	65.31	65.77	66.22	66.67	67.13	67.58
150	68.04	68.49	68.94	69.40	69.85	70.30	70.76	71.21	71.66	72.12
160	72.57	73.02	73.48	73.93	74.39	74.84	75.29	75.75	76.20	76.62
170	77.11	77.56	78.01	78.47	78.92	79.38	79.83	80.28	80.74	81.19
180	81.64	82.10	82.55	83.00	83.46	83.91	84.36	84.82	85.27	85.73
190	86.18	86.68	87.09	87.54	87.99	88.45	88.90	89.35	89.81	90.26
200	90.72	91.17	91.62	92.08	92.53	92.98	93.44	93.89	94.34	94.80

Example: To determine the kilogram equivalent of 43 pounds, read 40 pounds on the vertical scale, read 3 pounds on the horizontal scale, then add. 43 pounds equals 19.5 kilograms.

Appendix E: Common Nanda Diagnoses for Children and their Families

Activity intolerance

Activity intolerance, Risk for

Adaptive capacity, Decreased intracranial

Adjustment, Impaired

Airway clearance, Ineffective

Anxiety

Anxiety, Death

Aspiration, Risk for

Body image, Disturbed

Body temperature, Risk for imbalanced

Bowel incontinence

Breastfeeding, Interrupted

Breastfeeding, Effective

Breastfeeding, Ineffective

Breathing pattern, Ineffective

Cardiac output, Decreased

Caregiver role strain

Caregiver role strain, Risk for

Communication, Impaired verbal

Confusion, Acute

Confusion, Chronic

Constipation

Constipation, Perceived

Constipation, Risk for

Coping, Community, Ineffective

Coping, Community, Readiness for enhanced

Coping, Defensive

Coping, Family, Compromised

Coping, Family, Disabled

Coping, Family, Readiness for enhanced

Coping, Ineffective

Decisional conflict (specify)

Denial, Ineffective

Dentition, Impaired

Development, Risk for delayed

Diarrhea

Disuse syndrome, Risk for

Diversional activity, Deficient

Dysreflexia, Autonomic

Dysreflexia, Autonomic, Risk for

Energy field, Disturbed

Environmental interpretation syndrome, Impaired

Failure to thrive, Adult

Family processes, Dysfunctional: Alcoholism

Family processes, Interrupted

Fatigue

Fear

Fluid volume, Deficient

Fluid volume, Excess

Fluid volume, Risk for deficient

Fluid volume, Risk for imbalanced

Gas exchange, Impaired

Grieving, Anticipatory

Grieving, Dysfunctional

Growth and development, Delayed

Growth, Risk for disproportionate

Health Maintenance, Ineffective

Health-seeking behaviors (specify)

Home Maintenance, Impaired

Hopelessness

Hyperthermia

Hypothermia

Incontinence, Functional urinary

Incontinence, Reflex urinary

Incontinence, Stress urinary

Incontinence, Total urinary

Incontinence, Urge urinary

Incontinence, Urge urinary, Risk for

Infant behavior, Disorganized

Infant behavior, Readiness for enhanced

Infant behavior, Risk for disorganized

Infant feeding pattern, Ineffective

Infection, Risk for

Injury, Perioperative positioning, Risk for

Injury, Risk for

Knowledge, Deficient

Latex allergy response

Loneliness, Risk for

Memory, Impaired

Mobility, Impaired bed

Mobility, Impaired physical

Mobility, Impaired wheelchair

Nausea

Noncompliance (specify)

Nutrition, Imbalanced: Less than body requirements

Nutrition, Imbalanced: More than body requirements

Oral mucous membrane, Impaired

Pain, Acute

Pain, Chronic

Parent/infant/child attachment, Risk for impaired

Parental role conflict

Parenting, Impaired

Parenting, Impaired, Risk for

Peripheral neurovascular dysfunction, Risk for

Personal identity, Disturbed

Poisoning, Risk for

Post-trauma syndrome

Post-trauma syndrome, Risk for

Powerlessness

Protection, Ineffective

Rape-trauma syndrome

Rape-trauma syndrome, Compound reaction

Rape-trauma syndrome, Silent reaction

Relocation stress syndrome

Role performance, Ineffective

Self-care deficit,

Bathing/hygiene

Self-care deficit, Dressing/grooming

Self-care deficit, Feeding

Self-care deficit, Toileting

Self-esteem, Low, Chronic

Self-esteem, Low, Situational

Self-mutilation, Risk for

Sensory perception, Disturbed
(specify) (Visual, auditory,
kinesthetic, gustatory, tactile,
olfactory)

Sexual Dysfunction

Sexuality Patterns, Ineffective

Skin Integrity, Impaired

Skin Integrity, Impaired, Risk for

Sleep deprivation

Sleep pattern, Disturbed

Social interaction, Impaired

Social isolation

Sorrow, Chronic

Spiritual distress, Risk for

Spiritual well-being, Readiness for
enhanced

Suffocation, Risk for

Surgical recovery, Delayed

Swallowing, Impaired

Therapeutic regimen management,
Effective

Therapeutic regimen management,
Ineffective

Therapeutic regimen management,
Ineffective community

Therapeutic regimen management,
Ineffective family

Thermoregulation, Ineffective

Thought process, Disturbed

Tissue Integrity, Impaired

Tissue perfusion, Ineffective (specify
type) (Renal, cerebral,
cardiopulmonary,
gastrointestinal, peripheral)

Trauma, Risk for

Unilateral neglect

Urinary elimination, Impaired

Urinary retention Ventilation,
Impaired spontaneous

Ventilatory weaning response,
Dysfunctional

Violence, Risk for other-directed

Violence, Risk for self-directed

Walking, Impaired

Wheelchair, Transfer Ability,
Impaired

Source: North American Nursing Diagnosis Association. (2001). *Nursing Diagnoses: Definitions and Classification, 2001–2002.* Philadelphia, PA: Author.

Appendix F: Abbreviations

AA	Alcoholics Anonymous
AACAP	American Academy of Child and Adolescent Psychiatry
AAFP	American Academy of Family Physicians
AAMR	American Association of Mental Retardation
AAP	American Academy of Pediatrics
ABG	arterial blood gas
ACCH	Association for the Care of Children's Health
ACE	angiotensin-converting enzyme
ACHA	American College Health Association
ACIP	Advisory Committee on Immunization Practices
ACTH	adrenocorticotropic hormone
AD	atopic dermatitis
ADD	attention deficit disorder
ADH	antidiuretic hormone
ADHD	attention deficit/hyperactivity disorder
ADL	activities of daily living
AFDC	Aid for Families with Dependent Children
AGA	appropriate for gestational age
AGN	acute glomerulonephritis
AGS	adolescent growth spurt
AHA	American Heart Association
AIDS	acquired immune deficiency syndrome
AN	anorexia nervosa
ANA	American Nurses Association
ANA	antinuclear antibody
AOM	acute otitis media
APA	American Psychiatric Association
APPT	Adolescent and Pediatric Pain Tool
APSGN	acute poststreptococcal glomerulonephritis
ARDS	acute (or adult) respiratory distress syndrome
ARF	acute renal failure
ARF	acute rheumatic fever

250

AS	aortic stenosis
ASD	atrial septal defect
ASHA	American School Health Association
ASHA	American Speech-Language-Hearing Association
ASL	American Sign Language
ASO	antistreptolysin O
ATG	antithymocyte antibodies
A-V or AV	atrioventricular, arteriovenous
AVC	artrioventricular canal
AZT	Zidovudine, also known as ZDV
BAER	Brainstem Auditory Evoked Response
BIA	Brain Injury Association
BID	twice a day (Latin *bis in die*)
BLL	blood lead level
BMI	body mass index
BMR	basal metabolic rate
BN	bulimia nervosa
BP	blood pressure
BPD	bronchopulmonary dysplasia
BRAT diet	bananas, rice, applesauce, and toast or tea
BSE	breast self-examination
BSL	British Sign Language
BT shunt	Blalock-Taussig shunt
BUN	blood urea nitrogen
CARS	Childhood Autism Rating Scale
CAV	continuous arteriovenous
CBC	complete blood cell count
CBT	cognitive behavioral therapy
CCSC	Children's Coping Strategies Checklist
CD	Crohn's disease
CDC	U.S. Centers for Disease Control and Prevention
CDH	congenital diaphragmatic hernia
CF	cystic fibrosis
CFT	capillary filling time
CFU	colony forming units
CHB	complete heart block
CHD	congenital heart defect
CHF	congestive heart failure
CI	confidence interval
CIC	clean intermittent catheterization
CK	creatine kinase
CL	cleft lip
CMS	U.S. Centers for Medicare & Medicaid Services
CMV	cytomegalovirus
CN	cranial nerve

CNS	central nervous system
CO	cardiac output
COA	coarctation of the aorta
CP	cerebral palsy
CP	cleft palate
CPB	cardiopulmonary bypass
CPS	Child Protective Service
CPT	chest physiotherapy
CRF	chronic renal failure
CRP	C-reactive protein
CSF	cerebrospinal fluid
CSHCN	Children with Special Health Care Needs (Title V program)
CT	computerized tomography
CVA	cerebral vascular accident
CVP	central venous pressure
CXR	chest radiograph
d4T	Stavudine, also known as Zerit
DASE	Denver Articulation Screening Examinations
dB	decibel
DD	dysthymic disorder
ddC	Zalcitabine, also known as Hivid
DDH	developmental dysplasia of the hip
ddI	Didanosine, also known as Videx
DDAVP	desmopressin acetate
DDST	Denver Developmental Screening Test
DEET	diethyltoluamide
DEST	Denver Eye Screening Test
DHHS	U.S. Department of Health and Human Services
DIC	disseminated intravascular coagulopathy
DIT	Defining Issues Test
dl	deciliter
DMD	Duchenne muscular dystrophy
DMG	dimethylglycine
DNA	deoxyribonucleic acid
DRG	diagnosis-related group
DS	Down syndrome
DSM-IV	*Diagnostic and Statistical Manual of Mental Disorders*, Fourth Edition
DTaP	diphtheria, tetanus toxoid, and acellular pertussis vaccine
DTP	diphtheria, tetanus toxoid, pertussis
DTwP	DT with whole-cell pertussis
DWI	driving while intoxicated
EA	esophageal atresia
EBV	Epstein-Barr virus
ECF	extracellular fluid

ECHO	echocardiogram
ECI	early childhood intervention
ED	emergency department
EIA	enzyme immunoassay
EKG	electrocardiogram
ELISA	enzyme linked immunosorbent assay
ELM	Early Language Milestone Scale
EMG	electromyogram
EMLA	eutectic mixture of local anesthetics
EMS	emergency medical service
EPA	U.S. Environmental Protection Agency
EPSDT	early and periodic screening, diagnosis, and treatment
ESR	erythrocyte sedimentation rate
ESRF	endstage renal failure
ESSR	"enlarge, stimulate, swallow, rest"
ET	enterostomal therapist
ETT	endotracheal tube
FA	Fanconi's anemia
FAS	fetal alcohol syndrome
FDA	U.S. Food and Drug Administration
FFT	failure to thrive
FSH	follicle-stimulating hormone
GABHS	group A beta-hemolytic streptococci
GAD	generalized anxiety disorder
GER	gastroesophageal reflux
GFR	glomerular filtration rate
GH	growth hormone
GHT	gentle human touch
GI	gastrointestinal
GPA	grade point average
HAART	highly active antiretroviral therapy
HAV	hepatitis A virus
Hb A	adult hemoglobin
Hb F	fetal hemoglobin
Hb S	sickle hemoglobin (hemoglobin S)
HBV	hepatitis B virus
HCV	hepatitis C virus
HCFA	U.S. Health Care Financing Administration
HCG	human chorionic gonadotropin
HCl	hydrochloric acid
Hct	hematocrit
HD	Hirschprung's disease
HDL	high-density lipoprotein
hep B	hepatitis B vaccine
H-flu	*Haemophilus influenzae*

HIB (Hib)	*Haemophilus influenzae* type B
HIV	human immunodeficiency virus
HLHS	hypoplastic left heart syndrome
HMO	health maintenance organization
HP	Healthy People [2010]
HPS	hypertrophic pyloric stenosis
HPV	human papilloma virus
HR	heart rate
HSV-1	herpes simplex virus type I
HUD	U.S. Department of Housing and Urban Development
HUS	hemolytic uremic syndrome
Hz	hertz
IBD	inflammatory bowel disease
ICF	intracellular fluid
ICU	intensive care unit
IDEA	Individuals with Disabilities Education Act
IE	infective endocarditis
IEP	Individualized Educational Plan
IFSP	Individual Family Service Plan
IgA	immunoglobulin A
IgE	immunoglobulin E
IgD	immunoglobulin D
IgG	immunoglobulin G
IgM	immunoglobulin M
IHP	Individual Health Plan
IM	intramuscular
IMR	infant mortality rate
INR	international normalized ratio
IPV	inactivated polio vaccine
IQ	intelligence quotient
IRB	institutional review board
ITP	immune thrombocytopenic purpura
IV	intravenous
IVIG	intravenous immune globulin
IVP	intravenous pyelogram
JA	juvenile arthritis
JCA	juvenile chronic arthritis
JRA	juvenile rheumatoid arthritis
KD	Kawasaki disease
KOH	potassium hydroxide
LA	left atrium
LBW	low birth weight
LGMD	Limb-Girdle muscular dystrophy
LCP	Legg-Calve-Perthes disease
LDL	low-density lipoprotein

LES	lower esophageal sphincter
LGA	large for gestational age
LH	luteinizing hormone
LIP	lymphoid interstitial pneumonia
LPD	lymphoproliferative disease
LSD	lysergic acid diethylamide
LTB	laryngotracheobronchitis
LV	left ventricle
MCHC	mean corpuscular hemoglobin concentration
MCV	mean corpuscular volume
MD	muscular dystrophy
MDD	major depressive disorder
MDI	metered dose inhaler
MDMA	methylenedioxymethamphetamine
MHC	mean corpuscular hemoglobin
ml	milliliter
MMPI	Minnesota Multiphasic Personality Inventory
MMR	measles, mumps, rubella
MMWR	*Morbidity and Mortality Weekly Report*
MR	mental retardation
MRI	magnetic resonance imaging
NA	Narcotics Anonymous
NASN	National Association of School Nurses
NCPCA	National Committee to Prevent Child Abuse
NCV	nerve conduction velocity
NEC	necrotizing enterocolitis
NG	nasogastric
NHANES	National Health and Nutrition Examination Survey
NIAID	National Institute of Allergy and Infectious Disease
NICHCY	National Information Center for Children and Youth with Disabilities
NICU	neonatal intensive care unit
NIS-3	Third National Incidence Study of Child Abuse and Neglect
NJ	nasojejunal
NMDA	N-methyl-D-aspartate
NMPMC	nursing mutual participation model of care
NRTI	nucleoside reverse transcriptase inhibitor
NNRTI	non-nucleoside reverse transcriptase inhibitors
NOFTT	non-organic failure to thrive
NPA	National Pediculosis Association
NPO	nothing by mouth
NS	neophrotic syndrome
NS	normal saline
NSAIDs	nonsteroidal anti-inflammatory drugs
NVS	neurovascular status

OAE	otoacoustic emission test
OASPE	Office of the Assistant Secretary for Planning and Evaluation
OFFT	organic failure to thrive
OI	osteogenesis imperfecta
OM	otitis media
OME	otitis media with effusion
OPV	oral polio vaccine
ORS	oral rehydration solution
ORT	oral rehydration therapy
OSHA	U.S. Occupational Safety and Health Administration
PA	pulmonary artery
PCA	patient-controlled analgesia
PCC	Poison Control Center
PCR	polymerase chain reaction
PDA	patent ductus arteriosus
PERF	peak expiratory flow rates
PFO	patent foramen ovale
PGE	prostaglandin E
PHV	peak height velocity
PI	protease inhibitor
PICU	pediatric intensive care unit
PKU	phenylketonuria
PL	prolactin
PPD	purified protein derivative
PPI	parent-present induction
PPO	preferred provider organization
PQRST	mnemonic device for pain assessment format
PR	by rectum
prn (PRN)	as needed (pro re nata)
PS	pulmonary stenosis
PT	prothrombin time, also known as INR
PTSD	post-traumatic stress disorder
PTT	partial thromboplastin time
PVR	pulmonary vascular resistance
Q	every (quid)
QD	every day (quaque die)
RA	right atrium
RAPS	recurrent abdominal pain syndrome
RDA	recommended daily allowance
RDS	respiratory distress syndrome
REM	rapid eye movement
RF	rheumatoid factor
RICE	rest, ice, compression, elevation
RL	Ringer's lactate
RLQ	right lower quadrant

ROP	retinopathy of prematurity
RR	respiratory rate
RSV	respiratory syncytial virus
RSV-IGIV	RSV immune globulin intravenous (RespiGam)
RV	right ventricle
SA	sinoatrial
SAARDs	slow-acting anti-rheumatic drugs
SAD	separation anxiety disorder
SaO$_2$	oxygen saturation
SBHC	school-based health center
SBS	shaken baby syndrome
SC	subcutaneous
SCA	sickle cell anemia
SCFE	slipped capital femoral epiphysis
SCHIP	State Children's Health Insurance Program
SCT	sickle cell trait
SEE	Signed Exact English
SGA	small for gestational age
SIDS	sudden infant death syndrome
SLE	systemic lupus erythematosus
SLHC	school-linked health center
SPF	sun protection factor
SSI	Supplemental Security Income
SSRI	selective serotonin reuptake inhibitor
STAIC	State-Trait Anxiety Inventory for Children
STD	sexually transmitted disease
SUD	substance use disorder
SV	stroke volume
SVR	systemic vascular resistance
SVT	supraventricular tachycardia
TA	truncus arteriosus
TAC	tetracaine, adrenoline, cocaine
TB	tuberculosis
Td	tetanus and diphtheria
TEACCH	Treatment and Education of Autistic and Communication Handicapped Children
TEF	tracheoesophageal fistula
TEN	toxic epidermal necrolysis
TENS	transcutaneous electrical nerve stimulation
TGA	transposition of the great arteries
3TC	Lamivudine, also known as Epivir
TIBC	total iron binding capacity
TM	tympanic membrane
TOF	tetralogy of Fallot

TORCH	toxoplasmosis, other (e.g., hepatis), rubella, cytomegalovirus, and herpes simplex
TPN	total parenteral nutrition
TSH	thyroid-stimulating hormone
UA	urinalysis
UAP	unlicensed assistive personnel
UC	ulcerative colitis
UDT	undescended testis, also known as cryptorchidism
UGI	upper gastrointestinal
URI	upper respiratory infection Urine C&S urine culture with sensitivity
UTI	urinary tract infection
UV	ultraviolet
UVA	ultraviolet A
UVB	ultraviolet B
VCUG	voiding cystourethrogram
VLBW	very low birth weight
VSD	ventricular septal defect
VUR	vesicoureteral reflux
vWF	von Willebrand's factor
WBC	white blood cell count
WIC	Women, Infants, and Children
WPPSI	Wechsler Preschool and Primary Scale of Intelligence
WPPSI-R	Wechsler Preschool and Primary Scale of Intelligence-Revised
ZDV	Zidovudine, also known as AZT
ZPD	zone of proximal development

Appendix G: Preparation for NCLEX

The future belongs to those who believe in the beauty of their dreams.
(Eleanor Roosevelt)

A new graduate from an educational program that prepares registered nurses will take the NCLEX, the national nursing licensure examination prepared under the supervision of the National Council of State Boards of Nursing. NCLEX is taken after graduation and prior to practice as a registered nurse. The examination is given across the United States. Graduates submit their credentials to the state board of nursing in the state in which licensure is desired. Once the state board accepts the graduate's credentials, the graduate can schedule the examination. This examination ensures a basic level of safe registered nursing practice to the public. The examination follows a test plan formulated on four categories of client needs that registered nurses commonly encounter. The concepts of the nursing process, caring, communication, cultural awareness, documentation, self-care, and teaching/learning are integrated throughout the four major categories of client needs (Table G-1).

■ TOTAL NUMBER OF QUESTIONS ON NCLEX

Graduates may receive anywhere from 75 to 265 questions on the NCLEX examination during their testing session. Fifteen of the questions are questions that are being piloted to determine their validity for use in future NCLEX examinations. Students cannot determine whether they passed or failed the NCLEX examination from the number of questions they receive during their session. There is no time limit for each question, and the maximum time for the examination is 5 hours. A 10-minute break is mandatory after 2 hours of testing. An optional 10-minute break may be taken after another 90 minutes of testing.

Each test question has a test item and four possible answers. If the student answers the question correctly, a slightly more difficult item will follow, and

TABLE G-1   NCLEX Test Plan: Client Needs

Client Needs Tested	Percent of Test Questions
Safe, effective care environment:	
Management of care	7–13%
Safety and infection control	5–11%
Physiologic integrity:	
Basic care and comfort	7–13%
Pharmacological and parenteral therapies	5–11%
Reduction of risk potential	12–18%
Physiological adaptation	12–18%
Psychosocial integrity:	
Coping and adaptation	5–11%
Psychosocial adaptation	5–11%
Health promotion and maintenance:	
Growth and development through the life span	7–13%
Prevention and early detection of disease	5–11%

the level of difficulty will increase with each item until the candidate misses an item. If the student misses an item, a slightly less difficult item will follow, and the level of difficulty will decrease with each item until the student has answered an item correctly. This process continues until the student has achieved a definite passing or definite failing score. The least number of questions a student can take to complete the exam is 75. Fifteen of these questions will be pilot questions, and they will not count toward the student's score. The other 60 questions will determine the student's score on the NCLEX.

■ RISK FACTORS FOR NCLEX PERFORMANCE

Several factors have been identified as being associated with performance on the NCLEX examination. Some of these factors are identified in Table G-2.

■ REVIEW BOOKS AND COURSES

In preparing to take the NCLEX, the new graduate may find it useful to review several of the many NCLEX review books on the market. These review books often include a review of nursing content, or sample test questions, or both.

TABLE G-2   Factors Associated with NCLEX Performance

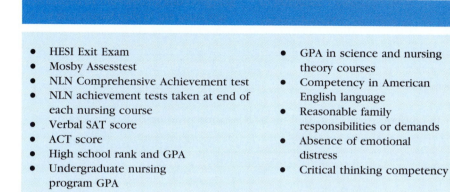

- HESI Exit Exam
- Mosby Assesstest
- NLN Comprehensive Achievement test
- NLN achievement tests taken at end of each nursing course
- Verbal SAT score
- ACT score
- High school rank and GPA
- Undergraduate nursing program GPA

- GPA in science and nursing theory courses
- Competency in American English language
- Reasonable family responsibilities or demands
- Absence of emotional distress
- Critical thinking competency

They frequently include computer software disks with test questions for review. The test questions may be arranged in the review book by clinical content area, or they may be presented in one or more comprehensive examinations covering all areas of the NCLEX. Listings of these review books are available at *www.amazon.com*. It is helpful to use several of these books and computer software when reviewing for the NCLEX.

NCLEX review courses are also available. Brochures advertising these programs are often sent to schools and are available in many sites nationwide. The quality of these programs can vary, and students may want to ask former nursing graduates and faculty for recommendations.

■ THE NLN EXAMINATION AND THE HESI EXIT EXAM

Many nursing programs administer an examination to students at the completion of their nursing program. Two of these exams are the NLN Achievement test and the HESI Exit Exam. New graduates will want to review their performance on any of these exams because these results will help identify their weaknesses and help focus their review sessions.

Students who examine their feedback from the NLN examination or the HESI Exit Exam have important information that can help them focus their review for the NCLEX. A strategy for examining this feedback and organizing this review is outlined in the following section.

■ ORGANIZING YOUR REVIEW

In preparing for NCLEX, identify your strengths and weaknesses. If you have taken the NLN examination or the HESI Exit Exam, note any content strength and weakness areas. Additionally, note any nursing program course or clinical content areas in which you scored below a grade of B. Purchase one or more of

TABLE G-3   Preparation for the NCLEX Test

Name: _____

Strengths: _____

Weak content areas identified on NLN examination or HESI Exit Exam:
_____
_____
_____

Weak content areas identified by yourself or others during formal nursing education pro-gram (include content areas in which you scored below a grade of B in class or any fac-tors from Table G-2):
_____
_____
_____

Weak content areas identified in any area of the NCLEX test plan, including the following:
Safe, effective care environment

Physiological integrity

Psychosocial integrity

Health promotion and maintenance

Weak content areas identified in any of the top 10 patient diagnoses in each of the following:
Adult health

Women's health

Mental health nursing

Children's health
(Consider the 10 top medications, diagnostic tools and tests, treatments and procedures used for each of the ten diagnoses.)

Weak content areas identified in the following:
Therapeutic communication tools

Defense mechanisms

Growth and development

Other

TABLE G-4 Organizing Your NCLEX Study

Note your weaknesses identified in Table G-3.

Take a comprehensive exam from one of the review books and analyze your performance. Then, depending on this test performance and the weaknesses identified in Table G-3, your schedule could look like the following:

Day 1: Practice adult health test questions. Score the test, analyze your performance, and review test question rationales and content weaknesses.
Day 2: Practice women's health test questions. Repeat above process.
Day 3: Practice children's health test questions. Repeat above process.
Day 4: Practice mental health test questions. Repeat above process.
Day 5: Continue with other weak content areas. Continue this process until you are doing well in all areas of the test.

the NCLEX review books. It is useful to review questions developed by different authors. Review content in the review books in any of your weak content areas.Take a comprehensive exam in the review book or on the computer software disk and analyze your performance. Try to answer as many questions correctly as you can. Be sure to actually practice taking the examinations. Do not just jump ahead to look at the section on correct answers and rationales before answering the questions if you want to improve your examination performance.

Next, once you have completed the comprehensive examination, review the answers and rationales for any weak content areas and take another comprehensive exam. Repeat this process until you are doing well in all clinical content areas and in all areas of the NCLEX examination plan.

Finally, do a general review of the top 10 patient diseases, medications, diagnostic tests, and nursing procedures in each major nursing content area, as well as defense mechanisms, communication tips, and growth and development. Practice visualization and relaxation techniques as needed. These strategies will assist you in conquering the three areas necessary for successful test taking—anxiety control, content review, and test question practice. Table G-3 will help organize your study.

■ WHEN TO STUDY

Identify your personal best time.Are you a day person? Are you a night person? Study when you are fresh. Arrange to study 1 or more hours daily. Use Table G-4 to organize your study if you have 1 month to go.

Students who use this technique should increase their confidence in their ability to do well on the NCLEX.

Glossary

absence seizures—Characterized by a transient loss of consciousness that may appear as cessation of current activity; a type of generalized seizure.

absorption—Process whereby a drug moves from site of administration into the bloodstream.

acceptance—When the griever is consciously aware of what has happened or what is most likely to occur. Kubler-Ross' fifth stage of grief.

accessory muscles—Muscles used to increase ventilation in individuals with labored breathing. Accessory muscles may include muscles in the neck, back, and abdomen.

accommodation—Modification of behavior and mental structures as a result of new experiences; the process of modifying existing schema to adapt to or incorporate new experiences, Piagetian term; the ability of the eye to focus clearly on objects at all distances.

acidosis—An acid-base imbalance indicated by a blood pH below 7.35.

acoustic feedback—A whistling sound in a hearing aid caused by improper fit into ear or too high a volume.

acquired immunity—Long term protection against a new infection that forms in response to exposure to antigens in nature or vaccines.

acrocyanosis—A condition characterized by blue discoloration, coldness, and sweating of the extremities, especially the hands.

acromion process—The lateral extension of the spine of the scapula, forming the highest point of the shoulder and connecting with the clavicle at a small oval surface in the middle of the spine. It gives attachment to the deltoideus and trapezius muscles.

active euthanasia—Giving a treatment that will directly and intentionally result in the death of a person.

acute pain—Pain generally lasting 3 to 5 days and attributed to a specific injury or cause.

adaptive immune system—Produces a specific reaction to infectious agents, remembers that agent, and prevents a later infection by the same agent.

addiction—Psychological and physiological need to use a medication for non-prescribed purposes.

A-delta nerve fibers—Mylineated nerve fibers that fire rapidly.

adolescence—The time of life that begins with puberty and ends when the individual is physically and psychologically mature and able to assume adult responsibilities.

adolescent growth spurt (AGS)— Rapid acceleration in weight and height gain; lasts about 4.5 years.

adrenarche—Pubic hair development.

advocate—Nursing role involved in pleading causes for and assisting others in making informed decisions in the child and family's best interest.

affective learning—One type of learning related to feelings and emotions.

age of majority—The age, determined by state law, at which a person is considered to have all the legal rights and responsibilities of an adult.

AIDS—A term used when the immune system has become compromised enough to allow advanced HIV disease to occur.

akinetic seizures—Total lack of movement; child appears frozen in a position.

alkalosis—An acid-base imbalance indicated by a blood pH above 7.45.

allergen—Antigen responsible for clinical manifestations of allergy.

alopecia—Hair loss.

alopecia areata—The sudden onset of asymptomatic, non-inflammatory, round bald patches. Traumatic alopecia, bald patches created by traction from braids, pony tails, corn rows.

amblyopia ("lazy eye")—A reduction of vision in one eye. The most common cause is strabismus; the brain suppresses the vision in the deviated eye to avoid the double image that it is receiving.

amniocentesis—The drawing out of a portion of amniotic fluid with a long aspirating needle for the purposes of direct examination, chemical testing, and cell culture.

anal stage—Anal activities become primary ways of gratifying the sexual instinct; Freud's second stage of psychosexual development.

analgesia—Pain control using medication or other interventions for relief.

anaphylaxis—An acute, life-threatening reaction to an antigen.

anastomosis—The surgical joining of two ducts, blood vessels, or bowel segments to allow flow from one to the other.

ancephaly—Absence of cranial vault with cerebral hemispheres either completely missing or greatly reduced in size.

anemia—Decrease in the hemoglobin content of the blood due to underlying disease or injury.

anencephaly—Congenital absence of major portions of the brain and malformation of the brainstem.

anergy—The inability to respond to infectious challenges.

anger—Feeling of rage, envy, and resentment. Kubler-Ross' second stage of grief.

angioedema—Swelling of the skin, subcutaneous, or sub-mucosal tissue.

anhedonia—Markedly diminished interest or pleasure in previously enjoyed activities.

animism—Belief that inanimate objects have human qualities.

aniridia—A congenital absence of the iris.

anorexia nervosa—A potentially life-threatening disorder characterized by voluntary refusal to eat and significant weight loss.

anthracycline—Chemotherapeutic agent known to cause cardiac toxicity.

anthropometric measurements—The science of measuring the human body as to height, weight, and size of component parts, including skinfolds, to study and compare the relative proportions under normal and abnormal conditions.

antigen—A foreign substance capable of stimulating an immune response.

anuric—Without urine output.

anxiety—A subjective feeling of apprehension or uneasiness caused by uncertain, nonspecific danger or threat.

aplastic anemia—A condition in which the bone marrow fails to produce adequate numbers of erythrocytes, leukocytes, and platelets because of injury to or abnormal expression of the stem cells.

aplastic crisis—A type of sickle cell crisis characterized by a decrease in erythropoiesis.

apocrine glands—Sweat glands concentrated in the axillae, scalp, face, abdomen, and genital area.

aqueduct of Sylvius—Canal between the third and fourth ventricle through which CSF flows.

aqueductal stenosis—Stenosis of the aqueduct of Silvius; a cause of hydrocephalus.

arachnoid mater—The second meningeal membrane under which the cerebrospinal fluid flows.

Arnold-Chiari malformation (ACM)—A brain defect in the posterior fossa that allows herniation of the cerebellum, medulla, pons, and fourth ventricle into the cervical spinal canal.

arrhythmia—Abnormal heart rhythm, caused by electrical abnormalities of the heart.

art therapy—Drawings and other art objects are used to help the therapist gain information about the child, her or his behaviors, concerns, and problems.

arteriovenous malformation—A web-like tangle of vessels providing a network between the cerebral arteries and veins.

assault—An unlawful, sudden, violent attack on another person; rape is considered a type of assault.

assent—When a child is explained the process of a procedure or treatment and agrees to cooperate with it.

assimilation—Incorporating new experiences into existing mental structures; Piagetian term.

astatic-akinetic seizures (see atonic seizures).

astigmatism—Blurry vision caused by abnormal curvature of the cornea or the lens.

atelectasis—Collapse of lung tissue.

atlantoaxial deformity—A spinal deformity resulting in instability of the upper cervical spine (associated with Down syndrome).

atonic seizures—Drop attacks; sudden loss of muscle tone with the head dropping forward for a few seconds.

atopy—A heredity predisposition to develop allergic disease.

atraumatic care—A philosophy of providing therapeutic care through the use of interventions that eliminate or minimize the psychological and physical distress experienced by children and families during hospitalization.

atresia—Complete occlusion of or lack of normal opening in a body part.

atrial septostomy—A procedure to enlarge the patent foramen ovale or to create an atrial septal defect. This allows mixing of blood at the atrial level.

attachment—Reciprocal, enduring, emotional and physical affiliation behaviors between a child and a caregiver.

attention deficit hyperactive disorder (ADHD)—The presence of impaired social interaction; impaired communication, and restricted repetitive and stereotyped patterns of behavior, interests, and activities.

aura—A somatic, sensory, or psychic warning that a seizure will occur; premonition, usually lights or sounds, experienced prior to the onset of a migraine headache.

authority and social order maintaining orientation—Laws should be obeyed because they are the laws; Kohlberg's fourth stage of moral development.

autism—A genetic developmental disorder, characterized by extreme difficulty communicating with and relating to the environment; manifested by bizarre behavior, delayed language acquisition, poor social relations, impairment of self-care skills, and altered sensory responses.

autogenous—Originating from within one's own body.

autograft—A permanent skin graft that requires transferring the child's own skin to cover the burned areas.

autoimmunity—An inability of the body to distinguish self from nonself, causing the immune system to respond against itself.

autoinoculation—Transfer of infection from one site to another on the same individual.

automatisms—Repeated nonpurposeful actions.

autonomy—The right of the client to freedom and self-determination.

autonomy versus shame and doubt—Psychosocial conflict where toddlers demonstrate independence and learn competencies related to self-care; Erikson's second stage of psychosocial development.

autopsy—Surgical and chemical analysis of the body to determine the cause of death.

average for gestational age (AGA)—Newborn lies between the 10th and 90th percentile of weight for gestational age.

avulsion—The tearing away of tissue either accidentally or surgically.

B lymphocytes—Lymphocytes produced in the bone marrow; differentiate into producers of one of five major classes of immunoglobulins

bacteremia—Bacteria in the blood.

bacteriuria—The presence of bacteria in the urine.

bad touch—Any physical contact in which the child is told "not to tell anyone."

bargaining—Attempt to postpone the occurrence of the event, by "making a deal." Kubler-Ross's third stage of grief.

barotrauma—Physical injury sustained as a result of exposure to increased environmental air pressure.

behavioral perspective—Posits that human actions and interactions come from learned responses to environmental stimuli.

behavioral therapy—Behavioral modification that uses stimulus and response to alter inappropriate behaviors. Appropriate behavior is reinforced while inappropriate behavior is extinguished and replaced with a more desirable one.

beneficence—Doing good for and to others.

bereavement—The process of mourning; an adaptation to a loss. The behavior one exhibits after a loss.

beta-thalassemia major (Cooley's anemia)—A type of thalassemia characterized by impaired beta hemoglobin synthesis that is associated with a life-threatening form of anemia.

bifid—Split into two parts.

binocularity—Fixation of two ocular images into one cerebral picture.

bioavailability—The proportion or fraction of an administered drug that reaches general circulation and is available at site of action.

bioethics—The application of moral reasoning to the life sciences, medicine, nursing, and health care.

biologic response modifiers (BRMs)—Agents and therapies used to stimulate the body's immune system to destroy cancerous cells.

biotransformation (metabolism)—Transformation or alteration of chemical structures from their original form.

blind—Vision allows only light perception; other senses are relied upon as a chief means of learning.

blindisms—Movements or behaviors that are repetitive and not purposeful, such as body rocking, eye rubbing, and head shaking. Used by blind children to compensate for inadequate stimulation.

body image—A mental conception of one's physical appearance.

bone age—Calculation of skeletal maturation utilizing an X ray of the hand and wrist or knee.

bone marrow transplantation—Replacement of hematopoietic stem cells into a person whose own bone marrow has been destroyed by disease or treatment for a malignant disease.

bottle-mouth caries (see nursing caries)

bradyarrhythmia—Abnormally slow heart rhythm.

brain death—An irreversible form of unconsciousness characterized by complete loss of brain function while the heart continues to beat.

brain stem—Area of the brain that is below the cerebellum; controls the vital centers.

bronchiectasis—A lung condition characterized by irreversible dilation and destruction of the bronchial walls.

brown fat—Increases cellular metabolic rates and oxygen consumption, resulting in heat; found primarily in the subscapular, axillary, adrenal, and mediastinal regions.

Brudzinski's sign—Sign of meningeal irritation; when child is supine, will automatically flex hips and knees if head is flexed forward.

buffer—A substance that either releases or absorbs hydrogen ions in order to maintain a stable blood pH.

bulimia nervosa—Characterized by episodes of binge eating followed by various methods purging to control weight gain.

BUN—The concentration of urea, an end-product of protein metabolism, formed in the liver and excreted by the kidney (as measured by blood urea nitrogen).

buphthalmos—Enlargement of the eyeball.

callus—Osseous material woven between the ends of a fractured bone that is ultimately replaced by new bone.

cancer—Group of diseases in which there is out-of-control growth and malignant cells.

candidiasis—Yeast infection caused by Candida species.

cao gao—Practiced by Southeast Asians; involves rubbing a coin or a spoon heated in oil on an ill child's neck, spine, and ribs; may create a burn or abrasion.

caput succedaneum—A localized pitting edema in the scalp of a fetus that may overlie sutures of the skull. It is usually formed during labor as a result of the circular pressure of the cervix on the fetal occiput.

cardiomegaly—Enlarged heart.

cardiomyopathy—Primary disease of the heart muscle caused by a multitude of etiologies (familial, infectious, ischemic) that results in poor pump function. There are three types: dilated, hypertrophic, and restrictive.

cardioversion—A process whereby an abnormal heart rhythm is converted to normal sinus rhythm. This can be accomplished by electrical cardioversion via a defibrillator, or by medication.

carditis—Inflammation of the heart.

caregiver—Nursing role involved in delivering direct nursing care to children and their families that is based on the nursing process; also a parent, guardian, or other person responsible for the child.

caregiver burden—The effect of the challenges and demands of caring for a child with a chronic condition.

care theory—A major theoretical orientation that bases ethical decision making on the individual's needs or concerns.

carriers—Persons who can harbor and spread the organism to others without becoming ill.

case management—A practice model initially developed to minimize fragmentation of services and maximize individualization of care by using a systematic approach ensuring optimal client outcomes.

cataract—Opacity (clouding) of the crystalline lens of the eye.

"catch-up" growth—A rate of growth greater than the expected rate for age.

cat's eye reflex—A whitish glow in the pupil, a sign of retinoblastoma.

causality—One of the four components of the concept of death according to Corr and Corr. The notion that death has an internal and external cause, which can be natural/unnatural or good/evil.

cavernous sinus thrombosis—A syndrome caused by an infection of the eye that results in venous congestion of the eye and paralysis of the extraocular muscles.

ceiling dose—Maximum dose of a medication thought to be effective; increasing the dose beyond this point will not increase the effectiveness.

cell mediated system—T cells; they specifically recognize antigens and interact with the B cells and other components of the innate system to inactivate the immune challenge.

cellular elements—The erythrocytes or red blood cells, the leukocytes or white blood cells, and the thrombocytes or platelets.

central hearing loss—Damage that interrupts sound transmission between the brainstem and the cerebral cortex.

cephalhematoma—Swelling caused by subcutaneous bleeding and accumulation of blood. It may begin to form in the scalp of a fetus during labor and enlarge slowly in the first few days after birth; subperiosteal bleeding over a cranial bone that is due to ruptured blood vessels from a traumatic delivery. The swelling does not cross suture lines.

cephalocaudal—Principle that growth proceeds from the head downward.

cerebellum—Found in the posterior fossa, controls motor coordination, posture, and equilibrium.

cerebral edema—An increase in intracellular fluid in the brain.

cerebral palsy (CP)—Nonprogressive motor dysfunction caused by damage in the motor areas of the brain.

cerebrum—Largest area of the brain that controls thinking, speech, vision, and hearing.

channel—The medium through which a message is transmitted; it may be visual, auditory, or kinesthetic.

chelating agent—A drug used to either prevent or reverse the toxic effects of a heavy metal or to accelerate the elimination of the metal from the body.

child abandonment—Caregiver's intentional withholding from a child, without just cause or excuse, the caregiver's care, presence, love, protection, maintenance, and opportunity for displaying affection for a child.

child abuse—A range of intentional behaviors by a parent or caregiver that can include neglect, physical, emotional, or sexual abuse.

child life program—An organized program conducted by child life staff in health care settings that are designed to promote optimum development of children and their families, to maintain normal living patterns, and to minimize psychological trauma (Child Life Council, [1995]. *Child Life Position Statement*. Author, Rockville, MD.)

child life staff—Specialists with expertise in child growth and development who provide children with opportunities in gaining a sense of mastery, for play, for learning, for self-expression, for family involvement, and for peer interaction.

child maltreatment—The intentional injury of a child.

child molestation—Sexual involvement (oral-genital contact, genital fondling and viewing, masturbation) involving a child.

child neglect—Caregiver inattention to the child's basic need for care, protection, or control, which results in the child experiencing serious injury or impairment.

chloromas—Localized collections of malignant cells.

choanal atresia—A congenital anomaly in which a bony or membraneous occlusion blocks the passageway between the nose and pharynx.

cholestasis—Interruption in the flow of bile.

chordee—Downward curvature of the penis.

chorea—Abnormal uncontrollable, involuntary, purposeless movements of extremities and the trunk.

chorionic villus sampling—A procedure for obtaining prenatal evaluation data in early pregnancy by withdrawing a chorionic villi sample from fetal membranes.

choroid plexus—Area within the ventricle that secretes cerebrospinal fluid.

chronic (cyclic) sorrow—Cyclical, never-ending grief response of caregivers of children with chronic conditions. Occurs at somewhat predictable times in the child's and family's life.

chronic condition—A physical, psychological, or cognitive condition that places limitations on day-to-day functioning or requires reliance on special treatments and is expected to last for at least several months.

chronic pain—Pain lasting for long periods of time or coming and going frequently over long periods of time.

Chvostek's sign—Twitching of the facial muscles after gently tapping over the facial nerves near the parotid gland.

circumcision—The surgical removal of the foreskin, the skin that covers the glans or head, of the penis.

classical conditioning—Learning occurs when a response that is already part of the organism's normal activities can be reproduced by an associated stimulus that previously would not have produced it.

classification—The ability to group items according to common characteristics.

clinical cure—Resolution of signs and symptoms of infection.

clinical nurse specialist—Usually a nurse with a master's degree who provides expert physical, social, and psychological support and care; consults with nursing staff and other health care personnel; educates clients and families in health care management; conducts practice outcome research; and serves as a role model for staff.

clinical pathways—Plans of care designed to achieve specific client outcomes in a defined time frame.

clinical trials—Carefully designed investigation of drug effects on human subjects.

cliques—Three to nine "buddies" or "mates" who exhibit a strong sense of cohesion.

closed adoption—An adoption where there is no contact between the birth and adoptive parents.

closed reduction—The alignment of the bone by manual manipulation or traction.

C-nerve fibers—Slow conducting, unmyelinated nerve fibers.

cognitive ability—The capacity to understand and then use phenomena in the world around us.

cognitive learning—One type of learning where describing or explaining something or answering questions occurs.

colic—Recurrent episodes of unexplained crying and inability to be consoled occurring in infant less then 3 months of age.

collaborative—Mutual sharing and working together to achieve common goals in such a way that all persons or groups are recognized and growth is enhanced.

collateral—Extra vessels that are formed to supply blood if the normal vessels are stenotic or absent.

color blindess—Color deficiency or color vision deficit.

coma—The most severe form of depressed consciousness; no response to intense painful stimuli.

comedone—Lesions associated with noninflammatory acne.Lesions may be closed (whiteheads) or open (blackheads).

commensal fungi—Fungi living on or within another organism and deriving benefit without causing harm or benefit to the host.

communicable diseases—Infectious illnesses that exhibit the potential to spread through the community.

communicating hydrocephalus—Hydrocephalus caused by an obstruction outside the ventricular system leading to decreased absorption of cerebrospinal fluid in the sub-arachnoid space.

communication—The process of creating common or shared meaning.

community health nursing—A synthesis of nursing and public health practice directed toward promoting, restoring, and preserving the health of a community or a total population.

compartment syndrome—Condition caused by increased pressure within a compartment, leading to impairment of circulation.

compensation—Body process used to restore blood pH to normal by changing the partial pressure of carbon dioxide (pCO^2) or the bicarbonic ion concentration.

complement—Twenty different proteins that when activated by an antigen-antibody contact respond, amplify, and "complement" antibody activity.

complex partial seizures—Partial psychomotor or temporal lobe episodes.

concrete operations—The mental ability to group objects, actions, and events.

concrete operations stage—Acquisition of logical operations and effective reasoning skills; Piaget's third stage of cognitive development; ages 7–11.

conductive hearing loss—A temporary or permanent hearing deficit that occurs when something (such as fluid) affects the progress of sound into the ear canal or across the middle ear system.

confusion—A form of depressed consciousness; although alert, disoriented to time, place, and person; unable to answer simple questions.

conjunctivitis ("pink eye")—An inflammation of the conjunctiva.

conscious sedation—Administration of central nervous system depressant drugs and/or analgesics which allows a child to be both pain-free and also sedated for a procedure.

conservation—The ability to acknowledge that a change in shape does not mean a change in amount.

consolidation phase—Second phase of leukemia therapy that aims at eradicating any residual leukemic cells.

contact burns—Burns that are the result of certain implements such as curling irons, steam irons, cigarette lighters, matches, hot pots, space heaters, or radiators.

contact dermatitis—Delayed hypersensitivity; occurs when an antigen is applied directly to the skin.

context specificity—Suggests there are differences in children related to cultural values, beliefs, and experiences.

continuity—Developmental change is orderly and built upon earlier experiences; a gradual and smooth process without abrupt shifts.

contusion—An injury resulting in damage to soft tissues, subcutaneous structures, small vessels, and muscles without disrupting the skin.

conventional level—According to Kohlberg's theory of moral development, the school-aged child is at the conventional level of moral development. During this level the child's conscience develops an internal set of "rules" that must be followed in order to "be good."

conventional morality—Societal values are internalized; moral judgments are based on a desire to uphold the law and

social order or gain approval; Kohlberg's third level of moral development.

coordination of secondary schemes phase—Infant understands concepts of space and object permanence, learns to direct actions toward an intended goal, and anticipates actions of others; Piaget's fourth phase of cognitive development.

cor pulmonale—Right-sided heart failure caused by pulmonary disease.

corporal punishment—Physical restraint or infliction of pain to the body by a person in authority.

crackles—An adventitious lung sound caused when air passes over airway secretions or collapsed airways are suddenly opened.

cradle cap (seborrhea)—A dry, scaly scalp condition.

cranioschisis—Defect in the skull through which neural tissue protrudes.

craniosynostosis—Premature ossification and closing of the sutures of the skull, often associated with other skeletal defects.

craniotabes—Benign congenital thinness of the top and back of the skull of a newborn.

crawling—Pulling self forward with abdomen on the floor.

creeping—Moving on hands and knees with abdomen off floor.

cremasteric reflex—A superficial neural reflex elicited by stroking the skin of the upper thigh in a male. This action results in a brisk retraction of the testis on the side of the stimulus.

crepitus—Grating sound heard on movement of the ends of a broken bone.

cretinism—Stunted physical growth and severe mental retardation caused by untreated thyroid deficiency.

critical period—A limited time span when a child is biologically prepared to acquire certain behaviors, but needs the support of a suitably stimulating environment.

crowd—An association of two to four cliques in which relations are less intimate than in the smaller groups.

cruising—Walking sideways while holding onto furniture for support.

cryptorchidism—A developmental defect characterized by failure of one or both of the testicles to descend into the scrotum. They are retained in the abdomen or inguinal canal.

crystalluria—Crystals in the urine that may be a source of urinary irritation.

cultural relativism—Differences in children are related to cultural values, beliefs, and experiences.

cultural sensitivity—Having an awareness and appreciation of cultural influences in health care and being respectful of differences in cultural belief systems and values.

cultured epithelial autograft—Sheets of skin grown in the lab from a small skin biopsy of the client; this is a permanent skin graft that is used in children with burns covering 80% of their body.

cupping (ventosos)—Practiced by Latin American and Russian cultures; occurs by creating a vacuum under a cup or glass when a small amount of burning material is placed on the skin.

cystitis—Inflammation of the bladder with symptoms including urinary frequency and dysuria, often accompanied by urgency and tenesmus.

cystogram—Radiograph of the bladder that examines the bladder, urethra, and ureters.

cytokines—Substances secreted by cells participating in the immune response.

cytoreduction—Conditioning regimen for bone marrow transplant in which lethal doses of chemotherapy, often combined with radiation, are used to eradicate all malignant cells and to suppress the child's immune system to prevent rejection of the transplanted marrow.

cytotoxic/killer T lymphocytes—Lymphocytes that attack infected or pathogenic cells.

dacrocystitis—An infection of the lacrimal sac caused by obstruction of the nasolacrimal duct, characterized by tearing and discharge from the eye.

Dandy-Walker syndrome—An obstruction in the foramina of Luschka and Magendie causing hydrocephalus.

date or acquaintance rape—Sexual intercourse with force or threat of force where the victim and perpetrator know one another either socially or professionally.

dating scripts—What is expected of dating partners.

debridement—Removal of dead skin tissue from a burn site.

decerebrate—Rigid extensor posturing secondary to trauma to the midbrain or pons; associated with poor prognosis.

deciduous teeth—The first 20 teeth to develop and erupt in a child; also referred to as primary or baby teeth.

decontamination—Decreasing absorption of an ingested poison from the GI tract.

decorticate—Flexor posturing; associated with bilateral cerebral hemisphere injury.

deficit-orientation model—Views of chronic conditions that depict them as pathological states with major negative consequences in most, if not all, aspects of life.

delayed hypersensitivity—A cellular reaction involving T cells and macrophages; there is a longer duration between exposure and reaction.

delayed primary closure—Wound closure performed 3–5 days after the injury.

delirium—Condition where anxiety, fear, and agitation are seen.

denial—Detachment; having lost hope for permanent reunion with caregiver. Third stage in adapting to hospitalization; when the grieving person does not accept the loss or believes it is true. Kubler-Ross's first stage of grief.

deontologic theory—A major theoretical orientation focused on rules, obligation, and commitment.

depot injection—An intramuscular injection of a medication that will be absorbed over a longer period of time.

depression—A great sense of loss or sadness. Kubler-Ross's fourth stage of grief.

depressive disorder—Disturbance in mood characterized by loss of interest or pleasure in normal activities.

dermatophytes—Keratin-loving fungi that are parasitic upon the skin.

dermis—The fibrous inner layer of skin just below the epidermis.

descriptive ethics—Identification of preferences in ethical situations.

despair—Withdrawal, refusal of food, diminished communication, and general loss of interest in the environment. Second stage in adapting to hospitalization.

desquamation—Shedding of the outer layer of the epidermis.

development—Physiological, psychosocial, and cognitive changes occurring over one's life span due to growth, maturation, and learning.

developmental delay—Achievement of developmental milestones later than expected.

dextrocardia—The location of the heart in the right hemithorax, either as a result of displacement by disease or as a congenital defect.

diagnosis-related group (DRG)—A classification system used to determine Medicare payments to hospitals and providers of medical services based on client diagnosis, procedures, age, and length of hospitalization.

dialysis—Treatment that acts as a filtration system outside the body to rid the body of waste products.

diaphysis—The shaft of the long bone.

diastasis recti—The separation of the two rectus muscles along the median line of the abdominal wall.

differentiated practice—A nursing practice model being implemented in some care settings, refers to a philosophy that delineates a nurse's role and functions according to experience, competence, and education.

diffusion—The movement of a solute from an area of higher concentration to an area of lower concentration until an equilibrium is reached.

DiGeorge syndrome—A congenital syndrome associated with hypoplasia or aplasia of the thymus and parathyroid gland; it is associated with congenital heart disease. There is lack of parathyroid with hypocalcemia, and deficits of cell mediated immunity caused by hypoplasia of the thymus.

direct services—Providing nursing care to individual clients.

disability—A functional limitation that prevents or interferes with a person's ability to perform age-expected activities.

discontinuity—Development is a series of discrete steps or stages that elevate the child to more advanced or higher levels of functioning with increased age.

dislocation—A displacement of two bone ends or of a bone from its articulation with a joint.

disseminated intravascular coagulation (DIC)—A coagulation disorder in which the stimulus for coagulation overwhelms the control mechanisms that normally confine coagulation to the area of bleeding.

distribution—Process whereby a drug moves from blood to interstitial spaces of tissues and from there into cells.

diurnal cycle—Sleeping through the night alternating with daytime wakefulness.

divorce decree—Legal document approved by the court that grants divorce, divides marital property, and specifies child custody.

domestic mimicry—One way of expressing an understanding of the differentiated sex-roles observed within the family/community. In imaginative play, the child enacts the role of "mommy," "daddy," and "baby."

Down syndrome—A congenital chromosomal disorder caused by an extra chromosome 21 characterized by varying degrees of mental retardation and a characteristic appearance.

drowning—Death from a submersion incident.

dry drowning—Drowning secondary to hypoxemia resulting from intense laryngospasm; fluid has not entered the lungs.

ductus arteriosus—Fetal connection between the aorta and pulmonary artery that closes shortly after birth.

ductus venosus—A shunt in the fetus that carries oxygenated blood from the umbilical veins to the inferior vena cava.

dura mater—The first meningeal membrane that adheres to the inner surface of the skull.

dysfluency—Impaired rate, rhythm, or general flow of speech.

dyshormonogenesis—Inborn error in the synthesis of a hormone.

dysmorphic—Abnormal or unusual features, commonly associated with various genetic syndromes.

dyspnea—Shortness of breath or difficulty in breathing.

dysuria—Difficult or painful urination.

ecchymosis—Black or blue discoloration of an area of skin caused by extravasation of blood into subcutaneous tissue as a result of trauma; bruise.

eccrine glands—Sweat glands distributed across the body and responsible for thermoregulation.

echolalia—Repeating the last word or words heard; sometimes initially mistaken for true speech.

ecological theory—Bronfenbrenner's view suggesting developing individuals are embedded in a series of environmental systems.

ecomap—A visual overview of the complex ecological system of a family, showing the family's organizational patterns and relationships.

ectasia—Larger than normal.

ectoparasites—Parasites living on the surface of the host's body.

educator—Nursing role involved in providing information to clients, families, and staff as indicated and needed.

effusion—The accumulation of fluid such as in the middle ear or pleural cavity.

ego—Freud's term for the rational component of the personality.

egocentrism—View the world only from own point of view.Cannot imagine that another may have a different perspective; when children and adolescents are unable to appropriately differentiate between themselves and the objects of their attention.

Electra complex—Complex described by Freud where preschool female child has strong feelings of attraction for the caregiver of the opposite sex and thus feels that she must compete with the caregiver of the same sex.

electrolytes—Charged particles that are found in body fluid. Most important body electrolytes are sodium (Na$^+$), potassium (K$^+$), calcium (Ca^{++}), and chloride (Cl$^-$).

electrophysiology—Study and treatment of heart rate, rhythm, and electrical abnormalities.

elicitation phase—Phase of a hypersensitivity reaction that occurs with reexposure to the antigen.

emancipation—The legal recognition that a minor lives independently and is legally responsible for his or her own support and decision making.

emotional abuse—See psychological abuse.

empathy—The ability to put one's self in the other person's shoes—to feel as well as to intellectually know what the other person is experiencing.

empyema—An accumulation of infected fluid in a body cavity.

encephalitis—Inflammation of the brain.

encephalocele—Protrusion of the brain and meninges into a fluid-filled sac through a defect in the skull.

endocarditis—Inflammation of the endocardial lining of the heart.

endocardium—Serous inner membrane of the heart.

enterocolitis—Inflammation of the small intestine and colon.

enucleation—Surgical removal of the eye.

enuresis—Urinary incontinence.

envenomation—The poisonous effects caused by venom following a bite or sting such as that from a spider, insect, or snake.

epidermis—The outermost layer of the skin.

epidural hematomas—Space-occupying lesions in the brain usually secondary to rupture of the meningeal artery.

epilepsy—A chronic seizure disorder often associated with central nervous system pathology.

epileptogenic focus—Area in the brain where seizures originate.

epiphora—Excessive tearing.

epiphyseal growth plate—Thin layer of cartilage located between the metaphysis and the epiphysis at the end of the long bones; controls long bone growth.

epiphysis—The proximal and distal ends of the long bone.

epistaxis—Nose bleed.

Epstein's pearls—Small white pearl-like epithelial cysts that occur on both sides of the midline of the hard palate of a newborn.

equilibrium—Harmonious relationships between thought processes (assimilation, accommodation, adaptation) and the environment; Piagetian term.

erythema marginatum—Fine, pink rash.

erythema multiforme—An erythematous, maculopapular, vesicular, urticarial rash; may include target lesions; 20% are caused by drugs.

erythema toxicum—A transient newborn rash characterized by a red macular base with a white vesicular center.

erythematous—Diffuse redness over the skin.

erythrocytosis—Increase in red blood cell production in response to chronic hypoxemia.

erythropoiesis—The production of red blood cells.

erythropoietin—A hormone released by the kidneys that stimulates the bone marrow to produce red blood cells.

eschar—Thick leather-like dead skin that forms as a result of a burn.

escharotomy—Incision made into constricting eschar to restore peripheral blood circulation.

esotropia—An inward turning of one eye relative to the other fixating eye.

esotropia (convergent) strabismus—One or both eyes turn toward midline.

ethics—The study of the nature and justification of principles that guide human behaviors and that are applied when moral problems arise.

ethnocentrism—The tendency for all individuals and cultures to believe their values are the best and the most correct.

eutectic mixture of local anesthetics (EMLA)—An anesthetic cream applied for one hour or more prior to procedures such as injections and venipunctures to minimize pain.

euthanasia—Ending life by passive or active means.

euthyroid—Normal thyroid hormone levels.

evulsed tooth—Tooth that has been knocked out or removed from socket.

exancephaly—Malformation where the brain is totally exposed or herniated through a defect in the skull.

excretion—Process whereby a drug or its metabolites move from the tissues back into the circulation and then to the organs of elimination.

exhibitionism—Exposing one's genitals to strangers.

exophthalmos—Bulging of the eyeballs.

exosystem—Bronfenbrenner's term for settings influencing individuals even though not experienced directly.

exotropia—A visual disorder in which the deviating eye looks outward. The eye often is blind or has defective vision.

exotropia (divergent) strabismus—One or both eyes turn away from midline.

exploitation—A category of sexual abuse that involves prostitution and child pornography.

expressive language—The ability to use gestures, words, and written symbols to communicate with others.

extensor surfaces—Surfaces of an extremity that do not come into contact when the extremity is flexed.

extracellular fluid (ECF)—Body fluid that is outside the cells and includes interstitial, intravascular, and lymphatic fluid; ECF contains large amounts of sodium, chloride, and bicarbonate.

extracorporeal membrane oxygenator (ECMO)—A device that oxygenates the blood outside the body.

extramedullary—Outside the bone marrow.

extravasate—The leaking out of the vein of a drug that is being administered.

exudate—Fluids, cells, or other substances released from body.

family—Two or more persons who are joined by bonds of sharing and emotional closeness and who identify themselves as members of the family.

family as client—The family considered as a set of interacting parts; assessment of the dynamics among these parts renders the whole family the client.

family as context—The family considered as the context within which individuals are assessed; emphasis is placed primarily on the individual, keeping in mind that she or he is part of a larger system.

family assessment—The process of collecting data about the family structure; relationships, and interactions among individual members.

family therapy—The therapist looks at the child's symptoms or problems as a reflection of the family's problems. Family therapy may include the child, the primary care-givers, siblings, and other people from the extended family, for example, grandparents, ex-partners, and step siblings.

family-centered care—A philosophy of care that recognizes the centrality of the family in the child's life and inclusion of the family's contribution and involvement in the plan for and the delivery of care.

Fanconi's anemia—The inherited from of aplastic anemia in which the bone marrow fails to produce adequate numbers of erythrocytes, leukocytes, and platelets.

fantasy stage (of career development)—Adolescents choose careers they are most impassioned about.

febrile seizures—A type of tonic/clonic seizure usually associated with rapid rise in temperature that reaches a minimum of 39° centigrade (102.2° Fahrenheit).

fecalith—A hard, impacted mass of feces in the colon.

feedback—Information from the receiver about the message sent.

ferritin—A stored form of iron.

fibrin—The end result of the coagulation cascade and the primary protein from which clots are formed.

fibrosis—The repair and replacement of injured or infected tissue with scar tissue.

fidelity—Keeping one's promise or word.

filtration—Movement of a solute based on the force exerted by the weight of the solution.

first-pass-effect—Effect of biotransformation of a drug by the liver before reaching systemic circulation.

flaccid areflexia—Absence of response; an indication of severe brain stem injury.

flexion burns—Occur when caregivers purposefully immerse a child in hot liquids and the body part immersed is held in a flexed position so that a "zebra" pattern occurs.

flexural surfaces—Surfaces of an extremity that come into direct contact when the extremity is flexed.

fomites—Inanimate objects on which disease-causing organisms may be conveyed.

Fontan—One of three staged palliative procedures for patients with single ventricle physiology. Goal of procedure is to connect inferior vena caval blood to the pulmonary artery.

fontanels—Soft spots found at junctions of suture lines of skull bones; allow for adaptation to the pelvis shape during delivery and growth of the brain over the coming year.

foramen ovale—Normal in utero communication between the right and left atrium that normally closes after birth. A patent foramen ovale is one that has not closed.

foreclosed—Individuals who demonstrate a strong sense of commitment, but have not experienced a crisis or exploratory period to establish commitment.

forensic examination—An examination performed for the purpose of collecting medical evidence when the health care provider suspects the client may be the victim of a crime.

formal communication—Organized communication with a particular agenda.

formal operations stage—Piaget's fourth and final stage of cognitive development; individuals from 11–12 and up begin thinking systematically and rationally about hypothetical events and abstract concepts.

fragile X syndrome—A chromosomally caused syndrome that includes mental retardation, unusual behaviors, and a characteristic appearance.

friendship dyad—The most fundamental peer relation, and the one most likely to be based on similar interests and emotional support.

gastric residuals—Feeding retained in stomach following tube feeding.

gate control theory of pain—Theory which explains how pain impulses travel and are interpreted in the body.

gender identity—The way we think about ourselves as either male or female; a culmination of biological makeup, personal experiences, social expectations, and recommendations about how males and females should think and behave.

generalized seizures—Tonic/clonic movements arising from both cerebral hemispheres; usually no aura, but always loss of consciousness.

genital stage—Freud's fifth stage of psychosexual development (puberty and onward); sexual desires reemerge, but are more appropriately directed toward opposite-sex peers.

genogram—A graph outlining a family's history over a period of time, usually over three generations.

Glenn shunt—A prodecure where the superior vena cava (SVC), which normally carries unoxygenated blood back to the right atrium (RA), is disconnected from the RA and sutured directly to the right pulmonary artery.

glial cells—Cells that provide the supporting structure of the brain.

glomerular filtration rate (GFR)—The amount of fluid that is filtered by the glomeruli (a semi-permeable membrane).

gluconeogenesis—Formation of glucose in the liver from fat and protein.

glycogenolysis—Formation of glucose from glycogen.

goiter—Enlargement of the thyroid gland.

goniotomy—A surgical procedure for glaucoma. A linear incision is made into the trabecular meshwork to increase drainage of the aqueous humor from the anterior chamber of the eye, therefore controlling intraocular pressure.

good touch—Any physical contact that helps the child in getting clean or taking care of bruises or abrasions and is done by the parent or a caregiver approved by the parent.

graft versus host disease (GVHD)—An immune response that occurs after bone marrow transplant when the donor white cells perceive the client's body as foreign material to be attacked and destroyed.

grief—An individual's response to a loss. Thoughts and feelings associated with a loss.

group therapy—Involves a group of children, usually 6 to 10, with a focus on interpersonal relationships.Socialization process occurs among group members whereby feedback and support come from peers rather than from the therapist alone.

growth—A physiological increase in size through cell multiplication or differentiation.

grunting—A sound produced by the premature closure of the glottis during early expiration. Grunting increases airway pressure and preserves or increases the functional residual volume.

guarding—A rigid contraction of the abdominal wall muscles. It usually occurs as an involuntary reaction to pain such as when an examiner attempts to palpate inflamed areas or organs in the abdominal cavity.

habituation—The ability to decrease responses to disturbing stimuli.

half-life—Time required for 50% of a drug to be excreted from the body.

hand-foot syndrome—A type of vaso-occlusive crisis in the bone marrow of the hands and feet that causes severe pain.

handicap—A barrier imposed by society, the environment, or one's self in response to perceived differences.

health-orientation model—View of chronic conditions that depicts them as a common variation in life and focuses on an individual's strengths.

hearing impairment—Impairment in processing linguistic information through hearing, with or without amplification.

heave—A lifting of the cardiac area secondary to an increased workload and force of the left ventricular contraction.

helper T cells—Cells that stimulate B lymphocytes to divide and mature into plasma cells.

hemarthrosis—A condition wherein bleeding occurs in the joints, causing pain and limited movement.

hematemesis—Vomiting of blood.

hematogenous—Originating or transported in the blood.

hematomas—Pockets of blood under the skin that result from excessive bleeding into the space following trauma.

hematuria—Presence of blood in the urine.

hemihypertrophy—A relative increase in size of one half of the body as compared to the other.

hemisensory—Loss or decrease of function of a sense organ on one side of the body.

hemodialysis—A hemofiltration system that occurs outside the body. It requires an arteriovenous fistula or shunt placed in a large vessel.

hemofiltration—A continuous form of dialysis by means of an arteriovenous or venovenous shunt. These shunts, like hemodialysis, require an extracorporeal circuit through which the blood flows into a filter system.

hemoglobin (Hb)—A protein within red blood cells that enhances the cells' ability to transport oxygen to the tissues.

hemoglobin S (Hb S)—An abnormal form of hemoglobin that undergoes sickling.

hemolysis—The destruction of red blood cells.

hemophilia A—The most common type of hemophilia, caused by a deficiency of factor VIII.

hemophilia B (Christmas disease)—A type of hemophilia caused by a deficiency of factor IX (Christmas factor).

hemophilia C—A type of hemophilia caused by a deficiency of factor XI.

hemophilias—A group of bleeding disorders in which a factor in the first phase of coagulation is deficient.

hemoptysis—Coughing up blood from the respiratory tract.

hemorrhagic cystitis—An abnormal bleeding of the bladder.

hemosiderin—An iron-rich pigment that is a product of red cell hemolysis, Iron is often stored in this form.

hemosiderosis—A buildup of excess iron in the body, eventually causing organ failure and death.

hemostasis—The control of bleeding in order to maintain blood volume, pressure, and flow through injured vessels.

hepatomegaly—Liver enlargement.

herd immunity—Reduction of the number of persons susceptible to a communicable disease by immunization, preventing the spread of disease in epidemic proportions.

heterograft—Type of temporary skin graft that comes from a donor of a different species, most often pigskin.

highly active antiretroviral therapy (HAART)—Anti-retroviral drugs, such as zidovudine and epivir, used to treat HIV/AIDS; administered during pregnancy and delivery or during the neonatal period.

hirsutism—Excessive body hair in a masculine distribution pattern.

HIV disease—An illness continuum, from asymptomatic to death, with an acquired immunodeficiency syndrome (AIDS) diagnosis usually occurring in the latter part of the continuum.

HIV infection—A multisystem disease known primarily for its effects on the immune system.

home health care—Skilled nursing and health-related services provided to individuals and families in their place of residence.

homeostasis—Dynamic equilibrium of the body that is maintained by dynamic processes of feedback and regulation.

homograft—Type of temporary graft of tissue that comes from a donor of the same species.

hormone—A chemical substance produced by an endocrine gland that is secreted into the bloodstream and produces a specific effect on a target organ.

humoral system—Consists of B lymphocytes.

hydrocele—A collection of fluid between the parietal and visceral layers of the tunica vaginalis.

hydrocephalus—An enlargement of the head without enlargement of the facial structures, due to an accumulation of CSF in the ventricles of the brain.

hydrolyze—To cause a substance to break down into its component parts by adding water.

hydronephrosis—Distension of the kidney caused by urine accumulating in the renal pelvis secondary to outflow obstruction.

hydrostatic pressure—Pressure of blood against the capillary walls generated by the contraction of the heart; hydrostatic pressure within the capillary bed pushes fluid across capillary membranes into the interstitial space and is balanced by osmotic pressure.

hypercapnia—An excess of carbon dioxide in the blood.

hypercyanotic spells—Spells commonly associated with tetralogy of Fallot, precipitated by agitation; result in extreme cyanosis and distress.

hyperopia (farsightedness)—Improper focusing of light on the retina; difficulty with near vision.

hyperplasia—Abnormal proliferation of normal cells.

hyperpnea—Deep, rapid respirations.

hypertonic dehydration—State in which the water loss is greater than the sodium loss.

hypertonic fluid—Fluid that is more concentrated (higher osmolality) than normal body fluid.

hypertrophy—An increase in the size of a cell or a group of cells resulting in an increase in the size of an organ.

hypertropia—Occurs when the eyes are out of vertical alignment.

hyphae—The branching outgrowths of a fungus or bacterium that invade tissue and establish an infection.

hyphema—A hemorrhage into the anterior chamber of the eye.

hypoalbuminemia—Low levels of albumin in the blood.

hypoplastic—Underdeveloped or incompletely developed organ or tissue.

hypotonic dehydration—State in which the sodium loss is greater than the water loss.

hypotonic fluid—Fluid that is less concentrated (lower osmolality) than normal body fluid.

hypoxia (hypoxic/hypoxemia)—Decreased oxygen to body tissues.

id—Freudian term for the inborn element of personality driven by selfish urges or instincts.

identity—Adolescents' definition of who they are based on their cumulative understanding of their inherent motivations, personal belief systems, and previous experiences.

identity achievement—Individuals who have experienced a crisis period and have achieved a sense of commitment to their resulting decisions.

identity diffusion—Individuals who have not experienced an identity crisis or made a commitment to any ideologic or occupational direction.

identity versus role confusion—Fifth stage of Erikson's psychosocial development whereby adolescents need to form a coherent self-definition or otherwise remain confused about life directions.

idiosyncratic—Peculiar to an individual.

imaginary audience—Adolescents' exaggerated sense that they are always on stage, the focus of others' attention.

immediate hypersensitivity—A reaction to an antigen; has a short duration between exposure and reaction.

immersion burns—Burns that are found on the arms, buttocks, or genitals that are sharply demarcated or circumferential due to either an accidental fall in hot bath water or from the child being held in hot water.

immune system—Spleen, lymph nodes, lymphoid tissue, white blood cells, phagocytes; natural killer cells; skin, mucus secretions, cilia, sebaceous gland secretions, stomach acid, normal intestinal flora that protect the human from disease.

immune thrombocytopenic purpura (ITP)—An autoim-mune disorder characterized by low platelet counts and exaggerated bleeding.

immunity—Processes used by the body to protect against harmful organisms.

immunoglobulins—Chemicals that "tag" or identify an antigen or pathogen for destruction by other immune cells.

immunosuppression—The reduction or prevention of the normally occurring reaction by the immune system to respond to antigenic stimuli.

immunotherapy—The use of synthetic or natural elements to stimulate or suppress the body's immune response.

incarceration—Strangulation of a portion of the bowel leading to circulation impairment and tissue necrosis.

incest—Sexual intercourse between closely related persons.

indirect services—Consulting with school and district to deliver services to meet a child's health needs.

individual health plan (IHP)—A document, based on the health assessment of a child, that outlines special health needs, goals, and strategies necessary to improve and maintain the health of the child and allow full participation in school experiences.

individual therapy—The focus is on the child's individual behavioral, developmental, and psychological issues and problems. The age, developmental level, and psychosocial alteration of the child determine the therapeutic interventions used.

individualized educational plan (IEP)—A written plan, spelling out the type and duration of services needed for a particular child.

induction—The initial phase of chemotherapy used to reduce the tumor burden to an undetectable level.

industry—The ability to be useful and productive.

industry versus inferiority—Erikson's fourth stage of psychosocial development whereby school-aged children learn to master important social and cognitive skills or otherwise feel incompetent.

infant mortality rate—The number of infant deaths during the first year of life per 1,000 live births.

infantile spasms—A type of seizure in which the head may suddenly drop forward while both arms and legs are flexed; eyes may roll upward or downward; infant may cry out and turn pale, cyanotic, or flushed.

infectious disease—One that can be transmitted from one person to another or from animal to human by either direct or indirect contact.

infiltrate—Exudate, blood, or other substances that pass into tissues.

inflammation—The protective response of body tissues to irritation or injury characterized by redness, heat, swelling, pain, and loss of function.

informal communication—When communication has no particular agenda or protocol.

informed consent—The duty of a health care provider to discuss the risk and benefits of a treatment or procedure with a client prior to giving care.

infratentorial—In the posterior third of the brain, primarily in the cerebellum and brain stem and below the tentorium.

initiative versus guilt—Erikson's third stage of psychosocial development whereby preschool-aged children learn to initiate new activities or otherwise become self-critical.

injury—Damage or harm to an individual resulting in destruction of health, disability, or death.

innate immune system—The first line of defense against infections; includes biochemical and physical barriers.

innate immunity—Physical barriers such as skin, mucous membranes, and cough reflex.

innate purity—Doctrine that suggests children are inherently good and born without an intuitive sense of right and wrong.

inotropes—Medications that increase the force of muscular contractions.

instrumental realistic orientation stage—Rules are obeyed to gain rewards or satisfy personal objectives; Kohlberg's second stage of moral development.

insufflation—Act of blowing air into a cavity.

intelligence quotient—The individual's functional age on the intelligence test divided by the chronologic age and multiplied by 100.

interferons—Chemicals that inhibit replication of many viruses; have anti-tumor effects; host specific rather than antigen specific; secreted by infected cells.

interleukins—Chemical mediators or messengers; also termed cytokines.

interpersonal concordance orientation—Behavior and decisions are evaluated on the basis of one's intent and concerns about others' reactions; Kohlberg's third stage of moral development.

interpersonal theory—Sullivan's view suggesting self-concept development, the key to personality development, is impacted by the home environment.

interstitial fluid—The portion of extracellular fluid that is between the cells and outside the blood and lymphatic vessels.

intertriginous—Skin surfaces that are apposing or form folds such as the interdigital, axillary, cubital, popliteal, and inguinal areas.

intertrigo—An erythematous skin eruption occurring on apposed skin surfaces.

intracellular fluid (ICF)—Body fluid that is located inside the cells; ICF contains large amounts of potassium, phosphate, sulfate, and proteins.

intracranial pressure (ICP)—The force exerted by the brain, blood, and cerebrospinal fluid within the cranial vault.

intrathecal—Administration of medication directly into the spinal canal for diffusion throughout the spinal fluid.

intravascular fluid—The portion of extracellular fluid that is in the blood vessels.

intravenous pyelogram (IVP)—Radiographic examination of the entire urinary tract; also called excretory urography.

intuitive phase—Characterized by sophisticated language, decreasing egocentrism, incessant questioning, reality-based play; Piaget's eighth phase of cognitive development.

iron deficiency anemia—An anemia caused by insufficient amounts of iron for adequate hemoglobin synthesis.

irreversibility—Knowledge that death is permanent.

isotonic dehydration—State in which the loss of sodium and water are equal.

isotonic fluid—Fluid that has the same concentration (osmolality) as normal body fluid.

Jacksonian seizures—Motor episodes beginning with tonic contractions of either the fingers of one hand, toes of one foot, or one side of the face, which then progress into tonic/clonic movements that "march" up adjacent muscles of the affected extremity or side of the body.

jaundice—The yellowish discoloration of the skin and eyes caused by excess bilirubin.

justice—Treating individuals equally or with fairness.

juvenile arthritis (JA); juvenile chronic arthritis (JCA); juvenile rheumatoid arthritis (JRA)—Term used for an inflammatory autoimmune disease causing many forms of arthritis in children.

karyotyping—Identification of the chromosomes' appearance, performed by growing cells from a blood or tissue sample, staining them during the metaphase stage of replication, and scanning them with a microscope.

kernicturus—A form of icterus neonatorum in which nuclear masses of the brain and spinal cord undergo pathologic changes accompanied by deposition of bile pigments within them.

Kernig's sign—Sign of meningeal irritation; child resists attempts to extend flexed leg or complains of pain on extension.

Kussmaul respiration—Abnormally slow, deep respiration characteristic of air hunger in acidotic states.

kyphosis—An abnormal thoracic curvature of the spine.

language—The meaningful use of words, phrases, and gestures to transmit meaning from one person to another.

large for gestational age (LGA)—An infant at greater than the 90th percentile of weight for gestational age, or >4,000 grams.

latchkey children—Children who are home alone after school for a period of time without adult supervision.

latency stage—Freud's fourth stage of psychosexual development; sexual drives are submerged, appropriate gender roles are adopted, the Oedipal/Electra conflict is resolved.

libido—Freudian term for psychic energy of basic biological instincts.

lichenification—Thickening and hardening of the skin with exaggeration of its normal markings.

limit setting—The caregiver defines boundaries and expectations for the toddler either by words, pictures, and/or role modeling. Setting boundaries requires consistency on the part of the caregiver in adhering to the limits set and following through on delivering consequences when the toddler exceeds the limits.

lipoatrophy—Indentation or atrophy of subcutaneous fat.

lipohypertrophy—Lumpiness or hypertrophy of subcutaneous fat.

lipolysis—The hydrolysis of fat.

listening—Providing verbal and nonverbal clues that communicate interest.

locomotion—The ability to move from place to place without assistance.

lordosis—Exaggerated curve of the lumbar spine, normal during the toddler years.

low birth weight—Weight of less than 2,500 grams—or 5 pounds, 8 ounces—at birth.

luxation—Complete dislocation of a joint, with no contact between articular surfaces of the joint.

lymphadenopathy—Enlargement of the lymph nodes.

lymphoblasts—Immature white cells, which when malignant are the leukemia cells that crowd out normal red cells, white cells, and platelets.

lymphokine—A substance that prevents or contains the migration of antigens.

Macewen's sign—A hollow or "cracked-pot" sound heard when percussing the head of a child with hydrocephalus.

macrosystem—Bronfenbrenner's term for the larger cultural or subcultural context of development.

maculopapular rashes—The most common form of cutaneous reactions to an antigen; symmetric, characterized by macules or papules.

mainstreaming—The placement of children with disabilities in a classroom with children without disabilities.

maintenance therapy—Phase of chemotherapy that follows consolidation in order to destroy residual cancer cells.

maldistribution—Abnormal distribution.

malignant brain edema (cerebral hyperemia)—Unique to children; a hyperemic or vascular reaction to head trauma because of the disruption in the blood-brain barrier; the mechanism to control cerebrospinal fluid absorption also is impaired.

malocclusion—An abnormality in the coming together of teeth, leaving the teeth uneven or crowded.

malpractice—Professional negligence.

managed care—A vehicle for cost-effective delivery of health care services.

manager/leader—Nursing role involved in being responsible for a group of clients or a group of staff.

mandated reporters—Individuals who are required to report to appropriate authorities suspicions of child abuse/neglect.

marginality—A situation in which a condition is less visible to others resulting in ambiguity about whether an individual is different from or like others. This results at times in inappropriate expectations.

matching hypothesis—Selection of a dating partner based on attractiveness.

maturation—Changes that are due to genetic inheritance rather than life experiences, illness, or injury.

mature minor doctrine—Some states have defined circumstances in which a child who has not reached the age of majority may make legal decisions, if that child can demonstrate adequate maturity.

meconium—First feces of a neonate, greenish black in color, tarry, and almost odorless.

medulla oblongata—Area of the brain stem that regulates the respiratory, cardiac, vasoconstrictor, sneeze, cough, and vomiting reflexes as well as cranial nerves IX, X, XI, and XII.

melanocytes—Cells within the epidermis that produce melanin, which gives pigment to the skin.

melena—Black or tarry stool indicating the presence of blood.

memory cells—T cells that remember an immune response.

menarche—The first menstrual period.

meninges—The three membranes covering the brain.

meningitis—Inflammation of the meninges.

meningocele—A sac-like herniation through the bony malformation that contains the meninges and cerebrospinal fluid.

meningomyelocele—A sac-like extrusion through the bony defect that contains the meninges, cerebrospinal fluid, and a portion of the spinal cord and/or nerve roots.

menorrhagia—Abnormally long and heavy menstrual periods.

mental combinations phase—One thinks before acting, uses memory for simple problem solving, imitates behavior of others, engages in symbolic, ritualistic play; Piaget's sixth phase of cognitive development.

mental retardation—A disorder characterized by subaverage general intellectual functioning with deficits in adaptive behavior.

mesosystem—Bronfenbrenner's term for the interrelationship between microsystems.

message—A verbal or nonverbal stimulus produced by a sender and responded to by a receiver.

metaphysis—A section of the long bone in which the diaphysis and epiphysis converge; it is responsible for growth until the child's adult height is attained.

microcephaly—A congenital anomaly characterized by a small brain with a resultant small head and a mental deficit.

microsystem—Bronfenbrenner's term for the immediate settings of a person's life (i.e., the family).

midbrain—Area of the brain stem that manages visual reflexes, tracking, and cranial nerves III and IV.

milia—A minute white cyst of the epidermis caused by obstruction of hair follicles and eccrine sweat glands. One variety is seen in newborns and disappears within a few weeks; small white papules on the nose, face, forehead, and upper torso caused by the plugging of the sebaceous gland.

minor—A person who has not yet reached the age at which he or she is considered to have the rights and responsibilities of an adult.

mixed conductive-sensorineural hearing loss—Results from interference with transmission of sound in the middle ear and along neural pathways.

modulation—The cascade of events that affect the firing of the pain nerve impulses or messages.

molding—The natural process by which a baby's head is shaped during labor as it is squeezed through the birth passage by the forces of labor.

molt—An arthropod's shedding of the exoskeleton to allow for growth.

mongolian spot—An irregularly dark pigmented area on the posterior lumbar region.

moral—Principle of right and wrong in behavior.

morality—Behavior in accordance with custom or tradition that usually reflects personal or religious beliefs.

morality of care—Gilligan's term for the dominant moral orientation of women; the individual emphasizes responsibility and concern for the welfare of others rather than abstract rights.

morality of justice—Gilligan's term for the dominant moral orientation of men;

moral dilemmas are seen as inevitable conflicts between the rights of two or more parties needing to be settled by laws.

moratorium—Individuals experiencing an occupational and/or ideologic crisis that has not yet been resolved, delaying the establishment of an ideologic or occupational commitment.

mosaicism—The presence of two differing cell lines in an individual or organism.

mourning—The process an individual undergoes in order to adapt to a loss.

mucositis—An inflammation of the oral mucosa ranging from mild redness to severe painful ulceration.

Munchausen syndrome by proxy—Mental disorder that causes caregivers to fabricate signs and symptoms of disease and/or expose their child to harmful medical interventions and painful invasive procedures.

Mustard procedure—Intra-atrial baffling performed for correction of transposition of the great vessels. This procedure has almost completely been replaced by the arterial switch procedure.

mycologic cure—Cure defined as the absence of fungal species.

mycoses—Diseases caused by fungi.

myelodysplasia—Malformation of the neural tube during the first 28 days of gestation.

myelosuppression—A transient decrease in blood cell production.

myocarditis—Inflammation of the myocardium, or middle muscular layer of the heart.

myocardium—The cardiac muscle, middle layer of the heart.

myoclonic seizures—Sudden repeated contractures of muscles of the head, extremities, or torso.

myopia (nearsightedness)—Improper focusing of light on the retina; difficulty with distance vision.

nadir—The lowest point of myelosuppression.

nasal flaring—The widening of nostrils during inspiration; indicates air hunger.

natural immunity—See innate immunity.

nature—Belief that development is predetermined by genetic factors and not altered by the environment.

near-drowning—Survival for more than 24 hours after a submersion episode.

nebulized—The production of spray or mist by forcing air through a liquid.

negativism—The toddler's quest for independence leads to rejection of the wishes and ideas of others.

negligence—When a person owes a duty to another and through failure to fulfill that duty causes harm.

nephrogenesis—Development or growth of the kidney.

neutropenia—A decrease in the number of neutrophils, putting one at risk of life-threatening bacterial infections.

nevus flammeus (port wine stain)—A hemangioma or vascular tumor that does not disappear with time.

N-methyl-D-aspartate (NMDA) receptors—Chemical receptors that make spinal column nerve receptors more responsive.

nociceptors—Nerve receptors specific to pain.

noncommunicating hydrocephalus—Hydrocephalus caused by an impediment of cerebrospinal fluid flow within the ventricular system, also called obstructive hydrocephalus.

nonfunctionality—All functions that make being alive stop, and there is no longer an ability to carry out functions needed to be alive.

nonmaleficence—Doing no harm to the client.

nonverbal communication—Communicating a message without using words.

normalization—Cognitive and behavioral strategies used by a family of a child with a chronic condition in order to view itself as normal.

normative ethics—Standards of justification for moral actions and choices.

nursing caries—Dental decay that occurs from frequent and/or prolonged exposure to the sugars present in milk, formula, or juice.

nursing interview—Discussion with caregivers that provides an opportunity for the nurse to establish helping relationships while learning essential information about child and family.

nursing mutual participation model of care—A collaborative approach used in nursing practice, based on the premise that optimal therapeutic interventions result from equal partnerships between nurses and caregivers.

nurture—Belief that environmental influences affect development.

object permanence—The ability to know that an object will continue to exist even when it cannot be seen.

obstructive hydrocephalus—See noncommunicating hydrocephalus.

Oedipal/Oedipus complex—Complex described by Freud where male child has strong feelings of attraction for the caregiver of the opposite sex and thus feels that he must compete with the caregiver of the same sex.

olecranon process—A proximal projection of the ulna that forms the point of the elbow and fits into the olecranon fossa of the humerus when the forearm is extended.

oligomenorrhea—Abnormally light or a reduction in menstruation.

oliguria—A decreased ability to form and excrete urine.

oncogene—Gene that is capable of causing normal cells to transform to a malignant state.

oncotic pressure—A force within the capillary beds that holds fluids in the capillaries and is caused by the amount of plasma proteins present in the vascular system.

on-demand feeds—Feeding the newborn when hungry instead of according to a pre-arranged time schedule.

open adoption—An adoption where there is contact between the birth and adoptive parents.

open reduction—Surgical procedure for reducing a fracture or dislocation by exposing the skeletal parts involved using wires, pins, bone screws, or plates.

operation—Mental action, according to Piagetian theory.

opisthotonus—Severe spasm of back muscles, causing back to arch acutely and head to bend back on neck.

opportunistic infections—Infections that take advantage of a suppressed immune system.

oral stage—Freud's first stage of psychosexual development; children gratify the sex instinct by stimulating the lips, gums, teeth, and mouth.

ordinary model—A health orientation model of chronic conditions in which awareness of the health condition follows a developmental sequence and is not central to identity and daily activities.

original sin—Belief that children are inherently evil and selfish egotists who must be controlled by society.

orthopnea—An increase in labored breathing when lying flat.

osmolality—The concentration of solute within a solution measured by the number of moles of particles per kilogram of water; used as a measure of fluid concentration.

osmolarity—The concentration of solute within a solution measured by the number of moles per liter of water.

osmosis—Movement of water across a semipermeable membrane from a solution that has a lower solute concentration to one that has a higher solute concentration.

osmotic pressure—A force within the capillary beds that tends to pull fluid into the capillaries and serves to balance hydrostatic pressures.

osteoblastic—Bone formation by osteoblasts.

osteoblasts—Cells of mesodermal origin concerned with formation of bone.

osteoclastic—Resorption of old bony tissue by osteoclasts in periods of growth or repair.

osteotomy—Surgical procedure in which the bone is redesigned to alter the alignment or weight-bearing stress areas.

palliative—Therapies or procedures performed to relieve or reduce the intensity of uncomfortable symptoms but do not result in correction of a defect or a cure.

palpebral fissures—The opening between the margins of the upper and lower eyelids.

palpitations—Sensation of abnormal, forceful, or rapid heart beats.

pancarditis—Inflammation of the entire heart.

pancytopenia—A marked reduction in the number of RBCs, WBCs, and platelets.

papilledema—An inflammation of the optic disk, evident by edema seen on fundoscopic examination.

parallel play—The ability to play side-by-side, yet totally independent of other children. There may be close physical proximity, but seldom talking or sharing of toys.

paraverbal cues—Tone, pitch, volume, inflection, and the speed of the voice used in communication; not considered language.

parenchyma—The functional tissue of an organ as distinguished from supporting or connective tissue.

parens patrie—A legal rule that allows the state to take the place of the caregivers when the actual caregivers are unable or unwilling to provide for the best interests of the child.

parentification—The process of assuming the role of a caregiver (parent) such as caring for siblings, organizing and performing household chores.

parenting—A dynamic process that provides guidance and nurturing to a child.

paresthesia—Numbness or tingling sensation.

paroxysmal—Coughing that is severe in nature.

passive euthanasia—Allowing a person to die by not treating him or her.

passive immunity—The passing or administration of pre-formed antibodies to a person without that antibody.

pathogens—Organisms that invade the body and produce disease.

patient-controlled analgesia—Means of delivering pain medication by client self-administration.

peak height velocity (PHV)—The period of greatest growth in height during the adolescent growth spurt (AGS).

peak weight velocity (PWV)—The period of greatest weight gain during the AGS.

pediatric nurse practitioner—Usually a nurse with a master's degree who functions independently or under the guidance of a physician and focuses on disease prevention and minor disease management.

pedophilia—An act by an adult where the adult directs his or her sexual interests primarily or exclusively toward children.

perception—The cognitive awareness of pain experienced at the end of the physiological pain cascade.

pericardial effusion—Abnormal collection of fluid in the pericardial sac; limits filling and decreases cardiac output.

pericarditis—Inflammation of the pericardium.

pericardium—Fluid filled sac that encases the heart.

peristalsis—Coordinated, rhythmic, serial contraction of the smooth muscle of the GI tract.

peritoneal dialysis—Requires the placement of a catheter into the peritoneal cavity for the purposes of removing excess fluids, solutes, and nitrogenous wastes. This placement may or may not require an open surgical procedure.

periungual—Located around the fingernail or toenail.

personal fable—Psychological state in which adolescents have an exaggerated notion of their own uniqueness.

petechiae—Small, pinpoint, nonraised, perfectly round, purplish red spots that are a result of an intradermal or submucosal hemorrhage.

phagocytosis—The ingestion and destruction of foreign particles by cells of natural immunity.

phallic stage—Freud's third stage of psychosexual development; children gratify the sex instinct by developing an incestuous desire for the parent of the opposite gender, or fondling their own genitals.

phantom limb pain—Pain perceived to be coming from the area of an amputated limb.

pharmacodynamics—Biochemical and physiologic effects of drugs and their mechanisms of action within the body.

pharmacokinetics—Movement of drugs throughout the body by the processes of absorption, distribution, biotransformation, and excretion.

pharyngitis—Infection or inflammation of the pharynx.

photoallergies—Delayed immune responses involving previous sensitization through exposure to a chemical substance and the appearance of a skin rash following exposure to UVA radiation.

photophobia—Light sensitivity.

phototherapy—The use of special high-intensity fluorescent lights, to reduce serum bilirubin levels and prevent kernicterus.

physical abuse—Bodily injury that appears to have been inflicted by other than accidental means.

physical dependence—Physical adaptation to the presence of a drug in the bloodstream.

physiologic anorexia—A decreased appetite and ritualistic interest in limited types of food; this usually accompanies a period of slowed physiological growth and is considered a normal occurrence of toddlerhood.

pia mater—The third meningeal membrane, which is attached to the brain itself.

pilosebaceous follicle—Unit consisting of the follicle, sebaceous gland, and vellus hair. These follicles are most widely distributed across the face, chest, and upper back and contribute to the development of acne.

plasticity—The ability of neural cells in a certain area of the brain to assume the functions of a different area.

platelets—Disk-shaped cytoplasmic fragments that facilitate blood coagulation.

play therapy—The child expresses him or herself through the use of toys, dolls, blocks, cars, or other play objects.The process of being with the therapist, toy selection, and interaction during the therapy session are part of the therapeutic process.

pneumatosis intestinalis—Air within the bowel wall.

pneumoperitoneum—Free air in the peritoneal cavity.

pneumothorax—A collection of air or gas in the pleural cavity.

polyarthritis—Inflammation of many joints.

polydactyly—A congenital anomaly characterized by the presence of more than the normal number of fingers or toes.

polydipsia—Excessive thirst.

polyhydramnios—An excess of amniotic fluid.

polymorphous—Appearing in many forms.

polyphagia—Excessive hunger.

polyuria—Excretion of abnormally large quantity of urine.

pons—Area of the brainstem that controls respiratory function and cranial nerves V, VI, VII, and VIII.

postconventional morality—Kohlberg's term for the third level of moral reasoning; moral judgments are based on an abstract understanding of universal principles of justice.

postpubertal—Late adolescence.

postvoid residual urine—A measurement of the amount of urine remaining in the bladder after voiding.

preconceptual phase—Increasing use of symbols, especially language, egocentric thought, symbolic play, mental imagery; Piaget's seventh phase of cognitive development.

preconventional morality—Kohlberg's term for the first level of moral reasoning; societal rules are not yet internalized, judgments are based on reward or punishment.

preconventional or premoral stage—Initial stage of moral development described by Kohlberg where right and wrong is determined by the rules that others place upon you; impulses rule behavior; unable to differentiate right from wrong.

precordium—The part of the front of the chest that overlays the heart and the epigastrium.

preoperational stage—Piagetian term for second stage of cognitive development; children between 2 and 7 years old think symbolically and have not mastered logical operations.

prepubertal—Early adolescence.

prepuce—Skin forming a hood over the glans, which is abnormally small ventrally and may be redundant dorsally.

primary circular reaction phase—Infant performs complex, repetitive behaviors appearing to be responses to initial chance events centering on the infant's own body; Piaget's second phase of cognitive development.

primary closure—Wound closure performed shortly after the injury in which the wound edges are approximated.

primary prevention—Involves interventions that promote health and prevent disease processes from developing.

processus vaginalis—A fold of peritoneum that precedes the testicle as it descends through the inguinal canal into the scrotum.

prodrome—The earliest phase or sign of a developing condition or disease.

professional boundaries—The spaces between the nurse's power and the client's vulnerability. The power of the nurse comes from professional position and access to private knowledge about the client. Establishing boundaries allows the nurse to control this power differential and allows a safe connection to meet the client's needs.

proprioception—Awareness of posture, movement, and changes in equilibrium and knowledge of position, weight, and resistance of objects in relation to the body. (*Taber's Cyclopedic Medical Dictionary*. [2001]. Philadelphia: F.A. Davis)

proptosis—A protrusion or forward displacement of the eyeball.

prostaglandins—A group of fatty acid substances present in many tissues. Extremely active biological substances responsible for a number of cellular interactions.

proteolysis—The hydrolysis of protein to simpler and soluble products.

proximodistal—Growth proceeds from the inside out.

pseudohermaphrodism—Ambiguous development of external genitalia.

pseudohypertrophy—Abnormal enlargement of an organ or body structure caused by an overgrowth of fatty and fibrous tissues.

pseudomenstruation—Blood observed on the diaper due to the withdrawal of the maternal hormones at the time of delivery.

pseudostrabismus—An appearance of strabismus caused by a fold of skin of the lower eyelid, which narrows the visible width of the sclera medial to the iris.

psychological abuse—Acts of omission or commission involving both the presence of hostile behavior as well as the absence of positive parenting behaviors.

psychomotor learning—One type of learning concerned with physical skills.

psychosexual theory—Freud's theoretical perspective emphasizing conflicts within the personality, unconscious motivations for behavior, and stages of development.

psychosocial theory—Theoretical perspective advocated by Erikson; stresses the complexity of interrelationships existing between emotional and physical variables during one's lifetime.

ptosis—A drooping of the eyelid.

pubertal—Middle adolescence.

puberty—The state of physical development when secondary sex characteristics begin to appear, sexual organs mature, reproduction first becomes possible, and the adolescent growth spurt starts.

pulsus paradoxus—Excessive variation in forcefulnes of arterial pulse during respiration demonstrated by a systolic reduction of more than 10 mm Hg.

punishment and obedience orientation stage—Behaviors, decisions, and conformity to rules are based on fear of punishment rather than respect for authority; Kohlberg's first stage of moral development.

pupil personnel team (service team)—A team of professionals who work together with teachers to provide interventions for students having difficulties.

purpura—Areas of blood underneath the skin or mucous membranes.

pyelonephritis—An inflammation of the kidney(s).

pyloromyotomy—Surgical procedure performed to relieve hypertrophic pyloric stenosis.

pyuria—White blood cells in the urine (a sign of bacterial or nonbacterial infection of the urinary tract).

rachischisis—Fissure in the vertebral column exposing the meninges and spinal cord.

radiation pneumonitis—Acute reaction caused by the swelling and sloughing of the endothelial cells of the small vessels of the lung, which allows fluid to accumulate in the interstitial tissues.

rape—Sexual intercourse with force or a threat of force, and without a person's consent.

rate of growth—A calculation of the amount of growth over a specific period of time.

realistic stage (of career development)—Young people begin to extensively explore and focus on available careers.

rebound tenderness—Sign of inflammation of the peritoneum elicited by a sudden release of a hand pressing on the abdomen.

receiver—The person intercepting the sender's message.

receptive language—The ability to understand spoken and written communication.

red blood cells (RBCs)—The blood cells whose primary function is to supply the tissues with oxygen.

reflexive phase—Predictable, innate survival reflexes becoming more efficient and generalized; first phase of Piaget's cognitive development.

refraction—The process by which the cornea and lens of the eye bend light rays so that they focus on the retina.

refractory seizures—Seizures lasting more than 60 minutes.

regression—Returning to a previous level of function or action. Often occurs when the toddler's routine and security are threatened (e.g., hospitalization, new baby enters family).

renal scanning—Examination of the urinary tract by ultrasound.

renal ultrasound—Radiographic examination of the kidney utilizing sound waves above the range of human hearing to formulate a two-dimensional image.

researcher—Nursing role involved in collecting, using, and evaluating evidence-based data in practice.

respiratory distress syndrome (RDS)—An inadequate production of surfactant in the lungs of premature infants, thereby reducing the surface tension of these surfaces, and interfering with the ability of the lungs to remain inflated during exhalation.

respite care—Involves having a person who relieves the usual caregiver of caregiving responsibilities for a period of time.

retractions—Inward movement of the soft tissues of the chest wall during inspiration; associated with increased respiratory effort.

retrograde—Moving backward.

reverse attention—Method of behavior management where attention is given to positive behaviors and negative behaviors are ignored.

reversibility—The ability to recognize that actions can move in reverse order.

Reye's syndrome—Acute, life-threatening, postinfectious encephalopathy.

rhizotomy—A procedure used to treat cerebral palsy, where a small secction of the spinal cord is cut.

ritualism—The repetition of sequences of occurrences, which produce structure and organization in the mind of a toddler. The repetition may involve a repeated action, phrase, and/or food/clothing choice and may continue for days or weeks.

rolandic or sylvian seizure—Tonic/clonic movements of the face with increased salivation and arrested speech; commonly occurs during sleep.

scald burns—Skin that is injured by hot water from the tap, coffee, tea, or hot cooking grease.

schema—Patterns of thought used to interpret or make sense of experiences, Piagetian term; One's own mental and/or physical structure developed through assimilation of new experiences..

school-age—The phase of development from 6 to 12 years.

school-based health clinics (SBHC)—Health centers within a school building set up and staffed by health care professionals other than the school nurse.

school-linked health clinics (SLHC)—Health centers set up and staffed by health care professionals to serve several schools, students, and other family members. May or may not be located within a school building.

scoliosis—A C-shaped or S-shaped curvature of the spine.

sebaceous glands—Glands that open into the hair follicles and secrete sebum, which helps lubricate the skin.

sebum—A complex lipid mixture produced by the sebaceous glands, which helps lubricate the skin.

secondary circular reaction phase—Infant learns from intentional behavior and begins to show some understanding of objects; Piaget's third phase of cognitive development.

secondary drowning—The rapid deterioration of respiratory function from several hours to days after successful resuscitation.

secondary intention—The natural process of wound healing that occurs when the wound edges cannot be approximated because of extensive tissue loss.

secondary prevention—Aims to detect disease in the early stages before clinical signs and symptoms manifest in order to intervene with early diagnosis and treatment.

self-competency—Adolescents' sense of how well they can function within a particular realm.

self-understanding—Adolescents' cognitive representation about themselves.

self-worth—The extent to which adolescents perceive themselves as individuals of worth.

sender—Generator of a message.

sensitive period—A time span that is optimal for certain capacities to emerge when the individual is especially receptive to environmental influences.

sensitization phase—Phase of a hypersensitivity reaction in which initial exposure to the antigen occurs.

sensorimotor stage—Piaget's first stage of cognitive development; during the first two years of life, the individual relies on motor behavior and senses to adapt to the world.

sensorineural hearing loss—Permanent hearing impairment that results from damage or malformation of the middle ear and/or auditory nerve.

separation anxiety—The behaviors demonstrated by an infant when separated from the caregiver.

sequestration crisis—A type of sickle cell crisis characterized by excessive pooling of blood in the liver and spleen.

sexual abuse—A sexual act, from fondling to vaginal or anal intercourse, imposed on a child who lacks the emotional, cognitive, or maturational development to deal with the actions.

shaken baby syndrome (SBS)—Vigorous manual shaking of a child, usually less than three years of age, that results in a subdural hematoma of the brain, occult bone fractures, and retinal hemorrhages.

sibling rivalry—Intense feelings of jealousy, envy, and stress toward a new infant sibling.

sickle cell anemia (SCA)—An anemia caused by the sickling of red blood cells caused by the presence of hemoglobin S.

simple partial seizures—Focal seizures characterized by local motor, sensory, psychic, and somatic manifestations.

sleep consolidation—Fewer periods of sleep with longer durations.

small for gestational age (SGA)—An infant who has a weight to gestational age ratio that is below the tenth percentile.

smegma—A collection of cells that shed from the outer layer of skin and gather under the foreskin of the penis.

social contract legalistic orientation—Just laws should be followed because they further human values and express the majority will; Kohlberg's fifth stage of moral development.

social learning theory—Bandura's theory; the individual learns behavior by observing behaviors of others.

social perspective taking ability—The understanding adolescents have about who they are in relation to those around them and their ability to understand the perspectives of others.

solute—A substance that is dissolved in a solution.

somnambulism—Sleepwalking.

somniloquy—Sleep talking.

somnolence syndrome—Subacute neurological toxicity seen 5-7 weeks postradiation therapy to the whole brain where drowsiness can be experienced up to 20 hours a day, and may be accompanied by fatigue, malaise, fever, dysphagia, ataxia, and transient papilledema.

span—Measurement obtained from measuring fingertip to fingertip.

speech—The physical production of sound using the oral mechanism (tongue, teeth, oral cavity, larynx).

spina bifida—A congenital, neural tube defect in the walls of the spinal cord caused by a lack of union between the laminae of the vertebrae.

spina bifida cystica—A defect in the closure of the posterior vertebral arch resulting in a protruding sac containing meninges (meningocele), spinal cord (myelocele), or both (meningomyelocele).

spina bifida occulta—A type of spina bifida where there is no herniation of the spinal cord or meninges.

splash burns—Occur when hot liquid is poured on a child; usually involves the back, lateral side of the face, or shoulder; the direction the hot liquid flows down the child's body assists in the diagnosis.

spongiosis—Inflammation of the skin's spongy layer.

sprain—A ligament that is stretched or torn from injury to a joint.

stage—The amount of spread of a malignancy, rated from stage I (1), with only local disease in one area or organ, to stage IV (4), with disseminated metastatic disease.

standard of care—Accepted action expected of an individual of a certain skill or knowledge level.

status epilepticus—A prolonged seizure or series of convulsions; loss of consciousness that may last for at least 30 minutes.

statutory rape—Consensual relations between a minor and an adult.

steatorrhea—Greater than normal amounts of fat in the feces, characterized by frothy, foul-smelling fecal matter that floats.

Stevens-Johnson syndrome—The most severe form of erythema multiforme caused by exposure to an antigen, usually a drug.

"stocking or glove" burns—Represent attempts by a child to prevent and protect himself or herself from being immersed in hot scalding tub water; burn has the appearance of a glove or stocking with an even edge.

strabismus—A condition in which each eye does not simultaneously focus on the same object in space because of lack of muscle coordination.

strain—The stretching or tearing of either a muscle or tendon from overuse, overstretching, or misuse.

stranger anxiety—The behaviors demonstrated by an infant with the appearance of a stranger and seen at approximately 8 to 12 months of age.

stratum corneum—The outermost layer of the epidermis, which is composed of several layers of dead skin cells.

stridor—A high-pitched sound produced by an obstruction of the trachea or larynx that can be heard during inspiration and/or expiration.

stupor—An unresponsive state; only responds to vigorous stimulation, and then returns to the original state once the insult is removed.

stuttering—A speech impairment in which an individual involuntarily repeats a sound or word, resulting in a loss of speech fluency.

subarachnoid villi—Area of the brain that reabsorbs CSF.

subdural hematomas—Space occupying lesions in the brain caused by rupture of the cortical veins bridging the subdural space.

subluxation—Incomplete or partial dislocation of the articular surfaces of a joint.

substance abuse—A maladaptive pattern of substance use manifested by recurrent and significant adverse consequences related to the repeated use of substance. (American Psychiatric Association. [1994]. *Diagnostic and statistical manual of mental disorders* [4th ed.]. Washington, DC: Author.)

substance P—A neuropeptide that sensitizes nerve endings to fire more rapidly.

sudden infant death syndrome (SIDS)—The sudden, unexplained death of an apparently normal and healthy infant under the age of 1 year even after a complete autopsy and review of history reveals no evidence of disease.

suicidal ideation—Thoughts about killing oneself.

suicide—The intentional or purposeful taking of one's own life. Suicide may be completed, attempted, or suicidal ideation.

sunblock—A sun protection product that reflects and scatters ultraviolet A and ultraviolet B radiation.

sunscreen—A sun protection product that absorbs the sun's rays. Protection against either or both ultraviolet A and ultraviolet B radiation may be provided.

superego—Freudian term for personality component consisting of internalized moral standards (conscience).

superior vena cava syndrome (SVC) —Syndrome caused by obstruction of the superior vena cava, resulting in edema of the face, neck, and upper trunk.

suppressor cells—T cells that reduce immunoglobulin production against a specific antigen.

suppurative—Pus forming.

supratentorial—A location in the anterior two-thirds of the brain, above the tentorium, primarily in the cerebrum.

synchronized cardioversion—Cardioversion of an abnormal rhythm to a normal rhythm using electrical shock (via a defibrillator) that senses the QRS and applies the energy in an appropriately timed manner in synchrony with the client's own rhythm. Can only be used in hemodynamically stable clients with normally upright QRS.

syncope—Fainting.

syndactylism—Congenital anomaly characterized by the fusion of the fingers or toes.

syndrome—A named condition characterized by a group of findings or attributes.

synovitis—An acute, nonpurulent inflammation of the synovial membrane of a joint; occurs most commonly in the hip joint.

T lymphocytes—The immune system's main defense against viruses; direct and regulate the immunologic response; secrete lymphokines; produced by the thymus gland.

tabula rasa—Doctrine that suggests children enter the world as a blank slate.

tachyarrhythmia—Abnormally fast heart rhythm.

tachypnea—Rapid respirations.

tamponade—An abnormal fluid collection around the heart in the mediastinal space that results in restricted filling of the heart and poor cardiac output. Can be life-threatening.

Tanner stages—The five stages of development of secondary sexual characteristics for males and females.

teething—The period of eruption of deciduous teeth.

telangiectatic nevi—A common skin condition of neonates, characterized by flat, deep-pink localized areas of capillary dilation that occur predominantly on the back of the neck, lower occiput, upper eyelids, upper lip, and bridge of the nose. The areas disappear permanently by 2 years of age.

telangiectatic nevi—Capillary hemangiomas commonly called "stork bites" that are sometimes found on the nape of the neck and the bridge of the nose.

telegraphic speech—Short sentences made up of only the key words.

teleologic theory—A major theoretical orientation that judges the rightness of actions by the ends achieved.

temper tantrums—An outward expression of the inner turmoil experienced by a toddler: openly angry and unpredictable. Usually disappears by preschool period.

temperament—The way in which a child behaviorally interacts with the surrounding environment.

tentative stage (of career development)—Adolescents begin to consider how they might fit in with the various career options they are considering.

tentorium—The dura mater located between the cerebrum and cerebellum supporting the occipital lobes.

teratogen—Any substance or process that interferes with normal prenatal development, causing developmental abnormalities in the fetus.

tertiary circular reactions phase—Characterized by interest in novelty and repetition, understanding causality, soliciting adult help, object permanence; Piaget's fifth phase of cognitive development.

tertiary prevention—Prevention directed toward children with clinically apparent disease.

thalassemias—A group of inherited autosomal recessive disorders, characterized by an impaired rate of hemoglobin chain synthesis.

therapeutic play—An intervention used by nurses and child life specialists where supervised play helps ill and hospitalized children express and understand their thoughts, feelings, and motivations.

thrill—A fine vibration, felt by an examiner's hand on a client's body over the site of an aneurysm or on the precordium, the result of turmoil in the flow of blood, indicating the presence of an organic murmur of grade 4 or greater intensity.

thrombocytopenia—A decrease in the platelet count below 150,000/ml.

tidal volume—The amount of air inhaled or exhaled with each breath.

time-out—A discipline strategy in which reinforcement for unacceptable behavior is removed to interrupt a pattern of negative behavior; a defined period of time in which the child is removed from activities and social interactions.

titration—Delivery of small doses of medication to achieve desired effect.

tolerance—Need to use increasing doses of a substance over time to achieve desired effect.

tonic/clonic seizures—Onset is usually abrupt and begins when the child loses consciousness and falls to the ground.

toxic epidermal necrolysis—An acute illness of fever, epidermal loss of more than 30% of the body surface area; 30–40% mortality rate caused by visceral involvement.

trabeculotomy—A surgical procedure for glaucoma; a direct opening between the canal of Schlemm and the anterior chamber of the eye, which controls intraocular pressure.

trajectory—The expected course of a health care alteration.

transduction—Beginning of the pain sensation when stimulus provokes electrical activity in pain receptors.

transductive reasoning—Unrelated events are linked to determine a reason for a particular event.

transferrin—An iron-transport molecule within the bloodstream.

transillumination—The use of a light to determine what structures are in the meningomyelocele.

transmission—Movement of impulses from peripheral site to terminals in spinal column dorsal horn.

trigone—A small triangular area at the base of the bladder where the ureters normally join the bladder.

trismus—Difficulty opening the mouth.

trisomy—The presence of three instead of two of a given chromosome.

tropic hormone—A hormone that causes a target organ to produce its hormone.

Trousseau's sign—Spasms of the carpals after pressure is applied to the upper arm nerves. Carpal spasms occur when the fingers contract and the individual is unable to open the hand. This is a sign of hypocalcemia.

trust versus mistrust—Erikson's first stage of psychosocial development; infants must learn to trust others to meet their needs so they learn to trust themselves.

tumor—Mass that may be either benign or malignant.

tumor lysis syndrome—Complication of initial cancer treatment; when tumor cells are killed by chemotherapy, purines are released from the lysed tumor cells, causing elevation of uric acid that can lead to renal failure.

tympanostomy—Surgical incision in the tympanic membrane for draining fluid.

uncertainty—Situations in which there is ambiguity about what can be expected. Typically results in stress.

unintentional injury—Injuries that occur without intent of harm.

universal ethical principle orientation—Right and wrong are defined on universal, comprehensive, consistent, yet personal ethical principles; Kohlberg's sixth stage of moral development.

universality—Belief that death is all inclusive, comes to every living thing; death is inevitable.

unlicensed assistive personnel (UAP)—Individuals who perform services for clients, such as first aid, medication administration, tube feedings, and catheterizations to students under the supervision of a registered nurse.

upper/lower body ratio—A ratio calculated from a measurement from the top of the head to the top of the synthesis pubis and from the synthesis pubis to the bottom of the feet.

uremia—A condition where excessive amounts of nitrogenous waste products, blood urea, and creatinine exist in the blood.

ureteropelvic obstruction—An obstruction at the junction of the ureters into the renal pelvis.

ureterovesical obstruction—An obstruction at the junction of the ureters into the bladder.

ureterovesical/vesicoureteral junction—Site where the ureter enters the bladder.

urethritis—Infection of the urethra.

urticaria—Wheal-like skin lesions seen in response to an antigen, often a drug; resolve fairly rapidly after discontinuing the drug.

values—Constructs that give meaning to our lives.

valvotomy—An incision into a cardiac valve to correct a defect.

valvulitis—Inflammation of the cardiac valves.

valvuloplasty—Procedure involving a balloon-tipped catheter used to dilate a cardiac valve.

vasculitis—Inflammation of blood vessels, including arteries or veins.

vaso-occlusive crisis—A type of sickle cell crisis characterized by the aggregation of sickled cells within a vessel, causing obstruction and infarction of the distal tissues.

vectors—Animals or insects that carry the infectious organism from one host to another.

vegetations—Abnormal growths inside body organs. In the heart they usually develop on heart valves.

vellus hair—Short, fine, often inconspicuous hair distributed across the body.

venous access device—Implanted device to facilitate the delivery of drugs, blood sampling and blood product administration, and the simultaneous administration of multiple drugs and intravenous fluids.

ventilation/perfusion (V/Q) ratio—The ratio of alveolar ventilation to capillary perfusion.

veracity—Telling the truth, particularly in health care, regarding diagnosis, treatment, or prognosis.

verbal communication—Messages using words and language.

vernix caseosa—A thick, cheesy, protective, integumentary deposit that consists of sebum and shed epithelial cells present on the newborn's skin.

verrucae—Benign epidermal tumors caused by the human papilloma virus, also known as cutaneous warts.

vertical transmission—The process of transmitting a disease from one generation to another.

vesicant—A chemotherapy agent that is a skin irritant and can cause discomfort, burning, and inflammation, if leaked outside the vein.

violent crime—Murder, forcible rape, robbery, and aggravated assault.

virilize—To develop sexual characteristics of a male. For example, a clitoris that is virilized will have the appearance of a penis.

virtue theory—A major theoretical orientation that focuses on the moral agent's intent, such as the virtue of truthfulness.

virulence—The degree or power of microorganisms to cause disease.

visual acuity—Clearness or sharpness of the image seen by the eye.

voiding cystourethrogram (VCUG)—Radiograph of bladder, urethra, and ureters during voiding.

von Willebrand's disease—A mild, congenital bleeding disorder caused by a deficiency of von Willebrand's factor.

von Willebrand's factor (vWF)—A protein that facilitates adhesion between platelets and injured vessel walls.

Waterhouse-Friderichsen syndrome—Fulminant meningococcemia.

weaning—A process of giving up one method of feeding for another.

wet drowning—Drowning caused by the aspiration of fluid into the lungs.

wheezing—A high-pitched musical sound produced by air flow through a narrowed airway.

white blood cells (WBCs)—The blood cells responsible for defending against invading microorganisms and removing debris.

windshield survey—A systematic assessment performed while the nurse travels through the community.

xanthelasma—Creamy, yellow plaque on eyelid due to hypercholesterolemia.

xanthomas—Slightly elevated yellow nodules that develop in the subcutaneous layer of skin.

xerostomia—Dryness of the mouth, which occurs from decreased or arrested production of salivary secretions.

zone of proximal development (ZPD)—Tasks that are too difficult for individuals to master alone but that can be mastered with the guidance and assistance of adults or more skilled adolescents.

Code Legend

NP	**Phases of the Nursing Process**	Ph/7	Reduction of Risk Potential
		Ph/8	Physiological Adaptation
As	Assessment		
An	Analysis		
Pl	Planning	**CL**	**Cognitive Level**
Im	Implementation	K	Knowledge
Ev	Evaluation	Co	Comprehension
		Ap	Application
		An	Analysis
CN	**Client Need**		
Sa	Safe Effective Care Environment	**SA**	**Subject Area**
		1	Medical-Surgical
Sa/1	Management of Care	2	Psychiatric and Mental Health
Sa/2	Safety and Infection Control		
He/3	Health Promotion and Maintenance	3	Maternity and Women's Health
Ps/4	Psychosocial Integrity	4	Pediatric
Ph	Physiological Integrity	5	Pharmacologic
Ph/5	Basic Care and Comfort	6	Gerontologic
Ph/6	Pharmacological and Parenteral Therapies	7	Community Health
		8	Legal and Ethical Issues

GROWTH AND DEVELOPMENT – COMPREHENSIVE EXAM

1. The nurse is planning to teach a class on the principles of growth and development. Which of the following should the nurse include in the class?

   1. Development becomes increasingly integrated and complex with each new learned skill

   2. Infants and children continue to respond to stimuli in the same way as first learned

   3. Physiological, psychological, cognitive, and moral aspects of development are independent of each other

   4. Children develop physiologically, psychologically, and socially on a preset timetable

2. A mother who compared her child with the neighbor's child of the same age is concerned that her child's language skills are not as advanced as those of the neighbor's child. The nurse assesses the child and determines the language skills are within the range of normal. The nurse should inform the mother that

   1. Speech develops more rapidly in children with siblings

   2. Development of language skills varies greatly in children

   3. Some children's talents lie in areas other than language skills

   4. The child should have psychological testing

3. The nurse is teaching parents about Erik Erikson's psychosocial theory of development. According to this theory, a child who is between 6 and 12 years of age is going through which of the following stages?

   1. Initiative versus guilt

   2. Industry versus inferiority

3. Identity versus role confusion

4. Autonomy versus shame and doubt

4. Considering Erikson's psychosocial theory of development, which of the following instructions is appropriate to give the parents of a hospitalized infant?

   1. Avoid visiting to prevent upsetting the infant when leaving

   2. Spend as much time as possible with the infant

   3. Schedule visits around nursing care

   4. Limit visits to official visiting hours

5. The nurse is caring for an adolescent client recently diagnosed with type 1 diabetes. Considering developmentally appropriate education, the technical skill most appropriate for this adolescent client is

   1. management decision skill.

   2. urine testing skill.

   3. blood testing skill.

   4. insulin injection skill.

6. The nurse is caring for a 2-year-old child admitted with pneumonia. Which of the following play activities is developmentally appropriate for this child?

   1. Encourage the child to play with the roommate

   2. Engage the child in group dress-up play

   3. Offer the child a pull toy to play with

   4. Provide the child with puzzles to play with

7. Ongoing nursing measures to include in the plan of care for a 6-year-old child hospitalized should include

   1. eight hours of uninterrupted nighttime sleep.

   2. three servings of whole milk daily.

   3. video games to occupy play time.

   4. bathing and dressing the child.

8. The nurse is assessing neonatal reflexes. As the nurse moves the neonate's head slowly to the right or left, the eyes move more slowly than the head and do not immediately adjust to the position of the head. The nurse documents this reflex as

   1. cat's eye.

   2. head-lag reflex.

   3. doll's eye.

   4. eye delay.

9. When administering phototherapy to a baby, which of the following should the nurse include?

   1. Check the baby's blood glucose before therapy

   2. Cover the baby with a sheet during therapy

   3. Shield the baby's eyes and protect the gonads

   4. Apply a special sunscreen to the baby's skin prior to the treatment

10. The nurse observes the mother of a newborn and four other children feeding the newborn in the infant seat with the bottle propped. The appropriate intervention for the nurse is to

    1. instruct the mother about the importance of holding and cuddling in the attachment process.

    2. congratulate the mother for finding a safe place for the baby to take the bottle.

    3. inform the mother that this procedure encourages independence in the newborn.

    4. encourage the mother to let the older children hold the bottle for the baby in the infant seat.

11. A mother asks the nurse when the soft spot on the front of the baby's head will close. The appropriate response by the nurse is

    1. "The anterior fontanel will close shortly after the posterior fontanel."

    2. "Both the anterior and posterior fontanels will close by the time the baby is a year old."

    3. "The anterior fontanel will close in 6 months."

    4. "The anterior fontanel will close by 12 to 18 months of age."

12. A mother asks the nurse to explain what fine motor skills are. She has heard that it has something to do with a school-aged child's ability to draw and color within the lines, and she wants to know what this means in an infant. The nurse would explain that fine motor development is the ability to

    1. write and draw and that infants do not have any fine motor skills.

    2. coordinate hand to eye movement in an orderly and progressive manner.

    3. pick up items and move them from place to place in a voluntary fashion.

    4. use all of the fingers and both hands equally well in a coordinated way.

13. The nurse is assessing the dressing skills of an 18-month-old child. Which of the following dressing skills does the nurse evaluate as normal for this child?

    1. Put on own shoes

    2. Tie own shoes

   3. Remove own shoes

   4. Tie others' shoes

14. The nurse is working with the parents of a 32-month-old child. They are very concerned that their child and one of the child's playmates were discovered undressed. On questioning the children, it was clear that these children had been comparing and inspecting their bodies. The nurse would advise the parents that based on their child's state of development and age, the best response should be

   1. timely and logical explanation of the consequences for unacceptable behavior.

   2. punishment severe enough to prevent recurrence of behavior.

   3. constant one-on-one supervision during all waking hours.

   4. matter-of-fact manner by caregivers in responding.

15. The parents of a toddler who has behavior that is intrusive and in need of redirection ask the nurse how to respond to the child. The most appropriate response by the nurse is

   1. speak firmly and loudly to let the child know the behavior is not acceptable.

   2. separate the child from others to think about how to interact appropriately with others.

   3. send the child to his or her room and set a time with the child to talk later.

   4. get at eye level with the toddler, gently touch the child on the shoulder to get the child's attention before speaking.

16. A mother is upset that a 34-month-old child has begun to wet the bed and thumb-suck after being admitted to the hospital. The mother asks the nurse to explain why this is happening. The nurse's best response is which of the following?

   1. "This behavior is a defense mechanism when normal routines are changed."

   2. "Your child probably does not like the nurse who has been assigned."

   3. "Your toddler is angry and this is a way of letting the unhappiness become known."

   4. "Bedwetting and thumb-sucking are the child's way of getting even for abandonment."

17. A father asks the nurse why a toddler engages in fantasy and make-believe in play. The most appropriate response by the nurse is

   1. "Some children use fantasy to escape a stressful world, so the more stressful life is, the more fantasy."

   2. "Fantasy helps toddlers cope with parents' expectations and conceptualize how they want their world to be."

3. "Your child probably does not have enough playmates to stay in reality-based play."

4. "Some children are just more imaginative and creative than others and engage in fantasy play."

18. The nurse evaluates a preschooler who believes that objects such as rocks have human qualities. The nurse should document this characteristic as _____ .

19. The nurse is working with an adolescent who complains of being lonely and lacking a sense of fulfillment with life. This adolescent shies away from intimate relationships at times, yet at other times appears promiscuous. Which of the following is the priority for the nurse to focus on with this adolescent?

1. Loneliness

2. Identity

3. Isolation

4. Lack of fulfillment

20. Which of the following should the nurse include in a plan of care to promote nighttime sleep in a preschooler?
Select all that apply:

[   ] 1. Avoid bathing the child before bedtime

[   ] 2. Encourage watching television to enhance sleep

[   ] 3. Read a bedtime story and establish a firm bedtime

[   ] 4. Provide bedtime snack such as a milkshake or ice cream

[   ] 5. Establish and adhere to a wake-up time

[   ] 6. Promote an appealing and cozy bedtime environment

21. A father asks the nurse why his 18-year-old son is so idealistic and is so often involved in political or social causes. The father is especially concerned because the son recently turned down a family outing to an amusement park in order to attend a rally to benefit indigenous people in a third-world country. Which of the following is the priority response by the nurse?

1. "When children do not have enough limits set at home, they often fall in with peer groups who engage in these activities."

2. "Your son has a talent for politics and this may be something he has chosen as a career profession."

3. "This is your son's way of being different from you and exerting independence from the family."

    4. "This is a normal phase that adolescents go through. They interpret the world in an excessively idealistic perspective and often engage in causes."

22. A mother expresses amazement that a school-age son, who was somewhat slow to crawl and walk, is now riding a bicycle and rollerblading. The nurse would explain that the child is able to do these new activities well because of which of the following?

    1. Taking longer to crawl and walk provides a much better balance and coordination system

    2. Improved balance and coordination are part of the growth and development of this age

    3. Children who are slower in developing initial skills seem to have more high-risk behaviors later

    4. This child has developed the muscles needed for bicycling and rollerblading

23. The nurse assesses the apical pulse of a school-age child and finds a rate of 95 beats per minute while the child is lying in bed. The priority nursing action is to

    1. chart the apical pulse of 95 beats per minute.

    2. recheck the apical pulse for a full minute.

    3. call the physician.

    4. have another nurse recheck the apical pulse.

24. The nurse is working with a prepubescent adolescent. The family asks the nurse to explain when the adolescent will go through puberty. Based on an understanding of puberty, the priority response by the nurse is which of the following? Puberty

    1. "varies individually and cross-culturally."

    2. "is about the same for all females."

    3. "is slightly different for males and females."

    4. "depends largely on the family environment."

25. Which of the following should the nurse include in the instructions given to a mother who is preparing to bottle-feed her infant?

    1. Avoid propping the bottle up while feeding the infant

    2. Heat the bottle in the microwave so the formula is warm

    3. Add fresh formula to an existing bottle when it gets low to prevent sucking air

    4. Administer the whole bottle before attempting to burp the infant

26. Which of the following nursing tasks may the registered nurse delegate to a licensed practical nurse?
    1. Instruct the parents on the normal motor skills of a toddler
    2. Monitor the fine motor skills of an infant
    3. Initiate play activities with a preschooler
    4. Inform an adolescent about the usual physiological changes

ANSWERS AND RATIONALES

1. **1.** Development that becomes increasingly integrated and complex with each new skill should be incorporated into a growth and development class. For example, drinking from a cup requires both hand-eye and hand-mouth coordination. Physiological, psychological, cognitive, and moral aspects of development are affected by each other. Children have their own unique timetables for physiological, psychological, and social development.
   NP = Pl
   CN = He/3
   CL = An
   SA = 4

2. **2.** Every child has a unique timetable for development. Some children can name four colors by the time they are 3 years old, whereas others cannot name four colors until they are $4\frac{1}{2}$ years of age.
   NP = Im
   CN = He/3
   CL = An
   SA = 4

3. **2.** According to Erikson's psychosocial theory of development, the major developmental task of the school-age years is industry versus inferiority. Industry involves mastery of social, physical, and intellectual skills, and orientation toward and competition with peers. Inferiority develops when school-age children are ridiculed by peers and do not measure up to adult or their own expectations, or lack certain skills. Initiative versus guilt occurs in children between the ages of 3 and 6 years. Identity versus role confusion occurs in children between the ages of 12 and 18 years. Autonomy versus shame occurs between ages $1\frac{1}{2}$ and 3 years.
   NP = An
   CN = He/3
   CL = Co
   SA = 4

4. **2.** During infancy trust is developing, which means that the infant depends on having basic needs consistently met by reliable, nurturing caregivers, usually the parents. When the child becomes ill, it is important for the primary caregiver to spend as much time as possible with the infant so trust continues to develop.
NP = Pl
CN = He/3
CL = Ap
SA = 4

5. **1.** According to Piaget, children 12 years of age and older are a part of the formal operations stage of cognitive development, characterized by systematic and abstract thought. These children have the ability to consider alternative solutions and choose the right answer. They are capable of developing deductive reasoning and can organize and construct theories about their ideas. Although adolescents are capable of self-administering insulin injections, management decision skills, such as urine and blood testing, are the most age-appropriate technical skills.
NP = An
CN = He/3
CL = An
SA = 4

6. **3.** Toddlers (12 to 35 months) prefer parallel play or playing alongside other children. They do not engage in interactive play. They frequently grab toys and may hit another child for a toy. A pull toy is appropriate for a toddler. Encouraging the child to play with the roommate and engaging the child in group dress-up play involve interactive play reserved for preschool age. Playing with puzzles is also a play act age-appropriate for preschoolers.
NP = Ev
CN = He/3
CL = Ap
SA = 4

7. **3.** Video games are an appropriate play activity for school-age children (ages 6 to 12). Although video games are sedentary play activity and should be limited, they make a good play activity for hospitalization. A 6-year-old child requires 10 hours of sleep every day. It is not until the child is 12 years of age that the child sleeps only eight hours. During the preschool years, the child should be switched to low-fat or skim milk to prevent obesity. School-age children also only need two to three servings of milk. Six-year-old children should be encouraged to bathe and dress themselves.
NP = Pl
CN = He/3

CL = Ap
SA = 4

8. **2.** Head lag is seen in newborns because they do not have sufficient muscular development to support the head. Eye delay refers to the infant's inability to follow a light. Cat's eye is not a reflex.
NP = Im
CN = He/3
CL = An
SA = 4

9. **3.** Phototherapy is generally an effective method of reducing serum bilirubin levels and preventing kernicterus. The newborn's eyes should be shielded during the therapy to prevent possible retinal damage. The genital area should also be covered with a surgical mask to provide protection to the gonads.
NP = Im
CN = He/3
CL = Ap
SA = 4

10. **1.** Feeding time is crucial to the development of caregiver-infant attachment, since it is a time for them to interact and learn about each other. If the newborn remains in the crib or if the bottle is propped, attachment will be delayed.
NP = Im
CN = He/3
CL = Ap
SA = 4

11. **4.** The posterior fontanel typically closes by 2 months of age and the anterior fontanel closes by 18 months of age.
NP = An
CN = He/3
CL = An
SA = 4

12. **2.** Gross motor development is the ability to use large muscle groups to maintain balance and postural control or locomotion. Fine motor development is the ability to coordinate hand-eye movement in an orderly and progressive manner.
NP = Im
CN = He/3
CL = Ap
SA = 4

13. **3.** By 18 months, the toddler should be able to walk upstairs with help, turn book pages, walk and pull toys, unzip zippers, stack up to four cubes, and remove shoes and socks.
NP = Ev
CN = He/3
CL = Ap
SA = 4

14. **4.** Young children are naturally curious about their environment and the differences between genders. If parents were to respond negatively to this natural curiosity, preschoolers would feel guilty about their behavior and initiative would be affected.
NP = Im
CN = He/3
CL = An
SA = 4

15. **4.** Toddler-age children do not have the cognitive ability to understand explanations and are not able to think about the consequences of their behavior. It is not necessary to talk loudly to get a child's attention. All one has to do is to touch him or her gently and bend down so the toddler's and the adult's eyes are at the same level.
NP = An
CN = He/3
CL = An
SA = 4

16. **1.** It is not uncommon for toddlers to regress when stressed by the hospital experience. The behaviors will disappear after the stress is reduced and the child returns to the home environment.
NP = An
CN = He/3
CL = An
SA = 4

17. **2.** Play is the "work" of childhood. Fantasy play helps children conceptualize what and how they wish the world to be, helps them cope with parental expectations, and aids them in denying aspects of reality they prefer to ignore.
NP = An
CN = He/3
CL = An
SA = 4

18. **animism.** Animism is the belief that objects have human qualities and is a characteristic of preschoolers' cognitive development.
NP = Im
CN = He/3

CL = Co
SA = 4

19. 2. The major task of adolescence is to resolve identity versus role confusion. Identity is adolescents' definition of who they are based on their cumulative understanding of their inherent motivations. It is based on their individual and group identifications, their ability to master each prior developmental task, and the establishment of their own ideology based on the social, political, and religious attitudes and values they have adopted.
NP = Pl
CN = He/3
CL = Ap
SA = 4

20. 3, 5, 6. It is important to establish a bedtime ritual for children so that they are more likely to go to sleep when put to bed. Reading, playing a quiet game, having a bedtime story read, or listening to soothing music may help the child relax and learn how to be calm, and these routines will make falling asleep much easier.
NP = Pl
CN = He/3
CL = Ap
SA = 4

21. 4. The ability to think abstractly allows the adolescent to recognize the distinction between how things are and how things could be (the difference between the real and the ideal). This results in a new sense of idealism and a new set of standards with which they begin to assess the world around them as they become involved in causes of interest.
NP = An
CN = Sa/1
CL = An
SA = 4

22. 4. Muscle strength and size increase during the school-age years, and six basic gross motor skills (balancing, catching, throwing, running, jumping, climbing) are refined. Improved balance and coordination enable the child to become adept at new activities such as rollerblading and bicycling.
NP = Im
CN = He/3
CL = An
SA = 4

23. 1. As the cardiac and respiratory systems become more efficient during school age, the pulse and respiratory rates slow down. The average apical

pulse rate for the school-aged child is 90 to 95 beats per minute while at rest. The average respiratory rate is 20 breaths per minute while at rest.
NP = Im
CN = Sa/1
CL = An
SA = 4

24. **1.** Puberty is the state of physical development between ages 12 and 16 for males and ages 10 and 14 for females when secondary sex characteristics begin to appear. Reproduction first becomes possible and the adolescent growth spurt starts. The age when puberty begins and how long adolescence lasts varies individually and cross-culturally.
NP = An
CN = Sa/1
CL = An
SA = 4

25. **1.** The bottle should never be propped up during the feeding. The bottle should never be heated in the microwave nor should formula ever be added to an existing bottle. No bottle should be in use for longer than one hour. The infant should be burped halfway through the bottle and again at the completion of the bottle.
NP = Pl
CN = He/3
CL = Ap
SA = 4

26. **3.** Skills that involve instruction and monitoring are skills that must be performed by the registered nurse. A licensed practical nurse may initiate play activities with a child.
NP = Pl
CN = Sa/1
CL = An
SA = 8

EYE, EAR, NOSE, AND THROAT DISORDERS – COMPREHENSIVE EXAM

1. A child is diagnosed with viral conjunctivitis. The nurse most likely would observe which of the following clinical manifestations in the child?

   1. Mucopurulent eye discharge

   2. Unilateral involvement

   3. Presence of upper respiratory tract infection symptoms

   4. Crusting of eyelids, which are edematous

2. A 17-year-old female is diagnosed with right bacterial conjunctivitis, and her physician has prescribed an antibiotic eyedrop. Which of the following instructions should the nurse include in the discharge teaching for this client?

   1. Do not wear glasses while the infection is present

   2. Discard and replace any eye makeup that has been opened

   3. Do not return to school until the eye infection has resolved

   4. Gently rub the eye regularly to remove excess discharge

3. The nurse is caring for a client with left bacterial conjunctivitis. Which of the following statements by the client indicates a need for further teaching?

   1. "I will administer corticosteroid eyedrops to my left eye."

   2. "I will administer Tobramycin antibiotic eyedrops to my left eye."

   3. "I will clean the eye from the inner canthus outward."

   4. "I will discard all my eye makeup."

4. At a 4-month well-baby exam, the nurse observes that the infant's occiput is flattened and the head appears misshapen. The fontanels, sutures, and occipital-frontal circumference appear to be normal. The nurse notifies the physician that this finding is consistent with which of the following cranial deformities?

   1. Plagiocephaly

   2. Craniosynostosis

   3. Microcephaly

   4. Hydrocephalus

5. Which of the following is a primary feature that the nurse assesses in a 9-month-old infant diagnosed with craniosynostosis?

   1. Large head size

   2. Hematoma not crossing the suture lines

   3. Flattened occiput

   4. Ridging of the suture line

6. A nurse is admitting a newborn infant who has swelling over the parietal area that crosses the suture line. The nurse notifies the physician that this finding is consistent with which of the following conditions?

   1. Cephalohematoma

   2. Caput succedaneum

3. Hyperbilirubinemia

4. Craniostenosis

7. A nurse is caring for a newborn who has developed a cephalohematoma. Based on the nurse's understanding of cephalohematoma, which of the following should be included in the discharge plan?

   1. Cephalohematoma typically resolves within a few days

   2. It is likely that the swelling will cross the suture lines

   3. There will be extensive bruising

   4. A bony prominence may develop over the affected area in time

8. The nurse implements which of the following hearing screening tests for a newborn infant?

   1. Pure tone audiometry

   2. Tympanography

   3. Startle test

   4. Voice-whisper test

9. The nurse is caring for a 2-year-old child for whom eardrops have been prescribed. Which of the following measures is recommended when administering eardrops to a child of this age?

   1. Pull the pinna up and back to facilitate administration

   2. Pull the pinna down and back to facilitate administration

   3. Insert firm pressure on the tragus immediately after administration

   4. Chill the eardrops before instilling

10. The nurse is planning the care of a newborn diagnosed with cleft lip and palate. Which of the following is a priority for the nurse to focus on in the period immediately following diagnosis?

   1. Assessment of newborn feeding

   2. Assessment of parental understanding of treatment options

   3. Referral to craniofacial malformation specialist

   4. Referral to counselor to assist with adjustment to diagnosis

11. The nurse is caring for a newborn with cleft lip and palate who has feeding difficulties. The parent asks the nurse how to feed the infant. Which of the following instructions are the most appropriate for the nurse to give the parent?

   1. Place the newborn supine to feed

   2. Obtain a newborn nipple with a small opening to facilitate sucking

3. Place the newborn in an upright position to feed

4. Burp infrequently to ensure that infant continues sucking

12. A nurse is caring for a child after surgery for repair of cleft lip and palate. Based on an understanding of the complications that are most likely to follow this surgery, the nurse should implement which of the following interventions?

1. Monitor child's hemoglobin

2. Withhold oral feedings until suture line is healed

3. Avoid restraining the child

4. Provide meticulous care of the suture line

13. A child is being evaluated for otitis media. The physician requests an otoscope with an insufflator. The nurse understands that the purpose of using the insufflator is to

1. better visualize the tympanic membrane.

2. visually assess tympanic membrane movement.

3. measure hearing loss.

4. perform tympanocentesis.

14. The nurse is preparing an infant for an evoked otoacoustic emissions hearing screening test. The parents request information regarding the test. Based on an understanding of the test, the nurse should respond with

1. "It is the preferred method of screening newborns for sensorineural hearing loss."

2. "The results of the test will indicate the severity of cochlear damage."

3. "The results are more accurate if the infant is awake."

4. "It will require placement of electrode wires on the infant's scalp."

15. A nurse performs a cross-cover test on a 4-year-old child. The right eye is observed to move as it is uncovered. The nurse documents these results as indicative of

1. normal alignment.

2. absent red reflex.

3. malalignment.

4. myopia.

16. A nurse administers the Denver Developmental Screening Test II to a 9-month-old infant. The nurse notes that the infant does not consistently track 180 degrees with the eyes. Based on an understanding of normal development, the nurse recognizes this

    1. visual finding is within normal limits.

    2. visual finding may indicate malalignment.

    3. reflects the infant's inability to focus for long periods.

    4. finding necessitates parental instruction on infant stimulation activities.

17. The nurse documents that the Hirschberg test on a 2-week-old infant is abnormal and reports this finding as consistent with

    1. ptosis of the lid.

    2. presence of the sunset sign.

    3. lacrimal duct stenosis.

    4. unequal corneal light reflexes.

18. A nurse is caring for a 6-month-old infant whose mother is worried about conjunctivitis. The mother describes constant tearing and occasional mucopurulent discharge from one eye for about four months. The nurse recognizes these findings as most indicative of which of the following conditions?

    1. Viral conjunctivitis

    2. Upper respiratory infection

    3. Nasolacrimal duct stenosis

    4. Allergic conjunctivitis

19. The nurse is providing discharge instruction to the parents of a 4-month-old infant with nasolacrimal duct stenosis without inflammation. Which of the following should be included in the discharge plan? Instruction on

    1. lacrimal duct massage.

    2. applying ice packs to the affected area three to four times per day.

    3. how to patch the affected eye.

    4. instillation of antibiotic eye ointment.

20. The nurse is informing the parents of a child with herpes simplex type 1 virus around the mouth that recurs on triggers. Which of the following would it be appropriate to include in the plan? Viral triggers include

    1. allergies.

    2. exposure to sunlight.

    3. exposure to citrus foods.

    4. antibiotic therapy.

21. The nurse assesses an infant to have white patches adherent to the buccal surfaces. The nurse documents this finding as diagnostic of what condition? _____

22. An 8-year-old child is seen for persistent cold symptoms. The mother describes a constantly runny nose and sniffling. The nurse notes a horizontal crease across the lower one-third of the nose. This is a finding that is most consistent with which of the following conditions?

    1. Upper respiratory infection

    2. Asthma

    3. Sinusitis

    4. Allergic rhinitis

23. An infant who has been treated repeatedly for oral thrush is to be treated with gentian violet. The nurse should consider which of the following when applying the gentian violet? Gentian violet

    1. is used as first-line treatment for oral thrush.

    2. is likely to stain clothing and surrounding skin.

    3. is applied immediately before eating.

    4. should be applied to plastic nipples and pacifiers.

24. The nurse is caring for a child with acute sinusitis. Which of the following findings would indicate the client's condition is deteriorating?

    1. Swelling around the eye

    2. Persistent rhinorrhea

    3. Tenderness over the involved sinuses

    4. Teeth pain

25. On examination of a child for a sore throat, the nurse notes the child also has a rash over the trunk—a sandpaperlike rash over the abdomen and to a lesser degree on the back. The nurse evaluates this related finding is most consistent with which bacterial pathogen?

    1. *Mycoplasma pneumoniae*

    2. *Streptococcus pneumoniae*

    3. Group A beta-hemolytic strep

    4. *Haemophilus influenzae*

26. The registered nurse is delegating nursing assignments to both registered nurses and licensed practical nurses on a pediatric unit. Which of the following assignments may the nurse delegate to a licensed practical nurse?

    1. Feed an infant with a cleft lip and palate in an upright position

    2. Perform an HOTV vision test on a 5-year-old child

    3. Assess the fontanels of a 9-month-old child

4. Develop a teaching plan for the mother of a 3-year-old child on prevention of bacterial conjunctivitis

ANSWERS AND RATIONALES

1. **3.** Viral conjunctivitis usually occurs with an upper respiratory tract infection, and it can be easily spread by the hands. It typically involves both eyes. Serous discharge is present rather than mucopurulent discharge. The eyelids may be edematous, but there is no crusting of the eyelids. A mucopurulent eye discharge and unilateral involvement is generally characteristic of bacterial conjunctivitis.
NP = As
CN = He/3
CL = Ap
SA = 4

2. **2.** Eye cosmetics can be contaminated, and their continued application will result in recurrent or persistent eye infections. Once the eye is infected, it is highly likely the cosmetic is also contaminated, even if it wasn't the cause of the infection. Additionally, this client should be instructed not to wear eye makeup until the eye infection has resolved. She should be instructed not to wear contact lenses, but she can continue to wear her glasses as long as she cleans them regularly. She may return to school 24 hours after beginning the antibiotic eyedrop. It is not recommended to rub the eye, as this will contribute to the spread of the infection.
NP = Pl
CN = He/3
CL = Ap
SA = 4

3. **1.** Corticosteroid eyedrops are not used to manage bacterial conjunctivitis, because they may make the eye more susceptible to infection. It would be appropriate to administer Tobramycin eyedrops as prescribed, clean the eye from the inner canthus outward, and discard all existing makeup to prevent recontamination.
NP = Ev
CN = He/3
CL = Ap
SA = 4

4. **1.** Plagiocephaly occurs when a portion of the skull flattens as a result of continued pressure against a surface. That is, molding with flattening of the occiput may occur when infants lie on their backs continually. This has

become more common since it was recommended that caregivers place infants on their backs to sleep. Craniosynostosis is premature closure of the sutures. Microcephaly refers to small brain and small head size. Hydrocephalus is not a cranial deformity but is a disruption of the cerebrospinal fluid system resulting in ventricular dilation.

NP = An
CN = He/3
CL = Ap
SA = 4

5. 4. In craniosynostosis (craniostenosis), a fontanel closes earlier than usual and the sutures fuse earlier than usual. This produces palpable ridging of the suture line. There may be a small head size but not a large head size. Hematoma is not present in craniosynostosis, but is a consistent finding in cephalhematoma. A flattened occiput may be seen but is more common with plagiocephaly. A more common physical finding than flattened occiput is frontal bossing (prominence of the forehead).

NP = As
CN = He/3
CL = Ap
SA = 4

6. 2. Caput succedaneum is caused by diffuse swelling of the soft tissues following birth trauma. As it occurs at the subcutaneous tissue level, it does cross the suture lines. Cephalohematoma is a subperiosteal collection of blood and does not cross the suture line. Hyperbilirubinemia may follow cephalohematoma but is not directly related to swelling in the parietal area. Craniostenosis may cause skull deformities due to early fusion of the sutures, but does not cause swelling in the parietal area.

NP = An
CN = He/3
CL = Ap
SA = 4

7. 4. Cephalohematoma is a periosteal collection of blood that slowly resolves over several weeks to months. As it calcifies, a palpable bony prominence may develop at the site. The swelling in cephalohematoma does not cross the suture line because it is confined to the periosteal space. Unlike caput succedaneum, there is usually no noticeable bruising associated with this.

NP = Pl
CN = He/3
CL = An
SA = 4

8. **3.** The startle test would be most appropriate to screen hearing in the newborn age group. The startle reflex is present at birth and should be observed. The newborn is not capable of performing pure tone audiometry or of responding to the voice-whisper test in a meaningful way. Tympanography is not used in this age group because of hypermobility of the tympanic membrane and because it does not directly measure hearing.
NP = Im
CN = Ph/7
CL = An
SA = 4

9. **2.** Pulling the pinna down and back in a child under age 3 will help straighten the ear canal and allow more effective instillation of eardrops. If the child were older than age 3, then the pinna would be pulled up and back. Pressure should not be exerted on the tragus after administering eardrops because this might cause pain. The area just anterior to the ear could be gently massaged to facilitate entry of the drops. The nurse could also loosely insert a wisp of cotton (cotton ball) for five minutes after instillation or gently tip the head away from the affected ear to facilitate retention of the drops. To avoid discomfort, the nurse should gently warm the eardrops in the hand before instilling them.
NP = Pl
CN = Ph/8
CL = Ap
SA = 4

10. **1.** Depending on the severity of malformation, a newborn with cleft lip and palate can have feeding difficulties due to structural abnormalities. Because of these abnormalities, the infant may be unable to generate negative pressure and create suction in the oral cavity, thus producing an ineffective suck. It would be essential for the nurse to evaluate the infant's feeding abilities immediately in order to promote and maintain adequate hydration and nutrition. Although assessing the parent's understanding of the treatment options and referrals to a craniofacial specialist and a counselor may all be appropriate interventions, they are not the priority for the nurse.
NP = Pl
CN = Sa/1
CL = Ap
SA = 8

11. **3.** An infant with a cleft lip and palate should be in an upright position to feed to utilize the effects of gravity. If the infant is placed supine, the feeding is likely to escape through the cleft palate and then through the nose. There is also greater likelihood of aspiration and choking if supine.

Nipples that work best tend to be relatively large with a large slit or crosscut slit to provide more passive feeding, overcoming the infant's diminished ability to suck. These infants are more likely to swallow air while feeding and should be burped frequently.

NP = Im

CN = He/3

CL = AP

SA = 4

12. 4. Meticulous care of the suture line following repair of a cleft lip and palate is required to prevent inflammation and infection. The occurrence of either of these will interfere with healing and potentially cause scarring and disruption of the cosmetic effect of surgery. The child's hemoglobin would be monitored, but bleeding is not a significant concern in this surgery. Oral feedings are typically resumed as soon as possible after surgery. It is essential that the nurse clean the child and suture line well after feeding. Depending on hospital and physician preference, the child may be restrained after surgery to avoid disruption or rubbing of the surgical site.

NP = Im

CN = He/3

CL = Ap

SA = 4

13. 2. An insufflator is a bulb attached via plastic tubing to the otoscope. After inserting the otoscope into the ear canal and establishing an airtight seal, the examiner squeezes the bulb, sending a whiff of air forward toward the tympanic membrane. The examiner can see the membrane move in response to the airflow and can assess its mobility. Use of an insufflator does not directly enhance visualization of the tympanic membrane. The device does not directly measure hearing loss and it is not used to perform tympanocentesis.

NP = An

CN = Ph/7

CL = An

SA = 4

14. 1. The evoked otoacoustic emissions (EOAE) hearing test is the preferred method of screening for sensorineural hearing loss in newborns. It does not provide information about the severity of cochlear damage, so a BAER (brainstem auditory evoked response) test is usually recommended as follow-up. The infant needs to be in a quiet sleep for testing. The BAER test requires the application of electrodes to the scalp, but the EOAE is performed via an ear probe.

NP = An
CN = Ph/7
CL = An
SA = 4

15. 3. The cross-cover test involves having a child focus on an object while one eye at a time is covered. As the cover is removed from the eye and quickly brought over to the other eye, the examiner watches for movement of the uncovered eye. Absent visual stimulation, weakened eye muscles will relax and the gaze will drift inward (esotropia) or outward (exotropia). This is indicative of malalignment of the eyes. Assessment for red reflex does not occur in this test. This is not an effective test for myopia.
NP = An
CN = Ph/7
CL = An
SA = 4

16. 2. Consistent eye alignment in an infant is observed between 4 and 6 months. By 9 months, it should definitely be consistent. This finding suggests malalignment, and the physician should be informed. While most infants at this age cannot focus for long periods, they are typically able to track an object moving 180 degrees. Parental instruction on infant stimulation is always recommended, but in this case it will not address the problem of the weakened eye muscles and resultant malalignment.
NP = An
CN = Ph/7
CL = An
SA = 4

17. 4. The Hirschberg test involves shining a light in an infant's eyes and assessing for the reflection of the light on the infant's pupils. The reflection should be symmetrical; an asymmetrical reflection indicates malalignment. The sunset sign is not associated with the Hirschberg test. It is found in a variety of disorders and may reflect variant lid placement. Lacrimal duct stenosis is a blockage of the lacrimal duct and has no correlation with the Hirschberg test.
NP = An
CN = Ph/7
CL = An
SA = 4

18. 3. Nasolacrimal duct stenosis is characterized by continual tearing and occasional episodes of mucopurulent discharge. A viral conjunctivitis is

usually bilateral and is unlikely to persist for a 4-month period. An upper respiratory infection could prompt a or bacterial conjunctivitis, but this finding is not most indicative of nasolacrimal duct stenosis. Allergic rhinitis does not present with mucopurulent discharge and is usually bilateral.

NP = An
CN = He/3
CL = An
SA = 4

19. **1.** Lacrimal duct massage may help maintain patency of the tract and promote drainage and resolution of the clinical manifestations of nasolacrimal duct stenosis. If a child does not present with inflammation, antibiotics are not required. The parent should be instructed on signs of inflammation and infection. Patching of the eye would not be appropriate, because this may encourage bacterial growth.

NP = Pl
CN = He/3
CL = Ap
SA = 4

20. **2.** Sunlight is a known trigger for herpes simplex type 1, especially when it presents with recurrent lesions around the mouth. The child should be instructed to minimize the time in direct sunlight and to use appropriate sunscreen and lip saver. Allergies and citrus foods may play a role in the development of aphthous ulcers (canker sores) but are not known to precipitate herpetic lesions. Antibiotic therapy does not trigger the development of herpetic lesions.

NP = Pl
CN = He/3
CL = Ap
SA = 4

21. **Oral thrush.** White patches adherent to the buccal surfaces are a classic finding in infant oral thrush and are diagnostic.

NP = An
CN = He/3
CL = Co
SA = 4

22. **4.** The horizontal nasal crease is a common consequence when a child with allergic rhinitis repeatedly rubs his nose (allergic salute). While the nasal manifestations may be found in any of the conditions, the nasal crease is most characteristic of allergic rhinitis.

NP = An
CN = He/3
CL = An
SA = 4

23. **2.** Gentian violet is applied to oral lesions that have not responded to other therapy. Because it frequently stains clothing, teeth, and surrounding skin a deep violet color, it should be applied carefully. Gentian violet should be applied after eating, or the infant should not eat for at least 20 minutes following application. It is not applied to plastic or plastic pacifiers. They can be boiled to sterilize.
NP = An
CN = Ph/6
CL = Ap
SA = 5

24. **1.** Periorbital swelling can progress to periorbital cellulitis, which is a serious complication of sinusitis. Persistent rhinorrhea and teeth pain are findings consistent with acute sinusitis but do not indicate complications. Because the sinuses are poorly developed in young children, tenderness over the sinuses is a not always a consistent finding in children.
NP = An
CN = He/3
CL = An
SA = 4

25. **3.** A scarlatiniform (sandpaper) rash is characteristic of a group A beta-hemolytic streptococcal infection. It may be seen in children who have a streptococcal pharyngitis. It is commonly found on the trunk. It is not characteristic of *Mycoplasma pneumoniae, Streptococcus pneumoniae, or Haemophilus influenzae organisms*.
NP = Ev
CN = He/3
CL = An
SA = 4

26. **1.** Performing a vision test, assessing the fontanels, and developing a teaching plan are all skills that should be delegated to a registered nurse. Feeding an infant with a cleft lip and palate in an upright position is a task that may be delegated to a licensed practical nurse.
NP = Pl
CN = Sa/1
CL = An
SA = 8

RESPIRATORY DISORDERS – COMPREHENSIVE EXAM

1. A client's father asks the nurse what the physician meant by the phrase "floating ribs." The nurse's response should be based on which of the following?

   1. Ribs 1 and 2 are not anchored as securely as the other rib pairs

   2. Ribs 11 and 12 are not attached at their anterior ends

   3. Ribs 8 through 10 are also called the false ribs

   4. The ribs are more horizontal in children than in adults

2. Which of the following should the nurse include when collecting a health history from the parent of an infant who has frequent episodes of otitis media?

   1. Volume of formula the infant ingests per feeding

   2. Hand washing practices of the primary care giver

   3. Sleeping position of the infant

   4. Second-hand smoke exposure

3. At a 2-week newborn exam, the nurse instructs a mother on the use of a bulb syringe for clearing the infant's nose of nasal mucus. The information is based on the nurse's understanding that infants under 4 months of age

   1. are obligatory nose breathers

   2. use abdominal breathing more than diaphragmatic breathing

   3. lack the neuromuscular control to sneeze

   4. often regurgitate feedings through their nose

4. The nurse should report which of the following as the primary clinical manifestation in an infant admitted to the hospital experiencing respiratory distress?

   1. Tachypnea

   2. Bradycardia

   3. Head bobbing with each respiration

   4. Decreased intake on feeding

5. When preparing a child for chest x-ray, it would be essential for the nurse to explain which of the following aspects of the procedure?

   1. Cooperation is required so the child will receive a mild sedative

   2. It will be necessary for the child to wear a lead shield

   3. The child will need to be NPO for four to eight hours prior to the procedure

   4. The child will be asked to cough during the procedure

6. A child has a pulmonary angiogram. It would be essential for the nurse to observe for which complication following the procedure?

   1. Constipation
   2. Abdominal pain
   3. Headache
   4. Hematoma

7. A child is scheduled for MRI (magnetic resonance imaging). It would be essential for the nurse to include which of the following in a prescreening history?

   1. Whether the child possesses any internal or external metal objects
   2. Family response to magnetic resonance imaging
   3. Past medical history of bleeding tendencies
   4. Allergy to shellfish

8. The nurse should prepare which of the following infants for a sweat chloride testing? An infant who has

   1. asthma.
   2. cystic fibrosis.
   3. tuberculosis.
   4. pertussis.

9. What are the two criteria a nurse should consider before restoring food and fluids for a child who has had a bronchoscopy and has taken nothing by mouth? _____

10. A nurse is caring for a child who just had a thoracentesis. The nurse should place the child in which of the following positions immediately after the procedure?

    1. Sitting position for at least one hour
    2. Supine position for at least one hour
    3. Unaffected side for at least one hour
    4. Affected side for at least one hour

11. The nurse is caring for a child who had an open thoracotomy. Which of the following nursing measures should receive priority in the client's plan of care?

    1. Auscultating breath sounds
    2. Monitoring level of activity
    3. Positioning the child comfortably
    4. Monitoring intake and output

12. A child's father asks the nurse how the physician could diagnose the client on the results of a neck x-ray that showed a "thumb sign." The nurse's

response should be based on the understanding that which of the following diseases is characterized by a ''thumb sign'' on neck x-ray?

1. Laryngotracheobronchitis
2. Epiglottitis
3. Acute spasmodic laryngitis
4. Bacterial tracheitis

13. The nurse is caring for an intubated child diagnosed with bacterial tracheitis. Which of the following nursing measures should receive priority in the client's plan of care?

1. Administration of antipyretics
2. Monitoring of the white blood cell count
3. Monitoring of fluid intake and output
4. Frequent endotracheal suctioning

14. The nurse is directed to administer the pneumococcal polysaccharide polyvalent vaccine to a 2-month-old infant. The mother doesn't understand why the infant needs this. The nurse's response would be based on the understanding that the pneumococcal polysaccharide vaccine

1. may be effective in preventing infections caused by *Staphylococcus aureus.*
2. is usually given at birth.
3. should be given annually in the winter.
4. may be effective in preventing infections caused by *Streptococcus pneumoniae.*

15. The nurse is caring for a child diagnosed with pertussis. Which of the following should the nurse include in the plan of care?

1. Encourage activity
2. Administer a bronchodilator
3. Administer erythromycin
4. Restrict fluids in the diet

16. The nurse is teaching a class on pediatric tuberculosis. Which of the following should the nurse include in the class?

1. Children ages 3 to 15 years are often diagnosed by positive skin test rather than by clinical manifestations
2. The highest incidence of tuberculosis occurs in middle childhood
3. Tuberculosis is not considered a reportable contagious disease in the pediatric population
4. Fomite transmission is the predominant means of infection

17. The nurse is evaluating four children with tuberculosis. Which of the following children in what situation should the nurse be concerned about?

    1. The child who stays indoors at recess because of fatigue
    2. The child who declines an invitation to play football
    3. The child who is exposed to another child with active varicella
    4. The child who is exposed to another child with asthma

18. The parents of a 5-year-old with active tuberculosis are concerned that the child not receive immunizations while being treated for tuberculosis. Based on current recommendations, the nurse should inform the parent that

    1. immunizations are not recommended for a child with active tuberculosis.
    2. a child with tuberculosis should continue the regular immunization schedule.
    3. the child may have only those vaccines that are not live viruses.
    4. the child may continue immunizations while on isoniazid (INH) but not while on rifampin.

19. Which of the following nursing interventions should the nurse include in the plan of care for a child with asthma?

    1. Instruct the child that asthma can occur with exercise
    2. Avoid permitting the child to take control of daily self-care measures
    3. Administer erythromycin
    4. Instruct the parents to avoid obtaining an annual influenza vaccine

20. A 12-year-old child is seen for an asthma exacerbation and reports that the peak flow rates have been in the yellow zone the past few days. The child describes feeling short of breath. On auscultation, the nurse hears diminished breath sounds but no wheeze or crackle. Based on an understanding of asthma, the nurse recognizes that

    1. this child might only have exercise-induced asthma.
    2. bronchospasm is so severe that breath sounds and crackles are not audible.
    3. the child is not using proper peak flow meter technique.
    4. the exacerbation has subsided.

21. A 13-year-old child with asthma records a peak flow volume that is in the yellow zone. The nurse evaluates that this is indicative of

    1. poor peak flow meter technique.
    2. severe airflow obstruction.
    3. control of the asthma.
    4. cautionary asthma status.

22. Which of the following should the nurse consider before planning the care of a child diagnosed with mild persistent asthma?

   1. Exacerbations that do not affect activity
   2. Nighttime clinical manifestations occur less than two times per month
   3. Clinical manifestations occur more than two times per week but less than one time per day
   4. There is a peak flow rate between 60 and 80%

23. A nurse is caring for a child with newly diagnosed asthma. When instructing on pharmacotherapy, which of the following measures would be essential to include in the child's discharge instructions?

   1. Use inhaled corticosteroids on an as-needed basis during upper respiratory infections
   2. Use a bronchodilator such as albuterol as a rescue drug
   3. Use an anti-inflammatory such as cromolyn sodium for acute exacerbations
   4. Use albuterol daily to prevent exacerbations

24. Which of the following clinical manifestations indicate a child who has cystic fibrosis has developed a pneumothorax?
   Select all that apply:
   [ ] 1. Wheezing
   [ ] 2. Tachypnea
   [ ] 3. Cough
   [ ] 4. Bradycardia
   [ ] 5. Dyspnea
   [ ] 6. Cyanosis

25. A public health nurse is assigned to visit a family following the loss of their 5-month-old infant to sudden infant death syndrome. Which of the following statements by the family indicates a need for further education?

   1. "We are going to have another baby as soon as possible to take the pain away."
   2. "We know nothing could have predicted this."
   3. "We are meeting with another family who lost a baby three years ago."
   4. "We let our 5-year-old daughter say goodbye to him too."

26. The registered nurse is preparing the clinical assignments for a pediatric respiratory unit. Which of the following nursing skills is appropriate to delegate to a licensed practical nurse?

1. Administer prescribed IV corticosteroids to a child having an acute asthma attack

2. Admit a child with pertussis to the hospital

3. Take a health history from the parents of a child suspected of having cystic fibrosis

4. Take the vital signs of a child with pneumonia

ANSWERS AND RATIONALES

1. **2.** Because, unlike the other ribs, ribs 11 and 12 are not attached at their anterior ends, they are called floating ribs. Ribs 8 through 10 are called false ribs, which is not synonymous with floating ribs. The ribs of infants are placed more horizontally than those of adults or older children, but this placement not indicative of "floating ribs."
NP = An
CN = He/3
CL = An
SA = 4

2. **4.** Smoke exposure is a known risk factor for recurrent otitis media in an infant. It should be included in the history for infants who have recurrent otitis media. It is a modifiable risk factor. Although hand washing and sleeping position are important, they are more general. The volume of infant formula ingested per feeding will likely not be a causative factor for otitis media.
NP = As
CN = He/3
CL = An
SA = 4

3. **1.** Infants under 4 months of age are obligatory nose breathers. Since their nasal passages are small and narrow, a small amount of nasal discharge can occlude the passageways. Use of a bulb syringe to gently remove discharge will help maintain patent nasal passageways and ease the work of breathing when congested. Infants do use abdominal breathing more than diaphragmatic breathing, but abdominal breathing is not a factor in using the bulb syringe to clear the nose. Infants sneeze reflexively at birth. Infants do regurgitate their feedings through their noses but this alone does not form the basis for using the bulb syringe to clear.
NP = An
CN = He/3
CL = An
SA = 4

4. **3.** Head bobbing with each respiration in a sleeping infant is a sign of respiratory distress. The infant is using accessory muscles to breathe, which in turn causes the head to bob with each respiration. Although tachypnea and decreased oral intake also occur in respiratory distress, these are not the primary manifestations and may occur in many other disorders as well. Tachycardia is more likely than bradycardia in respiratory distress.
NP = An
CN = Sa/1
CL = An
SA = 4

5. **2.** A lead shield is placed over the immature gonads to prevent radiation-induced anomalies during a chest x-ray. The client and family should be informed of this to reassure them and to prepare them for the additional weight of the shield. Children are not sedated for a chest x-ray because this would hinder full inspiration. The child does not need to be NPO for this procedure. Holding one's breath and remaining still during the procedure are requirements of the child.
NP = Pl
CN = Ph/7
CL = Ap
SA = 4

6. **4.** Hematoma and hemorrhage are possible at the catheter insertion site following a pulmonary angiogram, and the client should be monitored closely. Bed rest and cold compresses are typically applied after the procedure to help prevent this complication. Abdominal pain, headache, and constipation are not usual complications of this procedure.
NP = As
CN = Ph/7
CL = Ap
SA = 4

7. **1.** Magnetic resonance imaging (MRI) uses a large magnet and radio waves to produce a two- or three-dimensional image of soft tissue, the central nervous system, or the blood vessels. If the child possessed any metal objects, they would be pulled toward the large magnet, so it is essential to screen for that prior to the procedure. MRI is a noninvasive procedure, not requiring venipuncture or arterial puncture. There is no injection of dye, so shellfish allergy is not an issue for this procedure.
NP = Pl
CN = Ph/7
CL = Ap
SA = 4

8. **2.** Sweat chloride testing is the diagnostic test for cystic fibrosis, in which the sodium and chloride content of the sweat are analyzed and quantified. Elevated levels of sodium and chloride (dependent on lab standards) are indicative of cystic fibrosis.
NP = Pl
CN = Ph/7
CL = Co
SA = 4

9. **Two hours have elapsed and the gag reflex is restored.** Topical anesthetic spray, such as lidocaine, is typically sprayed into the throat before a bronchoscopy procedure to inactivate the gag reflex. The cough reflex is also diminished. The potential for aspiration would increase if clear liquids were resumed too early. The gag reflex is usually restored in about two hours and clear liquids should not be begun before then. The sore throat may persist 24 to 48 hours. The cough will be absent initially after the procedure because of the effects of the topical lidocaine. Return of the cough would indicate that the cough reflex is also restored.
NP = An
CN = Ph/7
CL = Ap
SA = 4

10. **3.** Placing the child who had a thoracentesis on the unaffected side for at least one hour will allow the pleural puncture wound to close and prevent potentially more serious complications.
NP = Im
CN = Ph/7
CL = Ap
SA = 4

11. **1.** Auscultating the child's lung sounds is a means to assess whether the affected lung is reexpanding fully following a thoracotomy. Auscultation of the lungs will alert the nurse to early signs of pneumothorax (diminished breath sounds over affected area). Monitoring the level of activity, positioning the child comfortably, and monitoring intake and output are all nursing measures that are important, but assessing for the development of pneumothorax takes priority.
NP = Pl
CN = Sa/1
CL = An
SA = 4

12. 2. In acute epiglottitis, the epiglottis appears thickened and bulbous, like a thumb, on lateral view of the neck during a neck x-ray. As a result of this, the "thumb sign" is diagnostic for acute epiglottitis. Normally, the epiglottis is thin and curved on x-ray.

NP = An
CN = Ph/7
CL = Ap
SA = 4

13. 4. While administration of antipyretics and monitoring the white blood cell count and intake and output are all necessary measures, the most crucial measure is to frequently suction the child. Frequent suctioning will help to prevent airway obstruction caused by the thick purulent tracheal secretions characteristic of bacterial tracheitis.

NP = Pl
CN = Sa/1
CL = An
SA = 8

14. 4. The pneumococcal polysaccharide vaccine was developed to prevent infections caused by *Streptococcus pneumoniae*. Since *Streptococcus pneumoniae* is one of the most common respiratory pathogens this vaccine would help prevent, otitis media and pneumonia may be decreased. To date, studies have found the vaccine to be effective in preventing pneumonia caused by *S. pneumoniae,* but it has been less effective in preventing otitis media. It is usually commenced at 2 months of age. It can be given any time of year. It is not effective in preventing *S. aureus* infections.

NP = An
CN = Ph/7
CL = An
SA = 4

15. 3. Erythromycin is the drug of choice that, when administered early in the paroxysmal stage of the disease, may limit the spread of the organism. It does not alter the course of the illness. Pertussis is caused by the bacteria Bordetella pertussis.It is a lengthy illness with four stages and can last 7 to 12 weeks. Most clients with pertussis do not require hospitalization, but can be managed with supportive care at home. Bed rest should be maintained until the fever is resolved. Bronchodilators are administered in asthma. Fluids are encouraged to maintain hydration.

NP = Pl
CN = He/3
CL = Ap
SA = 4

16. **1.** Children with tuberculosis may be asymptomatic or show a wide range of clinical manifestations. Because many children are asymptomatic, a positive skin test is often the method by which children are initially diagnosed. The highest incidence of tuberculosis occurs in infancy and again in puberty and adolescence. Tuberculosis is a reportable contagious disease in all age groups. The main method of transmission is by inhalation of microdroplets into the respiratory tract.
NP = Pl
CN = He/3
CL = Ap
SA = 4

17. **3.** Varicella shows great potential to develop into an infection in a body whose defense system is already compromised such as those who are fighting tuberculosis. A child with TB is encouraged to rest, so this would be a healthy coping response. The child with TB is also cautioned against participating in contact sports. Because asthma is not considered an infectious disease, it would not pose undue risk to a client with tuberculosis.
NP = Ev
CN = He/3
CL = An
SA = 4

18. **2.** Current recommendations regarding immunizations given to a child with active tuberculosis suggest continuing the regular immunization schedule for children with tuberculosis. Because of the child's already strained immune system, acquiring an infection that could possibly be prevented by an immunization would be an unnecessary risk.
NP = Im
CN = Ph/7
CL = An
SA = 4

19. **1.** Asthma can occur with exercise, but it can also be triggered by exposure to allergens, respiratory tract infections, and stress. Children with asthma should be encouraged to take control of their daily self-care measures. A bronchodilator is administered. The parents should be encouraged to obtain an annual influenza vaccine.
NP = Pl
CN = He/3
CL = Ap
SA = 4

20. **2.** If an obstruction with asthma becomes too severe, adventitious breath sounds may not be heard until after the airways are opened up by a

bronchodilator. For the nurse, this signifies the need to immediately report the child's status to the physician and to prepare to administer a bronchodilator such as albuterol per nebulizer. The child may have exercise-induced asthma, but it is clear that the asthma may be triggered by other things as well. It would be helpful to repeat the peak flow reading in the clinic both before and after the nebulization treatment and to assess for proper technique.

NP = An
CN = He/3
CL = An
SA = 4

21. 4. The green zone indicates good asthma control with the client achieving 80 to 100% of the personal best. The yellow zone is the cautionary zone with the client achieving 50 to 80% of the personal best. The red zone indicates airflow obstruction, with the client achieving less than 50% of the personal best. While the obtained volume may be related to poor peak flow meter technique, it cannot be assumed.

NP = Ev
CN = Ph/7
CL = An
SA = 4

22. 3. A diagnosis of mild persistent asthma is consistent with symptoms that occur more than two times per week, but less than one time per day. The exacerbations may affect activity. Nighttime symptoms typically occur more than two times per month and the peak flow rate is greater than 80% of predicted. These are characteristic of mild intermittent asthma. A peak flow rate between 60 and 80% is indicative of moderate persistent asthma.

NP = An
CN = He/3
CL = An
SA = 4

23. 2. Albuterol, a quick-acting beta-2 agonist, is an effective bronchodilator and is the rescue drug of choice for acute exacerbations of asthma. It should not be used regularly, but if its use is required regularly, moving up to the next step of therapy is recommended. Inhaled corticosteroids and inhaled cromolyn both have anti-inflammatory action and are recommended for persistent asthma as daily therapy. They are not rescue medications, nor should they be used only during exacerbations.

NP = Pl
CN = Ph/6
CL = An
SA = 5

24. 2, 5, 6. Pneumothorax is a collection of air or gas in the pleural cavity. It should be suspected in a child with cystic fibrosis who develops signs of acute respiratory distress. Clinical manifestations include tachypnea, tachycardia, dyspnea, pallor, or cyanosis.
NP = As
CN = He/3
CL = Ap
SA = 4

25. 1. Parents who lost a child to sudden infant death syndrome and want to replace the child as soon as possible are not expressing healthy response. They need to allow time to process their thoughts and feelings surrounding the birth, life, and death of the infant they have just lost. The nurse will need to facilitate the expression of their emotions and the fears they might have with any new pregnancies. The rate of sudden infant death for succeeding children is very low, but needs to be discussed. Providing additional information about sudden infant death syndrome will be helpful. Referral to a support center will also be helpful. Reinforcing the positive coping behaviors, such as meeting with a family who previously lost a child, is appropriate. It is also appropriate to let an older child say goodbye to the child who has died.
NP = Ev
CN = He/3
CL = An
SA = 4

26. 4. Nursing skills that involve administering IV medications, admitting a child to the hospital, and taking a health history all should be performed by a registered nurse. A licensed practical nurse may take the vital signs of a child with pneumonia.
NP = Pl
CN = Sa/1
CL = An

CARDIOVASCULAR DISORDERS - COMPREHENSIVE EXAM

1. Which of the following assessment findings does the nurse discover in a child with coarctation of the aorta?
   1. Cyanosis of the lips and nail beds
   2. Hypertension of the upper extremities
   3. Strong bounding pulses to the lower extremities

    4. A history of abdominal pain

2. When planning care for a child in congestive heart failure, the nurse should include which of the following interventions?

    1. Provide quiet diversional activities

    2. Encourage normal activities

    3. Administer large volumes of IV fluids

    4. Keep lower extremities elevated

3. Which of the following is a priority for the nurse to implement to prevent complications in a child with rheumatic fever?

    1. Push fluids

    2. Continue antibiotics as ordered

    3. Begin physical therapy as soon as possible

    4. Administer oxygen

4. The nurse caring for a client on a pediatric cardiac unit finds a child in cardiac arrest. Based on an understanding of how to perform chest compressions to a child, the nurse should administer chest compressions that are

    1. the same depth as in adults.

    2. the same rate as in adults.

    3. faster than in adults.

    4. deeper than in adults.

5. The nurse planning care for a child with Kawasaki disease should include which of the following interventions?
Select all that apply:

    [   ] **1.** Continuous cardiac monitoring

    [   ] **2.** Tepid baths

    [   ] **3.** Restrict fluids

    [   ] **4.** Skin care

    [   ] **5.** Soft foods

    [   ] **6.** Aspirin

6. A schoolteacher asks the school nurse what to do about a child with a cardiac disease who isn't keeping up with school work. Which of the following is the most appropriate response by the nurse?

    1. "Schedule a teacher-parent conference to evaluate the home environment."

    2. "Poor endurance is common in children with cardiac disease."

    3. "Evaluate the child's social skills with playmates."

4. "Question the child about nutrition intake."

7. The nurse monitors a child with acute rheumatic fever for which of the following clinical manifestations?
Select all that apply:

[ ] **1.** Polyarthritis

[ ] **2.** Hyperpnea

[ ] **3.** Hypertension

[ ] **4.** Carditis

[ ] **5.** Erythema marginatum

[ ] **6.** Subcutaneous nodules over the joints

8. The nurse should monitor what blood test for a client with Kawasaki disease who is receiving warfarin (Coumadin) to determine the degree of anticoagulation present?_____

9. The mother of a child with infective endocarditis asks the nurse how her child developed this condition. The nurse should respond based on an understanding of which of the following aspects of this disorder? "Infective endocarditis is

1. "a congenital disease."

2. "a genetic disorder."

3. "the result of an underlying structural heart disease."

4. "an idiopathic disorder."

10. The nurse is teaching a class on the physiology of patent ductus arteriosus. The nurse should inform the participants that which of the following normally causes closure of the ductus arteriosus shortly after birth?

1. Increased pulmonary vascular resistance

2. Increased systemic vascular resistance

3. Decreased pulmonary vascular resistance

4. Decreased systemic vascular resistance

11. A student nurse asks the nurse about the patent foramen ovale. Which of the following is the most appropriate response by the nurse as to the purpose of the patent foramen ovale in fetal life?

1. "It bypasses the liver."

2. "It increases the flow of oxygenated blood to the lungs."

3. "It decreases the flow of blood to the lungs."

4. "It decreases systemic circulatory pressure."

12. The registered nurse is preparing clinical assignments for a pediatric nursing unit. Which of the following should the nurse delegate to a licensed practical nurse?

    1.   Monitor the international normalization ration (INR) in a client with Kawasaki's disease who is receiving warfarin (Coumadin)

    2.   Help a child with congestive heart disease mark a menu

    3.   Inform the parents of a child with atrial septal defect to administer prophylactic antibiotics to prevent endocarditis

    4.   Instruct the parents of a child with patent ductus arteriosus about measures to decrease the cardiac workload of the child

13. The nurse is evaluating a hematocrit to be 50% in a 2-month-old infant with tetralogy of Fallot. Based on an understanding of hematocrit levels in children, the nurse recognizes this level as indicative of

    1.   polycythemia related to poor oxygenation.

    2.   pernicious anemia related to poor nutrition.

    3.   normal in a child.

    4.   iron-deficiency anemia.

14. During an admission interview with the mother of a child with a congenital cardiac disease, the mother expresses concern about the child's poor appetite, stating the child refuses to eat or eats very poorly. The nurse evaluates the poor appetite as

    1.   an attention-seeking behavior by the child.

    2.   indicating the mother needs instruction on nutrition.

    3.   an indication that the child is a picky eater.

    4.   common because of the dyspnea with the exertion.

15. When planning the nursing care for a 3-year-old child with cardiac disease, the mother expresses concern that the child is not playing with friends. Which of the following would be the appropriate nursing diagnosis?

    1.   Ineffective coping related to chronic disease

    2.   Activity intolerance related to hypoxemia

    3.   Ineffective breathing pattern related to pulmonary congestion

    4.   Interrupted family processes related to chronic illness

16. A 1-year-old child is admitted to the unit with crackles throughout both lung fields. The nurse assesses that the brachial pulses are strong, but the client's femoral pulses are weak. The priority nursing action is to

    1.   notify the physician immediately.

2. take upper and lower extremity blood pressures.

3. ask the parents to leave the room.

4. recognize this as a normal finding in young children.

17. The nurse assesses which of the following in an 8-year-old child with tetralogy of Fallot?
Select all that apply:

[   ] **1.** A ruddy, pink complexion

[   ] **2.** Overweight as a result of decreased activity levels

[   ] **3.** Clubbing of the fingers

[   ] **4.** Squatting

[   ] **5.** A history of frequent epistaxis

[   ] **6.** Difficulty in feeding

18. The nurse should monitor a child with Kawasaki disease for which of the following primary complications?

1. Hemorrhage

2. Central nervous system involvement and chorea

3. Migratory polyarthritis

4. Inflammatory microvasculitis

19. When planning the discharge instructions for the parents of a child recovering from rheumatic fever, the nurse should include

1. the need for prophylactic antibiotics.

2. the need for home oxygen.

3. instructions for home dressing changes.

4. the importance of avoiding active sports.

20. The nurse is evaluating the results of a hyperoxia test. Which of the following results should the nurse report as indicative of cardiac disease?

1. PaO_2 of 90 mm Hg

2. PaO_2 of 125 mm Hg

3. PaO_2 of 150 mm Hg

4. PaO_2 of 168 mm Hg

21. Which of the following should be in the care provided to a child scheduled for a cardiac catheterization?

1. Assess the brachial pulses preprocedure

2. Encourage ambulation postprocedure

3. Monitor the pulses of the affected extremity postprocedure

4. Administer an antipyretic preprocedure

22. The nurse should include which of the following dietary selections in the instructions given to the parents of a toddler who is going home on furosemide (Lasix) following a hospitalization for congestive heart failure? Select all that apply:

[   ] **1.** 1 cup of cantaloupe

[   ] **2.** 3/4 cup of blueberries

[   ] **3.** 1/2 cup of peach nectar

[   ] **4.** 1 banana

[   ] **5.** 1 cup of Kool-Aid

[   ] **6.** 1 cup of chocolate milk

23. Which of the following four children in the nurse's care should be suspected of having transposition of the arteries?

1.   A newborn with acute cyanosis who does not respond to oxygen

2.   An older child who is asymptomatic but has a murmur detected

3.   An infant of normal size who is asymptomatic but has a murmur

4.   A child who develops a hypercyanotic spell during crying

24. The nurse should instruct the parents of an infant with a congenital heart anomaly to monitor the infant for which of the following clinical manifestations suggestive of congestive heart failure? Select all that apply:

[   ] **1.** Poor feeding

[   ] **2.** Squatting

[   ] **3.** Decreased activity

[   ] **4.** Labored breathing

[   ] **5.** Weight loss

[   ] **6.** Flushed complexion

25. The nurse instructs the parents of a 2-month-old infant with congestive heart failure to increase caloric intake by

1.   adding sugar water between feedings.

2.   starting cereal feedings as soon as possible.

3.   increasing the volume of each feeding.

4.   using a formula with more calories per ounce.

ANSWERS AND RATIONALES

1. 2. Coarctation of the aorta is a stenosis, or narrowing, located generally within the thoracic aorta. Clinical manifestations include upper-extremity hypertension and a noticeable difference in the blood pressure between the arms and legs. There also are diminished pulses in the lower extremities. Hypertension of the upper extremities is caused by an increase in pressure related to the narrowing of the aorta at the coarctation site. This shunts blood back to the arteries supplying the head, neck, and upper extremities.

NP = As
CN = He/3
CL = Ap
SA = 4

2. 1. Congestive heart failure is the inability of the cardiovascular system to promote adequate cardiac output to meet the demands of the body. Rest and diversional activities should be planned for this client to decrease cardiac output. Fluids are restricted and diuretics are administered. A semi-Fowler's position is maintained. The extremities do not have to be elevated. Administering large volumes of IV fluids would increase the volume of blood flow through the pulmonary vasculature, potentially worsening the congestion in the lung caused by the heart failure. Encouraging normal activities and elevating the lower extremities increase the workload on the heart.

NP = Pl
CN = He/3
CL = Ap
SA = 4

3. 2. Acute rheumatic fever is thought to be an autoimmune response to untreated group A beta-hemolytic *Streptococcal pharyngitis*. Antibiotics are essential to prevent cardiac complications of rheumatic fever. Carditis with mitral involvement may occur. Oxygen is generally warranted only if the disease is complicated by carditis and manifests as congestive heart failure. Physical therapy is not necessary, although these clients may develop polyarthritis, which is migratory in nature and reversible. Oral fluids may be required during the course of treatment, but the priority intervention is to administer antibiotics.

NP = Im
CN = He/3
CL = Ap
SA = 4

4. 3. Because children's pulse rates are higher than those of adults, chest compressions on a child are faster than chest compressions on an adult.

The compressions on a child would also not be as deep as those performed on an adult.

NP = An

CN = He/3

CL = An

SA = 4

5. **2, 4, 5, 6.** Kawasaki disease is a multisystem vasculitis that affects the coronary arteries. Nursing interventions include tepid baths, adequate fluid intake, and good skin care. Aspirin is administered because of a fever. Soft foods are also encouraged because clients may have oral lesions. Monitoring the child's cardiac status is of primary importance in the acute phase of the disease. Children will experience vasculitis of the coronary arteries, which may lead to coronary artery aneurysms, thrombosis, or myocardial infarction. Temporary arthritis affects the larger joints primarily in the subacute phase. Tepid baths, good skin care, and aspirin may be helpful. Desquamation is generally not painful, but it is uncomfortable.

NP = Pl

CN = He/3

CL = Ap

SA = 4

6. **2.** Children with cardiac disease have a poor endurance and may not keep up either physically or socially in school activities. The cardiac disease leads to chronic hypoxemia, which leads to poor endurance and delayed growth.

NP = An

CN = He/3

CL = An

SA = 4

7. **1, 4, 5, 6.** Clinical manifestations of acute rheumatic fever include polyarthritis, erythema marginatum, carditis, and subcutaneous nodules over the joints. Hyperpnea is a manifestation of tetralogy of Fallot. Hypertension that occurs in children is usually indicative of another disorder, such as a renal or cardiac disorder.

NP = As

CN = He/3

CL = Ap

SA = 4

8. **International normalization ration (INR).** The international normalization ration (INR) is the blood test used to determine the amount of anticoagulation present in a client receiving warfarin (Coumadin).

NP = As
CN = Ph/7
CL = An
SA = 4

9. **3.** Infective endocarditis is a cardiac disease in pediatrics that is generally the result of an underlying heart disease. Children with a complex cyanotic heart disease, prosthetic cardiac valves, or a previous history of endocarditis are at most risk for developing infective endocarditis.
NP = An
CN = He/3
CL = An
SA = 4

10. **3.** The ductus arteriosus is a direct connection between the main pulmonary artery and the aorta necessary to the survival of the fetus. Before birth, blood flows from the superior vena cava into the right ventricle and out through the pulmonary artery. Much of this oxygenated blood (coming from the umbilical vein) is shunted to the aorta through the ductus arteriosus. When the infant takes a first breath, the hemodynamics change and systemic resistance increases while pulmonary resistance decreases, reversing blood flow through the shunt. If the ductus arteriosus remains patent after birth, a left-to-right shunt develops.
NP = Pl
CN = He/3
CL = An
SA = 4

11. **4.** In fetal circulation, oxygenated blood from the umbilical vein enters the right atrium through the superior vena cava and is shunted directly across the foramen ovale to the left atrium. From there, it enters the left ventricle and is pumped into the aorta and to the systemic circulation. This allows most oxygenated blood flow to the areas in greatest need of it during fetal development.
NP = An
CN = He/3
CL = Ap
SA = 4

12. **2.** Clinical assignments that involve skills of monitoring, informing, and instructing are all nursing tasks that should be performed by the registered nurse. A licensed practical nurse may help a client mark a menu because the initial instruction has taken place.
NP = Pl
CN = Sa/1

CL = An
SA = 8

13. **1.** Tetralogy of Fallot consists of a ventral septal defect, right ventricular hypertrophy, pulmonary stenosis, and an overriding aorta. A hematocrit of 50% is abnormally high. The normal hematocrit level in a 2-month-old infant is between 28% and 42%. A high hematocrit is not classified as anemia. The circulatory system of a child with polycythemia adapts to chronic hypoxemia by increasing the production of red blood cells.
NP = Ev
CN = Ph/7
CL = An
SA = 4

14. **4.** Children with congenital heart disease develop a hypoxemia that often manifests as dyspnea with exertion. Dyspnea during eating often causes a poor appetite and caloric intake less than the body requires.
NP = Ev
CN = He/3
CL = An
SA = 4

15. **2.** The most plausible reason a child with cardiac disease avoids playing with friends is that the child fears being unable to keep up with peers. This activity intolerance is related to the heart's inability to pump enough oxygenated blood to accommodate an increase in activity.
NP = Pl
CN = He/3
CL = An
SA = 4

16. **2.** Although it may be appropriate to notify the physician, the priority is to gather more information before calling the physician. The nurse should recognize that a difference in brachial and femoral pulses is an indication of coarctation of the aorta. This is not a normal finding in children. It is not necessary for the parents to leave the room when the nurse is taking the blood pressure and may actually produce separation stress in the child.
NP = Im
CN = Sa/1
CL = An
SA = 4

17. **3, 4, 6.** Tetralogy of Fallot is comprised of a ventral septal defect, pulmonary stenosis, right ventricular hypertrophy, and an overriding aorta. Clinical manifestations include cyanosis and ''blue spells'' or ''tet spells.'' ''Blue spells'' are spells of acute hypoxia usually occurring during

crying or exertion such as defecation or feeding when the oxygen demand is greater than supply. Children with cyanotic heart defects have diminished appetites related to dyspnea with eating. Clubbing of the fingers is a common manifestation due to the chronic hypoxia. The child may be noticed squatting in an attempt to get more air.

NP = As
CN = He/3
CL = Ap
SA = 4

18. **4.** Kawasaki disease is a multisystem vasculitis with a proclivity to affect the coronary arteries. Hemorrhage and central nervous system involvement are not found. The arthritis found in Kawasaki disease is not rheumatoid in nature and is temporary.

NP = As
CN = He/3
CL = An
SA = 4

19. **1.** Prophylactic antibiotics are necessary to prevent a recurrence of a systemic bacterial infection that could damage the already weakened mitral valve. Home oxygen and home dressing changes are not likely to be part of the care for a child with rheumatic fever. The ability to participate in active sports depends on the degree of damage to the heart valve and remaining cardiac function.

NP = Pl
CN = He/3
CL = Ap
SA = 4

20. **1.** A PaO_2 less than 100 mm Hg is indicative of inadequate pulmonary perfusion and is cardiac in nature. A PaO_2 at 150 mm Hg or higher is indicative of lung disease, which makes it difficult for the oxygen to move from the alveoli into the pulmonary capillaries.

NP = Ev
CN = Ph/7
CL = An
SA = 4

21. **3.** A cardiac catheterization is an invasive procedure in which a radiopaque catheter is inserted into the heart through a peripheral venous or arterial blood vessel for the purpose of obtaining direct measurements of pressure changes and oxygen saturation levels in the heart chambers and the great vessels. It also measures cardiac output. The pedal pulses should be assessed preprocedure. A fever or infection may delay the procedure. Ambulation is

discouraged postprocedure; the child should be kept quiet and flat generally for six hours postprocedure. The child's pulses, color, and temperature should be monitored postprocedure.

NP = Pl
CN = Ph/7
CL = Ap
SA = 4

22. **1, 4, 6.** High-potassium foods include bananas; a single banana contains between 196 and 390 mg of potassium. Very high-potassium foods include cantaloupe and chocolate milk, both of which have more than 390 mg of potassium. Low-potassium foods include blueberries, peach nectar, and Kool-Aid, which contain 1 to 120 mg of potassium.

NP = Im
CN = Ph/5
CL = Ap
SA = 4

23. **1.** A newborn who has acute cyanosis that does not respond to oxygen should be evaluated for transposition of the great arteries. An infant with mild pulmonary stenosis is generally of normal size but has a murmur. An older child who is asymptomatic but has a murmur is suspected to have coarctation of the aorta. A child who develops a hypercyanotic spell, or "tet spell," during crying, feeding, or defecating is exhibiting characteristics of tetralogy of Fallot.

NP = Ev
CN = He/3
CL = An
SA = 4

24. **1, 3, 4.** Clinical manifestations of congestive heart disease include poor feeding, labored breathing, and decreased activity. These indicate a worsening of the cardiac condition and pulmonary congestion. Squatting is characteristic of tetralogy of Fallot. An infant with congestive heart failure would demonstrate a weight gain related to sodium and water retention. The infant would also be pale.

NP = Im
CN = He/3
CL = Ap
SA = 4

25. **4.** Because infants with congestive heart failure often manifest with poor feeding, the ideal way to increase caloric intake is to increase the concentration of calories per ounce of formula. Increasing volume is too difficult for infants who have labored breathing. Sugar water is void of nutrients, and a 2-month-old infant is too young for solid foods.

NP = Im

GASTROINTESTINAL DISORDERS - COMPREHENSIVE EXAM

1. A 12-month-old is admitted to the hospital with a diagnosis of failure to thrive (FTT). The child's weight is below the third percentile, development is retarded, and neglect is evident. In considering this assessment, what other behaviors would support the possibility of parental deprivation? Select all that apply:

   [ ] **1.** Is easily comforted by being held

   [ ] **2.** Is unresponsive

   [ ] **3.** Becomes very irritable when touched

   [ ] **4.** Rarely cries

   [ ] **5.** Not interested in surroundings

   [ ] **6.** Cries to be held

2. Which of the following interventions would be appropriate for the nurse to plan in the care of an infant following a cleft lip repair?

   1. Instruct the mother that the infant may only be bottle fed

   2. Suction the infant as needed

   3. Place the infant in a side-lying position

   4. Inform the mother that she should not feel guilty for causing the cleft lip

3. The parent of a child with a bilateral cleft lip repair asks, "Why does my infant have to wear these arm restraints?" The nurse's best response is that the restraints

   1. protect infants from getting their arms in the crib rails.

   2. prevent infants from rubbing the incision site with their hands.

   3. enable infants to rest better in a strange environment.

   4. prevent infants from pulling on the IV line.

4. When assessing a child suspected of having appendicitis, which of the following is a priority to ask this child to support the diagnosis?

   1. "Do you have abdominal pain?"

   2. "Are you constipated?"

   3. "Are you hungry?"

   4. "Do you have tenderness in your abdomen?"

5. A 2-year-old has undergone a successful repair of a tracheoesophageal fistula (TEF), and the parents will need discharge teaching and anticipatory guidance related to signs of esophageal constriction at the

repair site. Which of the following clinical manifestations of esophageal constriction should the nurse include in the teaching plan?

1. Dysphagia
2. Constipation
3. Recurrent otitis media
4. Decreased salivation

6. The nurse should assess for which of the following clinical manifestations in a newborn suspected of having an esophageal atresia and tracheoesophageal fistula?
Select all that apply:

[ ] 1. Rattling respirations
[ ] 2. Diarrhea
[ ] 3. Choking
[ ] 4. Coughing
[ ] 5. Lethargy
[ ] 6. Cyanosis

7. The nurse receives report on a child presenting with a clinical picture suggestive of necrotizing enterocolitis (NEC). Which of the following clinical manifestations would confirm the diagnosis?
Select all that apply:

[ ] 1. Hypertension
[ ] 2. Abdominal distention
[ ] 3. Tachycardia
[ ] 4. Increased urine output
[ ] 5. Temperature instability
[ ] 6. Bloody stools

8. Which of the following would be the priority for the nurse to include when evaluating the fluid status of an infant with short bowel syndrome?

1. Maintain intravenous rate
2. Monitor skin integrity
3. Calculate daily caloric needs
4. Evaluate bowel elimination

9. When providing care for an infant in the early stages of necrotizing enterocolitis (NEC), which of the following nursing diagnoses has priority?

1. Imbalanced nutrition: less than body requirements
2. Fluid volume deficient

3. Ineffective breathing pattern

4. Anticipatory grieving

10. In planning the care for a child postpyloromyotomy, which of the following is the priority nursing diagnosis?

    1. Acute pain

    2. Imbalanced nutrition: less than body requirements

    3. Fluid volume deficient

    4. Impaired urinary elimination

11. After a child's pyloromyotomy, the parents ask, "What are the special feeding instructions the surgeon mentioned?" Which of the following statements by the nurse would be the best response to the parents' question?

    1. "Clear liquids will be given because they contain no large curds and are therefore better tolerated."

    2. "Thickened feedings will be avoided because they could put pressure on the incision line in the pylorus muscle."

    3. "Easily digested fluids will be given in large quantities to prevent dehydration and malnutrition."

    4. "Thickened feedings will be given to mechanically aid in the passage of food through the pylorus muscle."

ANSWERS AND RATIONALES

1. **2, 4, 5.** Failure to thrive is indicated by growth failure; weight and height usually fall below the third to fifth percentile. The child also shows signs of neglect, is expressionless, apathetic, and listless. A child who becomes irritable when touched may be exhibiting signs of stranger anxiety. A normal child would be easily comforted when held and cries to be held.
NP = As
CN = He/3
CL = Ap
SA = 4

2. **3.** Following repair of a cleft lip, the child should be placed on the side to facilitate drainage. An infant who has a cleft lip may be breast-fed. These infants will not have any more difficulty than other infants having successful breastfeeding. The breast itself may be an advantage because the breast may fill in the defect in the lip. Suctioning is contraindicated in this infant because it would cause trauma to the palate and suture line. It is important that the nurse comfort the mother that she did nothing wrong during her pregnancy to cause this defect.

NP = Pl
CN = He/3
CL = Ap
SA = 4

3. **2.** Arm or elbow restraints are used to protect the suture line following a cleft lip repair from being traumatized from rubbing or picking with the fingers. Restraints are used to prevent children from harming themselves.
NP = An
CN = He/3
CL = An
SA = 4

4. **3.** Appendicitis is an inflammation of the vermiform appendix. Although the child will have abdominal tenderness and pain, the priority question to ask this child is, "Are you hungry?" If the child responds yes, it is likely that the child does not have appendicitis. A child with appendicitis typically does not feel hungry once the clinical manifestations begin.
NP = As
CN = He/3
CL = Ap
SA = 4

5. **1.** In a tracheoesophageal fistula, a fistula forms between the trachea and the esophagus. It generally occurs with an esophageal atresia in which an incompletely formed esophagus terminates before the stomach. Dysphagia or difficulty swallowing is the main indication that an esophageal stricture is occurring. Constipation is the result of reduced enteral intake or slow motility of the bowel. Ear infections are common with bottle-fed infants. Decreased salivation occurs as an anticholinergic response to some drugs.
NP = Pl
CN = Ph/7
CL = An
SA = 4

6. **1, 3, 4, 6.** The classic clinical manifestations of tracheoesophageal fistula are rattling respirations, choking, coughing, and cyanosis.
NP = As
CN = He/3
CL = Ap
SA = 4

7. **2, 5, 6.** Necrotizing enterocolitis is a necrosis of the mucosa of the small and large intestines that creates a surgical emergency for neonates. As blood is shunted from the gut, the bowel becomes inflamed, and obstruction occurs, resulting in abdominal distention and bloody stools. Temperature instability is the result of compounding stress on the newborn's body. Other clinical manifestations include bradycardia, decreased urine output, and hypotension.

NP = As
CN = He/3
CL = Ap
SA = 4

8. **2.** A short bowel syndrome is a condition characterized by an inadequate surface area of the small intestine generally occurring after surgical resection of the intestine in conditions such as necrotizing enterocolitis, volvulus, or Crohn's disease. Medical management focuses on maintaining optimal nutrition. Change in skin integrity related to dehydration is the priority in the care of this child. Maintaining intravenous fluids, calculating daily caloric needs, and evaluating bowel elimination are all important interventions, but they do not provide much information related to the actual hydration status of the child.

NP = Ev
CN = He/3
CL = An
SA = 4

9. **3.** Necrotizing enterocolitis is a necrosis of the small and large intestines, generally the distal ileum and proximal colon. It is a life-threatening condition in preterm neonates and is a surgical emergency. An ineffective breathing pattern related to altered hemodynamics is the result of blood loss from the occurrence of NEC leading to poor respiratory and cardiac function. The child will develop respiratory acidosis secondary to decreased perfusion.

NP = Pl
CN = He/3
CL = An
SA = 4

10. **3.** Pyloromyotomy is the surgical procedure for a pyloric stenosis. The circular muscle fibers are released, opening the passage from the stomach into the duodenum. Fluid volume deficit is the priority diagnosis because of the fluid, acid-base, and electrolyte imbalances. Fluid, acid-base, and electrolyte imbalances must be corrected for 24 to 48 hours preoperative. Pain is important but is not a priority over a life-threatening condition such as imbalance in fluid status. Impaired urinary elimination is a not a priority.

NP = Pl
CN = He/3
CL = An
SA = 4

11. 4. A pyloromyotomy is the surgical procedure to correct pyloric stenosis. The circular muscle fibers are released to open the passage from the stomach into the duodenum. Thickened feeding will be given for approximately two weeks to allow for muscle healing. If clear liquids or easily digested liquids are given, they will contribute to dumping syndrome. Predigested formula such as Pregestimil is not used with this condition.
NP = An
CN = He/3
CL = An
SA = 4

Practice Test 2

1. In evaluating the status of a child with pyloric stenosis, which of the following lab data would confirm that the child's condition has deteriorated?

    1. K 6.5 mEq/L, urine specific gravity 1.015, and BUN 10 mg/dl

    2. Na 120 mEq/L, urine specific gravity 1.001, and BUN 10 mg/dl

    3. Na 125 mEq/L, urine specific gravity 1.015, and BUN 13 mg/dl

    4. K 3 mEq/L, urine specific gravity 1.030, and BUN 20 mg/dl

2. The nurse's priority in the care of a neonate diagnosed with esophageal atresia is the risk for impaired gas exchange related to

    1. fluid overload.

    2. change in hemodynamics.

    3. excessive oropharyngeal secretions.

    4. altered bowel elimination.

3. The nurse should ask the mother of an infant suspected of gastroesophageal reflux if what two primary clinical manifestations are present? _____

4. When preparing a 3-year-old child with Hirschsprung's disease for a temporary colostomy, the nurse should

    1. talk to the parents only because the child is too young to understand.

    2. use simple terms to explain the surgery and read a story about a child with an ostomy.

    3. use simple terms to talk to the child and allow the child to play with a doll with an ostomy.

4.   provide the child with a coloring book that has pictures of ostomy supplies and people with an ostomy.

5. Which of the following statements by the parents of a neonate newly diagnosed with Hirschsprung's disease indicates that the parents understand the disease?

1.   "Our baby has an inflamed area in the bowel that can be controlled by medication."

2.   "This condition is inherited and requires a special diet for life."

3.   "Our baby will outgrow this condition over time."

4.   "This condition is due to some missing nerves in the bowel, and surgery is required."

6. During the administration of phenobarbital to an infant diagnosed with biliary atresia, the father asks, "Why is my baby having to take that medication? He doesn't have epilepsy." The nurse's most appropriate response would acknowledge phenobarbital's use for seizures, but also explain, "It is used to

1.   increase the movement of the bowel."

2.   slow the movement of bile."

3.   make the stomach empty faster."

4.   increase the bile flow."

7. Which of the following assessment findings in a neonate with gastroschisis should be immediately reported to the physician?

1.   Pale pink to grayish bowel loops

2.   Dark pink bowel loops

3.   Yellowish-serous liquid covering majority of the bowel

4.   Serous liquid covering or 2 inches above the bowel

8. Which of the following comments by parents who received instructions regarding celiac crisis would indicate that further teaching is necessary?

1.   "A celiac crisis is a very serious problem."

2.   "My child must avoid exposure to infections."

3.   "It is okay for my child to skip a meal."

4.   "I cannot give my child an antihistamine for a runny nose."

9. Which of the following care instructions should be included in the parents' discharge instructions for a 2-month-old with gastroesophageal reflux (GER)?

1.   Breastfeeding should be stopped because breast milk is too thin and easily leads to reflux

2.   Place the infant on the abdomen in a flat or head-elevated position following feeding and at night

3. Gradually increase the infant's intake of fruit or citrus juices

4. Increase the feeding volume right before bedtime because the stomach retains more food at this time

10. When working with a nursing student in the care of a neonate with gastroschisis, the student asks the nurse about the function of the Silastic "silo." The nurse's best response is, "The silo is utilized to

   1. decompress the stomach prior to surgery."

   2. monitor the bowel tissue prior to surgery."

   3. prevent increased cardiac output as the abdominal contents are gradually returned to the abdominal cavity."

   4. prevent respiratory dysfunction as the abdominal contents are gradually returned to the abdominal cavity."

11. Which of the following interventions should the nurse make before placing a neonate, who has pathologic jaundice, on phototherapy?

   1. Completely undress the neonate, place the child prone then place the "bili" lights approximately 18 inches from the child

   2. Undress the child except for the diaper, protect the eyes with patches, then place the "bili" lights over the child

   3. Obtain parent consent for the procedure, undress the child, then place the child under the "bili" lights

   4. Obtain serum bilirubin level, put the dressed child in an isolette, and position the "bili" lights over the child

12. A mother expresses her disappointment about the disruption in breastfeeding while her infant is on phototherapy. Which would be the nurse's best response to this mother's concern?

   1. "I know this is disappointing for you, but you can breast-feed your next infant."

   2. "I know that this is disappointing for you, but it is best for your infant to completely stop breastfeeding."

   3. "Phototherapy will not disrupt your breastfeeding of your infant."

   4. "There is an enzyme in breast milk that causes jaundice to increase. Be sure to pump to maintain your milk supply until the feedings are restarted."

13. The nurse has just received total bilirubin levels on four neonates. Which of the following infants' levels should be reported to the physician first?

   1. A 27-hour-old full-term newborn with transient tachypnea and a 9 mg/dl total bilirubin

   2. A 30-hour-old premature with suspected cleft palate and a 10 mg/dl total bilirubin

3. A 24-hour-old full-term newborn with meconium aspiration and a 10 mg/dl total bilirubin

4. A 20-hour-old premature with biliary atresia and a 6 mg/dl total bilirubin

14. In the neonate being treated with cholestyramine (Questran) for biliary atresia, which of the following findings should the nurse report immediately?

1. Progressive abdominal distention

2. Periodic apneic episodes

3. Irritability

4. Intense scratching

15. The registered nurse is delegating nursing tasks on a pediatric gastrointestinal unit. Which of the following tasks may the nurse delegate to a licensed practical nurse?

1. Administer total parenteral nutrition to a child with ulcerative colitis

2. Obtain a food history from the parents of a child who is experiencing diarrhea

3. Administer prescribed H_2 antagonist to a child with gastroesophageal reflux

4. Evaluate the serum bilirubin level in a child who has hepatitis

ANSWERS AND RATIONALES

1. **4.** Hypertrophic pyloric stenosis causes a hypertrophied pyloric sphincter, resulting in a narrowed opening and gastric outlet obstruction. Projectile nonbilious vomiting is the primary clinical manifestation. As the vomiting continues, hydrogen and chloride ions are lost, leading to dehydration and hypochloremic metabolic alkalosis. Serum potassium of 3 mEq/L, urine specific gravity of 1.030, and a BUN of 20 mg/dl would be plausible lab data. Serum potassium of 6.5 mEq/L, urine specific gravity of 1.015, and a BUN of 10 mg/dl is reflective of hyperkalemia but not of dehydration. Serum sodium of 125 mEq/L, urine specific gravity of 1.015, and a BUN of 13 mg/dl is indicative of hyponatremia. Serum sodium of 120 mEq/L, urine specific gravity of 1.001, and a BUN of 10 mg/dl indicates overhydration or water intoxication.
NP = Ev
CN = Ph/7
CL = An
SA = 4

2. **3.** Esophageal atresia is an incomplete formation of the esophagus, which terminates before it reaches the stomach. A fistula usually occurs between the

trachea and the esophagus and a blind pouch develops. Because maintaining a patent airway always takes priority, accumulation of secretions secondary to the presence of a blind pouch is a major concern with esophageal atresia. Pulmonary edema related to altered hemodynamics is the result of the obstruction of the airway with secretions. Fluid overload is the result of overhydration or rapidly infusing intravenous fluids.

NP = Im
CN = He/3
CL = An
SA = 4

3. **Vomiting and regurgitation.** Gastroesophageal reflux results from a defect in the nerve transmission, causing an inappropriate relaxation of the lower esophageal sphincter. The two primary clinical manifestations are vomiting and regurgitation.

NP = As
CN = He/3
CL = Ap
SA = 4

4. 3. It is important to explain the surgery or temporary colostomy to the toddler, using developmentally appropriate language. The toddler should be told in simple terms about the surgery and should be given the opportunity to play with the ostomy doll prior to surgery. Reading a story or providing a coloring book is appropriate for a preschool child who has the ability to think in concrete terms.

NP = Im
CN = He/3
CL = Ap
SA = 4

5. 4. Hirschsprung's disease is caused by an absence of the parasympathetic ganglion cells in the colon. An aganglionic segment results, generally in the rectosigmoid area. The normal part of the bowel hypertrophies and dilates and may be referred to as a megacolon. The aganglioned bowel results in obstruction, and surgery is required to relieve the obstruction and remove the affected bowel. The condition is not inherited, the bowel is not inflamed, and a special diet will not alleviate the problem.

NP = Ev
CN = He/3
CL = Ap
SA = 4

6. 4. Although an anticonvulsant drug, phenobarbital is also used to increase the bile flow. This drug has no effect on stomach activity or bowel movements.

NP = An
CN = He/3
CL = An
SA = 4

7. **1.** Gastroschisis is a defect in the abdominal wall that permits extrusion of the abdominal contents, generally the small and large intestine, without involvement of the umbilical cord. Pale pink to grayish bowel loops are an abnormal finding suggestive of ischemia. The bowel loop should be pink to dark pink, indicating adequate blood perfusion through the gut. Serous or yellow-serous fluid covering or above the bowel is a normal finding.
NP = An
CN = Ph/7
CL = An
SA = 4

8. **3.** Celiac disease is a gluten-sensitive enteropathy that results in malnutrition and failure to thrive. A gluten-free diet must be maintained for life. The omission of a meal can cause irritation to the bowel, leading to celiac crisis.
NP = Ev
CN = He/3
CL = Ap
SA = 4

9. **2.** With gastroesophageal reflux, positioning the infant on the abdomen with the head of the bed flat or slightly elevated aids in stomach emptying and decreases the potential for aspiration. Breastfeeding is not contraindicated with GER. Increased volume of feeding will contribute to GER and potential for aspiration. Solid food is usually not introduced until 5 to 6 months of age. In addition, citrus juices are not introduced until around 12 months of age.
NP = Pl
CN = He/3
CL = Ap
SA = 4

10. **4.** The purpose of the silo used in surgery for a gastroschisis is to elevate the abdominal contents above the newborn's abdomen. This enables a decrease in organ edema and uses gravity to gradually return the contents to the abdomen. This reduces the risk of respiratory distress related to increased pressure against the diaphragm. Observation of the gut and returning the stomach to the abdominal cavity prior to surgery is not the only purpose of the silo. Increased cardiac output is always a concern, but the silo cannot prevent this condition.
NP = An
CN = He/3

CL = An
SA = 4

11. **2.** As much of the body as possible needs to be exposed to the "bili" lights to help with conversion and excretion of bilirubin. Eye patches must be used to prevent damage to the retina from the lights. A diaper is worn to protect the gonads. Serum bilirubin levels are used to monitor the effect of the light treatment. The parents are informed of the purpose of the "bili" lights, but their consent is not necessary.
NP = Im
CN = He/3
CL = Ap
SA = 4

12. **4.** Breastfeeding is encouraged, but when the bilirubin increases rapidly or goes above 15 to 16 mg/dl, then breastfeeding is held. The mother is encouraged to pump to maintain the milk supply, since the breast milk can be given in a bottle. In addition, breastfeeding will be restarted once the bilirubin levels drop to within normal limits.
NP = An
CN = He/3
CL = An
SA = 4

13. **3.** A bilirubin that has increased by 7 mg/dl in less than 24 hours as well as bilirubin being present in meconium should be reported. The aspiration stresses the newborn's immature system therefore contributing further to the child's inability to handle the increased bilirubin.
NP = An
CN = Ph/7
CL = An
SA = 4

14. **1.** Biliary atresia is a congenital anomaly of the bile ducts. Cholestyramine is an antihyperlipidemic. Progressive abdominal distention is an adverse reaction to cholestyramine (Questran), but can also be due to ascites and must be reported immediately. Periodic apneic episodes, irritability, and intense scratching are all expected findings in a neonate with biliary atresia.
NP = An
CN = Ph/6
CL = An
SA = 5

15. **3.** Administering total parenteral nutrition, obtaining a food history, and evaluating the serum bilirubin level are all nursing tasks that require the

skills of a registered nurse. A licensed practical nurse may administer an oral drug such as an H_2 antagonist.

NP = Pl

CN = Sa/1

CL = An

SA = 8

METABOLIC AND ENDOCRINE DISORDERS - COMPREHENSIVE EXAM

1. The mother of a child starting on growth hormone asks, "How long will the growth hormone be needed?" The nurse's response should be based on the understanding that the need for growth hormone will

   1. be lifelong.

   2. continue until the epiphyseal growth plates fuse.

   3. continue until the child reaches the preferred height.

   4. be discontinued when the child reaches puberty.

2. The nurse is admitting a child who has had a change in behavior, falling grades in school, an inability to sit still and focus. Which of the following clinical manifestations would the nurse interpret as indicative of hyperthyroidism?

   Select all that apply:

   [ ] 1. Weight loss

   [ ] 2. Cold intolerance

   [ ] 3. Sleepiness

   [ ] 4. Anorexia

   [ ] 5. Fine tremors

   [ ] 6. Tachycardia

3. The nurse is planning the care of a child diagnosed with acquired hypothyroidism. Which of the following should receive priority in the client's plan of care?

   1. Administer a prescribed thyroid drug based on the weight of the child

   2. Educate the parents and child about the disease process

   3. Increase fiber and fluids in the diet to prevent constipation

   4. Assess the child for the presence of a goiter

4. The nurse is admitting a child suspected of having chronic adrenocortical insufficiency (Addison's disease). Which of the following assessments would confirm the diagnosis?
Select all that apply:

[   ] **1.** Positive Trousseau's and Chvostek's signs

[   ] **2.** Hyperpigmentation of the skin

[   ] **3.** Hypertension

[   ] **4.** Weight gain

[   ] **5.** A salt craving

[   ] **6.** Hypokalemia

5. As the nurse is preparing to administer a growth hormone injection to a 7-year-old child with short stature, the child begins crying and asks if the injection will hurt. Which of the following is the priority nursing intervention?

   1. Ask a parent to hold the child so the injection can be given

   2. Assure the child that the injection will be given as quickly as possible

   3. Inform the child that a small needle is used and the injection will pinch

   4. Instruct the child how to self-administer the injection

6. The parents of a newborn ask the nurse why the blood test for phenylketonuria (PKU) cannot be done before the infant has the first feeding. The nurse's reply is based on knowledge that

   1. it is important that the infant have a full stomach.

   2. newborns must be fed immediately after birth.

   3. a calcium intake is important to ensure accurate test results.

   4. the newborn must have ingested a source of protein.

7. Parents of a child with a blood test positive for phenylketonuria (PKU) ask what will happen to their infant. Which of the following is the appropriate response by the nurse?

   1. "The complications of PKU are decreased with medication."

   2. "A diet low in protein will help prevent mental retardation."

   3. "Prognosis is guarded."

   4. "Special dietary restrictions will be lifelong."

8. The registered nurse is preparing the client assignments for the day. Which of the following client assignments would be appropriate for the registered nurse to assign to a licensed practical nurse?

   1. Conduct a complete history and assessment on a child suspected of precocious puberty

2. Develop a daily insulin injection, blood glucose testing, diet, and activity plan for a child with type 1 diabetes

3. Administer the prescribed cortisol replacement to a child who has congenital adrenal hyperplasia and a high fever

4. Perform the preoperative education on a subtotal thyroidectomy to the parents and child who has hyperthyroidism

9. The nurse is caring for a child with hypoparathyroidism. Which of the following clinical manifestations indicates a need for emergency intervention?

   1. Jittery movements and tingling

   2. Extreme lethargy and poor feeding

   3. Headaches and vomiting

   4. Dry, coarse, and scaly skin

10. The nurse should monitor a child who received regular insulin for type 1 diabetes at 0700 for an insulin reaction at which of the following times?

    1. 0730

    2. 0800

    3. 0900

    4. 1200

11. A woman who was treated for phenylketonuria (PKU) at birth now finds she is pregnant. She expresses great concern that her newborn will have the disorder and asks the nurse what she should do. The appropriate response by the nurse is

    1. "Avoid increases in dietary phenylalanine during pregnancy that increase the risk of having a child who is mentally retarded."

    2. "It is recommended that the pregnancy be terminated as soon as possible."

    3. "You were successfully treated at birth for phenylketonuria and do not need to worry."

    4. "Your newborn can be treated immediately upon birth as you were and avoid the complications."

12. The nurse is caring for a child with type 1 diabetes mellitus. Which of the following indicate that the child is experiencing hypoglycemia? Select all that apply:

    [ ] 1. Tachycardia

    [ ] 2. Shakiness

    [ ] 3. Flushed face

[   ] **4.** Dry skin

[   ] **5.** Dizziness

[   ] **6.** Rapid respiratory rate

13. The nurse is admitting a client in diabetic ketoacidosis. Which of the following nursing measures should receive priority in this client's plan of care?

1. Administer an intramuscular injection of regular insulin

2. Instruct the parents on the causes and treatment of diabetic ketoacidosis

3. Administer isotonic fluids gradually over 24 to 48 hours

4. Monitor the child's vital signs and neurological function every four hours

14. The nurse has been assigned to care for four newly admitted children. Which of the following children is a priority for the nurse to assess first?

1. A child receiving propylthiouracil (PTU) for hyperthyroidism who is experiencing arthralgia, loss of taste, and has a noticeable skin rash

2. An infant with a failure to thrive history who been vomiting, has a fever, and a specific gravity of 1.001

3. An infant with a large posterior fontanel, jaundice, a T_4 level of 6.0 µg/dl, and a TSH of 4.8 µU/ml

4. A child who is dehydrated, has a serum glucose of 210 mg/dl, an arterial pH of 7.28, and a serum bicarbonate of 13 mEq/L

15. Which of the following should the nurse include when caring for a child having a provocative growth hormone test (growth stimulation test)?

1. Inform the child and parents that the test is painless

2. Monitor the child for signs of hypoglycemia during the test

3. Instruct the child and parents that there are no dietary restrictions prior to the test

4. Encourage the child to increase fluids after the procedure

16. Which of the following is a priority for the nurse to include in the admission assessment of a 7-year-old female child with accelerated breast and genital maturity?

1. Assess the psychosocial development

2. Perform a complete physical examination

3. Inform the parents that an injection of gonadotropin-releasing hormone is the usual treatment

4. Ask about the child's use of skin lotions or hair products

17. A mother informs the nurse that her small child has begun drinking water excessively and was observed drinking water from a toilet bowl. The nurse should notify the physician of what endocrine disorder? _____

18. A child with hypoparathyroidism is receiving intravenous calcium gluconate. It is a priority for the nurse to

   1. administer the calcium as a bolus.

   2. assess for burning and stinging at the injection site.

   3. monitor the blood pressure and heart rate.

   4. observe for extravasation at the IV site.

19. The nurse should prepare a child suspected of having Cushing's syndrome for which of the following diagnostic tests?

   1. Serum T_3 and T_4 tests

   2. Adrenocorticotropin hormone stimulation test

   3. Serum 17-hydroxyprogesterone

   4. Dexamethasone suppression test

20. When planning the care for a 7-year-old child with type 1 diabetes mellitus, which of the following skills is appropriate for the nurse to teach this child?

   1. Insulin injection technique

   2. Nutrition decision skills

   3. Blood testing

   4. Management decision skills

21. Which of the following should the nurse include in the medication instructions for the parents of a child with congenital hypothyroidism who is to start on L-thyroxine (Synthroid)?

   1. Thyroid function tests should be done every three months

   2. The thyroid replacement will be discontinued when the thyroid tests return to normal

   3. Avoid giving the child soy-based formula while taking this drug

   4. Gradually start the drug by giving it every other day for one week

22. The nurse should monitor a child started on growth hormone for which of the following adverse reactions?
   Select all that apply:

   [   ] 1. Weight gain

   [   ] 2. Hypotension

   [   ] 3. Painful hip joints

   [   ] 4. Diarrhea

[   ] **5.** Anorexia

[   ] **6.** Headaches

23. The nurse should prepare a child with diabetes insipidus for which of the following diagnostic tests?

1. Serum sodium and osmolality

2. Serum 17-hydroxyprogesterone

3. Serum glucose and urine ketones

4. Serum cortisol

24. The nurse is reviewing the laboratory results on four children. The nurse reports which of the following laboratory results that requires further investigation?

1. A 6-year-old child with a serum sodium of 135 mEq/L

2. A 5-year-old child with a urine specific gravity of 1.000 and osmolarity less than 200 mOsmol/kg H_2O

3. An 8-year-old child with a T_4 of 6.8 µg/dl and TSH 4 µU/ml

4. A 13-year-old child with serum potassium of 3.8 mEq/ml

25. The nurse should monitor a child receiving NPH insulin at 0800 for an insulin reaction at which of the following times?

1. 0900

2. 1000

3. 1200

4. 1500

ANSWERS AND RATIONALES

1. **2.** There is no need to continue the growth hormone after the epiphyseal growth plates fuse. It is not needed lifelong. There is no indication for the growth hormone to allow attainment of preferred height.

NP = An

CN = He/3

CL = An

SA = 4

2. **1, 5, 6.** Hyperthyroidism results from a hyperfunction of circulating thyroid hormones. Clinical manifestations of hyperthyroidism include weight loss despite a good appetite, heat intolerance, insomnia, fine tremors, tachycardia, emotional instability, and ophthalmic changes.

NP = As

CN = He/3

CL = Ap
SA = 4

3. 1. Acquired hypothyroidism is generally autoimmune in cause and results in decreased serum T_4 levels and a concurrent increase in TSH (thyroid-stimulating hormone) levels. The priority of treatment in acquired hypothyroidism is replacing the thyroid hormone that is inadequate. The replacement thyroid hormone, L-thyroxine, must be carefully titrated in children based on the child's weight and the severity of the disease. A goiter is found in hyperthyroidism. Although educating the parents about the disease process and increasing fiber and fluids in the diet may be appropriate interventions, they are not the priority.
NP = Pl
CN = Sa/1
CL = An
SA = 8

4. 2, 5. Chronic adrenocortical insufficiency, or Addison's disease, is the insufficient production of aldosterone and cortisol affecting the sodium balance in the body. It leads to a salt craving and a hyperpigmentation of the skin. Weight gain and hypertension are clinical manifestations of excess cortisol. Electrolyte imbalances such as hyperkalemia and hypernatremia are present in Addison's disease. Positive Trousseau's and Chvostek's signs are indications of hypoparathyroidism.
NP = As
CN = He/3
CL = Ap
SA = 4

5. 3. The most appropriate response to a child who asks if an injection will hurt is honesty. The nurse should reassure the child that the injection will pinch but the smallest needle will be used and reiterate the fact that the injection will help to increase growth. Although plausible interventions such as asking the parent to hold and comfort the child when the injection is given are valid, they are not the priority. The injection should also be given quickly to avoid any unnecessary discomfort to the child but again this is not the priority. The child asked a direct question as to whether the injection will hurt, and that question should be addressed. At a later time, the child may be instructed to self-administer the injection depending on the child's readiness.
NP = Im
CN = Sa/1
CL = An
SA = 8

6. 4. Phenylketonuria (PKU) is caused by a deficiency in an enzyme needed to convert phenylalanine to tyrosine as part of protein metabolism. The existence of the disease results in elevations of phenylalanine after ingestion of a protein source. The test is most accurate if the infant has ingested a protein source before being tested. A full stomach is not necessary. Calcium is not a part of testing for PKU.
NP = An
CN = He/3
CL = An
SA = 4

7. 2. Phenylketonuria (PKU) is caused by a deficiency in an enzyme needed to convert phenylalanine to tyrosine as part of protein metabolism. The existence of the disease results in elevations of phenylalanine after ingestion of a protein source. A diet low in protein is necessary, but only until adolescence when full brain development is complete. Prognosis is good when dietary restriction of protein is adhered to. Medication is not needed.
NP = An
CN = He/3
CL = Ap
SA = 4

8. 3. A licensed practical nurse (LPN) cannot assess, plan, develop, or educate a client. These activities are reserved for the registered nurse. A licensed practical nurse can carry out an existing order such as administering a medication.
NP = Pl
CN = Sa/1
CL = An
SA = 8

9. 1. Reduced amounts of parathyroid hormone in hypoparathyroidism can cause jitteriness, tingling, and seizures, indicating the possibility of impending tetany and requiring immediate nursing intervention. Lethargy, poor feeding, headaches, vomiting, and dry scaling skin may occur but do not pose an emergency.
NP = An
CN = He/3
CL = Ap
SA = 4

10. 3. The onset of regular insulin is 20 to 30 minutes and the peak is 2 to 4 hours. A reaction would most likely occur within the peak time frame. A child who received insulin at 0700 would most likely have an insulin reaction between the hours of 0900 and 1100.

NP = As
CN = Ph/6
CL = An
SA = 5

11. **1.** Phenylketonuria (PKU) is caused by a deficiency in an enzyme needed to convert phenylalanine to tyrosine as part of protein metabolism. The disease results in elevations of phenylalanine after ingestion of a protein source. A woman of child-bearing age needs to be aware that an increase in dietary phenylalanine during pregnancy will increase the risk of producing a child who has mental retardation.
NP = An
CN = He/3
CL = An
SA = 4

12. **1, 2, 5.** Clinical manifestations of hypoglycemia include shakiness, dizziness, pallor, headaches, fatigue, and tachycardia. Flushed face, dry skin, and rapid respiratory rate indicate hyperglycemia.
NP =An
CN = He/3
CL = Ap
SA = 4

13. **3.** Diabetic ketoacidosis (DKA) is a potentially life-threatening complication of type 1 diabetes mellitus. Classic features include hyperglycemia, severe insulin deficit, acidosis, and ketosis. The first priority in the treatment of diabetic ketoacidosis is a slow fluid replacement. Isotonic fluids are replaced gradually over 24 to 48 hours, not exceeding a volume of four liters daily. A dehydrated client cannot absorb a subcutaneous or intramuscular injection of regular insulin. The method of insulin administration for DKA is regular insulin by intravenous infusion. Educating the parents on the causes and treatment is always important to prevent further episodes of DKA, but it is not the priority. Monitoring the child's vital signs and neurological function is also important to assess the response to treatment but, again, is not the priority.
NP = Pl
CN = Sa/1
CL = An
SA = 8

14. **4.** Adverse reactions of propylthiouracil (PTU) include skin rash, loss of taste, and arthralgia. These adverse reactions, although mild, should be reported for a dose adjustment or so an alternative drug can be ordered. An infant with a failure to thrive history, fever, and a urine specific gravity of less than 1.005 should be investigated for diabetes insipidus. An infant

with congenital hypothyroidism is usually asymptomatic at birth. An infant who presents with a large posterior fontanel, prolonged jaundice, a T_4 less than 6.5 μg/dl (normal is 6.5 to 13 μg/dl), and a TSH less than 5 μU/ml should be investigated for congenital hypothyroidism. In a child, dehydration, serum glucose over 200 mg/dl, arterial pH less than 7.30, and serum bicarbonate less than 15 mEq/L indicates diabetic ketoacidosis and must be considered an emergency and assessed first.
NP = As
CN = Sa/1
CL = An
SA = 8

15. **2.** The child should be monitored for signs of hypoglycemia during and after a provocative growth hormone test, also called growth stimulation test. Venous samples of blood are taken at scheduled intervals, usually at the beginning of the test, and at 60 and 90 minutes after an injection of insulin. The child should be NPO after midnight prior to the test. The test takes approximately two hours. There is no radioactive dye used, so there is no need to increase fluids. There is discomfort associated with the test, because an IV line is inserted and hypoglycemic effects may be felt from the insulin.
NP = Pl
CN = Ph/7
CL = Ap
SA = 4

16. **4.** It is a priority to question the child and parents about the child's use of skin lotions or hair products. Many of these products contain estrogen or placenta extracts, which the child absorbs, and they contribute to the development of secondary sex characteristics. Although the child's psychosocial development should be assessed, it is generally age-appropriate. A complete physical examination will confirm the presence of secondary sex characteristics and confirm the diagnosis of precocious puberty. An injection of gonadotropin-releasing hormone is the usual treatment to regulate pituitary secretions.
NP = Pl
CN = Sa/1
CL = An
SA = 4

17. **Diabetes insipidus.** Diabetes insipidus is a disorder of water regulation. There is a deficiency in the antidiuretic hormone that results in the excretion of large amounts of dilute urine. It is characterized by polyuria and polydipsia. Small children need to be monitored closely for their water

source because they may resort to unlikely sources, such as toilet bowls or plants, to alleviate the severe fluid deprivation.

NP = An

CN = He/3

CL = Ap

SA = 4

18. **3.** Hypoparathyroidism is a deficit in the parathyroid hormone, which maintains the serum calcium. Calcium gluconate is necessary in acute cases when seizures or tetany are present. The priority when administering intravenous calcium gluconate to a child with hypoparathyroidism is to closely monitor the child for the presence of cardiac arrhythmias, hypotension, and bradycardia that may occur from too rapid an administration. The calcium gluconate should be given by a slow infusion and never as a bolus.

NP = Im

CN = Sa/1

CL = An

SA = 8

19. **4.** Dexamethasone suppression test is used to diagnose Cushing's syndrome and distinguish it from other conditions. Serum T_3 and T_4 are used in the diagnosis of thyroid disorders. The ACTH stimulation test diagnoses an adrenal insufficiency. Serum 17-hydroxyprogesterone is also used to confirm an adrenal insufficiency.

NP = Pl

CN = Ph/7

CL = An

SA = 4

20. **3.** A technical skill that is age appropriate to teach a 7-year-old child with type 1 diabetes mellitus is blood testing. A child must be 8 to 10 years of age to teach insulin injections. Nutrition decision skills should not be taught until 10 to 14 years of age. Management decision skills would not be appropriate to teach before the age of 12 to 18 years of age.

NP = Pl

CN = He/3

CL = An

SA = 4

21. **3.** L-thyroxine (Synthroid) is a thyroid product used to treat hypothyroidism. Soy-based formulas should be avoided when an infant is taking Synthroid because the absorption of the drug is adversely affected. Thyroid function tests should be monitored every two weeks initially after starting treatment. Lifelong thyroid replacement is required to maintain

normal metabolism. The goal of therapy is to normalize thyroid function as soon as possible. A dose of 10 to 15 mEq/kg is given daily to start with.

NP = Pl
CN = Ph/6
CL = An
SA = 5

22. **1, 3, 6.** Growth hormone deficiency is caused by a failure of the pituitary to produce the growth hormone. It is characterized by poor growth and short stature. The goal of treatment is to administer the growth hormone. A sudden and rapid weight gain, painful hips, and headaches are adverse reactions to growth hormone.

NP = As
CN = Ph/6
CL = Ap
SA = 5

23. **1.** Diabetes insipidus is a disorder of water regulation caused by a deficiency of the antidiuretic hormone. Serum sodium and osmolality are diagnostic tests that measure the sodium level and concentration of osmotically active particles in the serum. They would be elevated in diabetes insipidus. Serum 17-hydroxprogesterone is used to diagnose an adrenal insufficiency. Serum glucose and urine ketones are diagnostic in diabetes mellitus. A serum cortisol is a diagnostic test used to evaluate the adrenal gland and associated disorders.

NP = Im
CN = Ph/7
CL = An
SA = 4

24. **2.** A urine specific gravity of 1.000 and osmolarity less than 200 mOsmol/kg H_2O require further investigation. Normal urine specific gravity for a child is 1.016 to 1.030. Normal osmolality is 275 to 295 mOsmol/kg H_2O. A child with diabetes insipidus has a urine specific gravity of less than 1.005 and an osmolality of less than 200 mOsmol/kg H_2O. Normal serum sodium for a child is 138 to 145 mEq/L. Normal T_4 is 6.4 to 13.3 μg/dl and TSH is 2 to 10 μU/L. Normal serum potassium for a child over the age of 12 years is 3.5 to 5.0 mEq/L.

NP = An
CN = Ph/7
CL = An
SA = 4

25. **4.** NPH insulin is an intermediate acting insulin. The onset is 1 to 4 hours and the peak is 6 to 10 hours. A child who receives NPH insulin at 0800 is most likely to have an insulin reaction between the hours of 1400 and 1800.

NP = As
CN = Ph/7
CL = Ap
SA = 4

NEUROLOGICAL DISORDERS - COMPREHENSIVE EXAM

1. The nurse is admitting a neonate diagnosed with an arteriovenous malformation. For which of the following initial clinical manifestations should the nurse assess the neonate?
   Select all that apply:

   [   ] **1.** Altered state of consciousness

   [   ] **2.** Congestive heart failure

   [   ] **3.** Jaundice

   [   ] **4.** Cardiomegaly

   [   ] **5.** Significant difference in blood pressure (BP) on left and right arms

   [   ] **6.** Cerebral bruit

2. The nurse is caring for a 6-month-old infant just admitted to the unit who is irritable, has bulging fontanels, and has for the last six hours vomited after feedings. The nurse should report these clinical manifestations as which of the following?

   1. Increased intracranial pressure

   2. Hypertension

   3. Skull fracture

   4. Myelomeningocele

3. Which of the following should the nurse include in the teaching given to the parents of a child who has generalized seizures?

   1. The child will have the seizures only in the first year of life

   2. The seizures are due to an abnormal activity in a small area of the brain

   3. There is a loss consciousness

   4. The clinical manifestations of the seizures are most often motor or sensory in nature

4. Which of the following should the nurse include in the teaching given to the parents of a child who is experiencing simple partial seizures?

   1. There is no aura

   2. The seizures are associated with loss of consciousness

3. The seizures are sensory in nature

4. The seizures may last several seconds to hours

5. Which of the following should the nurse include in the discharge instructions to the parents of a child admitted for febrile seizures?

1. They are a type of tonic-clonic seizure

2. They usually occur in children who are 5 to 10 years of age

3. They are often associated with central nervous system clinical manifestations

4. They have a postictal period that lasts for more than 15 minutes

6. The nurse is caring for a child who was not wearing a helmet, fell off a bicycle, and sustained a head injury. Which of the following clinical manifestations would indicate the child is experiencing increased intracranial pressure?

1. Symmetrical pupils

2. Widened pulse pressure

3. Hypotension

4. Tachycardia

7. A 12-year-old fell while rock climbing and sustained a spinal cord injury at C7. Upon assessment in the emergency department, which of the following clinical manifestations would indicate spinal shock?

1. Spastic extremities

2. Loss of deep tendon reflexes

3. Tachycardia

4. Increased peripheral vascular resistance

8. The nurse is caring for a child who has a glazed facial look after a fall down some stairs. A spinal cord injury is suspected. After determining the child has a patent airway, which of the nursing interventions is the priority?

1. Assist the child to a comfortable position

2. Assess the child's ability to flex and extend all extremities

3. Avoid moving the child

4. Instruct the caregiver to pick the child up to provide comfort

9. Which of the following should the nurse include in the long-term care instructions for a ventriculoperitoneal shunt in a child who has hydrocephalus?

1. Constant parental supervision until the child reaches adulthood

2. Monitor the child for mental retardation

   3. Begin immediate treatment for shunt malfunction or infection

   4. Restrict most of the usual childhood activities

10. The nurse instructs another nurse that the best method of evaluating a toddler's level of consciousness is the motor scale of the Glasgow Coma Scale because a toddler

   1. will be able to localize pain.

   2. will cry in response to stimuli.

   3. will not obey commands.

   4. cannot control reflexes.

11. The nurse should include which of the following in the teaching given to parents of a child with infantile seizures?

   1. The seizures occur in children between 6 months and 5 years of age

   2. They are not accompanied by a loss of consciousness

   3. There may be neurological abnormalities

   4. They ascend up the body

12. The parents of a 3-year-old who has a history of seizures, including momentary loss of consciousness, loss of muscle tone, and falling to the ground, recognize these as akinetic atonic seizures and ask the nurse how long the seizures will persist. Which of the following is the appropriate response by the nurse?

   1. There will be a remission in adolescence

   2. They may progress to adult seizures

   3. Medication will control these attacks

   4. They disappear by 6 years of age

13. The nurse is collecting a nursing history from the parents of a child who has encephalitis. Which of the following should the nurse assess? Select all that apply:

   [ ] **1.** Recent immunizations

   [ ] **2.** Exposure to oral or injectable polio vaccine

   [ ] **3.** History of insect bites

   [ ] **4.** Use of antibiotics

   [ ] **5.** Recent travel

   [ ] **6.** Use of antiviral agents

14. Which of the following should the nurse include in a class on noncommunicating or obstructive hydrocephalus?

1. There is no difference in incidence between communicating and noncommunicating hydrocephalus

2. Hydrocephalus is caused by an imbalance between the production and absorption of cerebrospinal fluid

3. The clinical manifestations of hydrocephalus do not vary according to age

4. Both communicating and noncommunicating hydrocephalus are caused by similar factors

15. When planning the plan of care of a 8-month-old who has an asymmetric tonic neck reflex, which of the following is the priority?

    1. Further neurological and developmental testing

    2. Schedule a reevaluation for when the child reaches 1 year of age

    3. Obtain a serum bilirubin

    4. Perform a needs assessment

16. The parents of a child who has sustained a head injury ask the nurse the purpose of comparing the child's current neurological status with the previous status. The most appropriate response by the nurse is to

    1. assess the Glasgow Coma Scale score.

    2. assess the level of consciousness.

    3. determine the need for medication.

    4. assess improvement, stability, or deterioration.

17. A mother asks the nurse why a child hospitalized for observation following a submersion injury cannot be discharged. Which of the following is the most appropriate response by the nurse?

    1. "It is important to determine how long the child was immersed."

    2. "Hypoxemia is the major injury associated with drowning."

    3. "Life-threatening complications may not be evident for at least 12 hours."

    4. "The child has to be afebrile and eating."

18. Which of the following should the nurse include in an accident prevention class for the parents of toddlers? Toddlers are more at risk for head injuries because

    1. the fontanels and sutures have closed.

    2. their abdomens protrude with lumbar lordosis.

    3. they are unsteady on their feet.

    4. their heads are large in proportion to their bodies.

19. The nurse is caring for a young infant who has been admitted with a possible diagnosis of meningitis. Which of the following assessment findings should the nurse report?

    1. Constipation
    2. Subnormal temperature
    3. Change in feeding pattern
    4. Generalized floppiness

20. The nurse is caring for a child who has just been diagnosed with meningococcal meningitis. Which of the following statements is the priority to communicate to close contacts and family members?

    1. "Your child will need to be hospitalized for treatment."
    2. "Your child will need to be isolated for 10 days."
    3. "Your child will be treated with prophylactic steroids."
    4. "Everyone in close contact with your child will be given prophylactic antibiotics."

21. The parents of a child with Reye's syndrome ask the nurse how their child got the disease. The appropriate response by the nurse is that "Reye's syndrome generally follows

    1. bacterial meningitis."
    2. an acetaminophen overdose."
    3. strep throat."
    4. a mild viral infection."

22. Which of the following is the priority for the nurse to assess in the plan of care for a child who had a closure of a neural tube defect?

    1. The presence of a urinary tract infection
    2. An alteration in the bowel function
    3. An increased intracranial pressure
    4. An alteration in the motor function in legs

23. The nurse should inform the parents of a child who suffered a submersion injury that the initial injury is the result of

    1. hypoxemia.
    2. cardiac arrest.
    3. alkalosis.
    4. pulmonary edema.

24. The nurse should document the involuntary writhing movements a child with cerebral palsy exhibits as _____ .

25. Which of the following should the nurse include in the teaching about latex allergy given to a child's parents?
Select all that apply:

[   ] 1. The child frequently experiences nausea, vomiting, and diarrhea

[   ] 2. A child with spina bifida is more likely to have a latex allergy

[   ] 3. All product labels should be checked

[   ] 4. Urticaria, wheezing, and rash are common manifestations

[   ] 5. Anaphylaxis from a latex allergy is rare

26. The registered nurse is preparing the clinical assignments for a pediatric neurological unit. Which of the following is appropriate for the nurse to delegate to a licensed practical nurse?

1. Instruct the parents of a child with seizures about a ketogenic diet

2. Monitor the level of consciousness in a child who sustained a head injury

3. Inform the parents of a child with ancephaly of the grave prognosis

4. Prepare a child for a spinal tap

ANSWERS AND RATIONALES

1. **2, 4, 6.** Initial clinical manifestations of an arteriovenous malformation include congestive heart failure, cardiomegaly, and cerebral bruit. A difference in BP between extremities is a sign of coarctation of the aorta. An altered state of consciousness and jaundice are not manifestations of an AV malformation.
NP = As
CN = He/3
CL = Ap
SA = 4

2. **1.** Clinical manifestations of increased intracranial pressure in infants include lethargy, irritability, bradycardia, tachycardia, apnea, bulging fontanels, setting-sun eyes, vomiting, and hypertension. Myelomeningocele is a neural tube defect seen on the back. Skull fractures may be asymptomatic or accompanied by other pathology that might be visible or invisible. Setting-sun eyes are not seen in hypertension.
NP = An
CN = He/3
CL = Ap
SA = 4

3. 3. Consciousness is lost with generalized seizures.
   NP = Pl
   CN = He/3
   CL = Ap
   SA = 4

4. 1. Simple partial seizures have no aura, rarely last several hours, and consciousness is not lost.
   NP = Pl
   CN = He/3
   CL = Ap
   SA = 4

5. 1. Febrile seizures are generally tonic-clonic, are usually associated with a rapid rise in temperature, and occur between 6 months and 5 years of age. There may be a positive family history of seizures, and the seizures are frequently accompanied by infectious processes (URI, pneumonia, pharyngitis, shigella, UTI, OM, roseola, meningitis). They often are self-limiting, with a postictal period that lasts less than 15 minutes.
   NP = Pl
   CN = He/3
   CL = Ap
   SA = 4

6. 2. Signs of increased intracranial pressure in children include headache, vomiting, asymmetrical pupils, generalized seizures, cranial nerve palsies of VI and VII, hypertension, wide pulse pressure, and bradycardia.
   NP = An
   CN = He/3
   CL = Ap
   SA = 4

7. 2. Signs of spinal shock include hypotension; bradycardia; decreased peripheral vascular resistance; impaired temperature control; warm, flushed, dry skin; flaccid paralysis; loss of deep tendon reflexes; no sensory response; loss of sphincter control with urinary retention; and priapism.
   NP = An
   CN = He/3
   CL = Ap
   SA = 4

8. 3. Whenever there is a concern about the presence of a spinal cord injury, the child should not be moved or asked to move any extremities until stabilized. Any such movement might cause further damage to the cord, or

damage to the cord itself if the injury was accompanied by a vertebral fracture.
NP = Im
CN = Sa/1
CL = An
SA = 4

9. 3. Children who have ventriculoperitoneal shunts should be allowed to participate in normal activities as much as their condition warrants and should not be overprotected. Mental retardation does not always accompany this condition. Any sign of shunt malfunction or infection needs to be reported immediately to the physician.
NP = Pl
CN = He/3
CL = Ap
SA = 4

10. 4. Using the motor scale of the Glasgow Coma Scale is especially appropriate when evaluating toddlers, because they cannot control their reflexes. Sometimes they have difficulty localizing pain, will not obey commands, especially if they do not know the person giving the command, and will cry whether or not they have received a stimulus.
NP = An
CN = He/3
CL = An
SA = 4

11. 3. Infantile (salaam) seizures begin at 3 months of age and are associated with children who have a history of gestational difficulties and exhibit developmental delay or other neurological abnormalities. During the seizure, the infant's head may suddenly drop forward while both arms and legs are flexed. The eyes may roll upward or downward. There may be a loss of consciousness.
NP = Pl
CN = He/3
CL = Ap
SA = 4

12. 4. Akinetic atonic seizures are usually seen between 2 and 5 years of age and are manifested by sudden loss of muscle tone with head dropping forward for a few seconds. More significant events occur when the child loses consciousness and falls to the ground (often face down). Amnesia is often seen, and the seizures may cause repetitive head injuries if the child's head is not protected by a football or hockey helmet. Many children who experience akinetic atonic seizures have underlying brain abnormalities and are mentally retarded.

NP = An
CN = He/3
CL = An
SA = 4

13. **1, 3, 5.** Encephalitis can be caused by bacteria, viruses, fungi, or protozoa. Encephalitis also can be caused by arthropod bites or may follow vaccines for tetanus, measles, rubella, diphtheria, or pertussis. Children who have traveled recently may also be at risk, if one of the causes of encephalitis is endemic to the geographic area to which they traveled.
NP = As
CN = He/3
CL = Ap
SA = 4

14. **2.** Causes of hydrocephalus and clinical manifestations differ according to age, since the condition is manifested by signs of increased intracranial pressure (ICP), which vary according to age. Noncommunicating hydrocephalus is more common than communicating hydrocephalus.
NP = Pl
CN = He/3
CL = Ap
SA = 4

15. **1.** The presence of any neonatal reflexes in an 8-month-old indicates the need for further and immediate neurological and motor evaluation, because this situation is an indication of cerebral palsy. It would do no good to delay the evaluation until the child is 1 year old. Serum bilirubin has no relation to asymmetric tonic neck reflex.
NP = Pl
CN = Sa/1
CL = An
SA = 8

16. **4.** Glasgow Coma Scale score and level of consciousness are determined at the time of the evaluation only. The need for medications is also evaluated at one point in time to determine if there is a need for changing or ordering them.
NP = An
CN = He/3
CL = An
SA = 4

17. **3.** In any submersion, the child's clinical picture may change within the first 24 hours after the event. Life-threatening events that occur later may include cerebral edema, pulmonary edema, shock, and pneumonia.

NP = An
CN = He/3
CL = An
SA = 4

18. 4. Toddlers are top-heavy and can easily topple forward because their heads are large in proportion to their bodies. Because their neck muscles are not well developed and may not be able to support their large heads, they have a tendency to fall.
NP = Pl
CN = He/3
CL = Ap
SA = 4

19. 3. Many clinical manifestations of meningitis in young infants are nonspecific, but a change in feeding pattern (eating less at each feeding, eating less often) is common. Other clinical manifestations are fever, vomiting, and diarrhea.
NP = As
CN = He/3
CL = Ap
SA = 4

20. 4. Meningococcal meningitis is easily spread by droplets to close contacts. Therefore, all close contacts including family members should be treated with the prophylactic antibiotic rifampin.
NP = An
CN = Sa/1
CL = An
SA = 8

21. 4. Reye's syndrome is a life-threatening encephalopathy with accompanying microvascular fatty deposits in the liver and kidney. It often follows a mild viral infection such as a upper respiratory infection, varicella, or gastroenteritis.
NP = An
CN = He/3
CL = An
SA = 4

22. 3. After closure of a neural tube defect, many infants develop hydrocephalus manifested by signs of increased intracranial pressure. Intracranial pressure should be measured at least every shift and any increase reported immediately.
NP = As
CN = Sa/1

CL = An
SA = 4

23. **1.** The initial injury following a submersion injury is the result of hypoxemia. Cardiac arrest, acidosis, and pulmonary edema may occur after the hypoxemia.
NP = Im
CN = He/3
CL = An
SA = 4

24. **athetosis.** Athetosis is a constant involuntary writhing motion affecting the entire body, but more severe distally.
NP = An
CN = He/3
CL = Co
SA = 4

25. **4.** Latex allergy is 41% more common in spina bifida. Product labels should be checked for latex. Urticaria, wheezing, watery eyes, and rash are common. Anaphylaxis may occur.
NP = Pl
CN = He/3
CL = Ap
SA = 4

26. **4.** A licensed practical nurse can prepare a child for a spinal tap. Instructing the parents on a ketogenic diet and monitoring the level of consciousness in a child are tasks that should be performed by a registered nurse. Informing the parents of a child of a grave prognosis is the responsibility of the physician.
NP = Pl
CN = Sa/1
CL = An
SA = 8

INTEGUMENTARY DISORDERS - COMPREHENSIVE EXAM

1. A child's mother asks the nurse how to tell if her child has head lice (pediculosis capitis). The nurse replies

    1. "Lice and nits will wash away with shampoo and water."

    2. "Nits look like dandruff but are firmly attached to the hair shaft."

    3. "The scalp will itch primarily at night."

    4. "Hair loss is sign of lice."

2. The mother asks the nurse how to prevent the lice from spreading to other family members. Which of the following is the nurse's most appropriate response?

    1. "Lice can't survive off the scalp."

    2. "Wash all clothes and linens in hot water and dry in a hot dryer."

    3. "Dispose of all household items that have come in contact with the affected child."

    4. "Adults cannot get lice."

3. Permethrin 5% (Elimite) has been prescribed for a 10-year-old child with scabies. Which of the following instructions should the nurse include?

    1. Treat all family members and close contacts

    2. Treat only the affected child

    3. Leave Elimite on for two hours

    4. Avoid applying to intertriginous zones

4. The mother of a 12-year-old basketball player calls to schedule surgery for excision of a congenital nevus. What postoperative care information should the nurse give to the mother?

    1. Physical activity should be avoided for two to four weeks

    2. Going to school is not permitted for one week

    3. The sutures will be removed in seven days

    4. There will be daily dressing changes

5. A 16-year-old female client presents with inflammatory papules and pustules on the face and is to begin oral antibiotics. Which of the following should the nurse tell her?

    1. It will take two weeks to see an improvement

    2. There are no adverse reactions from the antibiotics

    3. Antibiotics can decrease the effectiveness of oral contraceptives

    4. There will be scar formation after antibiotic therapy

6. Which of the following should the nurse include in a class on acne given to adolescents?

    1. Chocolate and fried food cause acne

    2. Vigorous scrubbing will improve acne

    3. Squeezing pimples will help to clear acne faster

    4. If using cosmetics, they should be water-based and oil-free

7. An 18-year-old female adolescent with severe cystic acne that has not responded to antibiotic therapy is scheduled to begin treatment with

isotretinoin (Accutane). Which of the following is the priority intervention the nurse should include in this client's plan of care?

1. Monitor the client for clinical manifestations of depression

2. Instruct the client that two forms of birth control must be used

3. Inform the client that there are no dietary restrictions

4. Monitor monthly liver, lipid, and CBC levels

8. An 8-year-old client presents with a chief complaint of dry, itchy skin. When assessing the client's skin, the nurse evaluates which of the following characteristics consistent with atopic dermatitis?

1. Dry red patches on the antecubital spaces and the popliteal fossae

2. Dome-shaped, flesh-colored papules

3. Irregularly shaped reddish-purple macular vascular lesions

4. Scaly, well-demarcated plaques

9. A 6-year-old child with atopic dermatitis returns for a follow-up visit. The mother states that the child has not improved despite following the plan of care. In reviewing the plan of care, which of the following indicates the mother does not understand the treatment?

1. The mother is bathing the child daily for a maximum of 10 minutes

2. The mother is applying the emollient followed by the steroid ointment

3. The mother is applying emollients frequently during the day

4. The child is wearing cotton clothing

10. An 8-year-old child presents in the clinic with papules and vesicles on the wrists, waistline, and interdigital spaces. The rash is intensely pruritic at night. Based on the clinical manifestations, the nurse prepares the child for which of the following tests?

1. KOH

2. Mineral oil prep

3. Punch biopsy

4. Wood's lamp examination

11. Which of the following medications instructions should the nurse give the parents of a child infested with scabies who is to begin on permethrin 5% cream (Elimite)?

1. Take a warm bath or shower prior to applying the medication

2. Apply the cream directly to each lesion

3. Leave the cream on for four hours and then wash off

4. Apply the cream from the neck down in a thin layer

12. A mother brings a child to a clinic complaining that the child has been losing hair. The answers to which of the following questions asked by the nurse would be most helpful in assessing the condition?

1. "Does your child have any sores on the scalp?"

2. "How long has your child been experiencing dandruff?"

3. "What type of shampoo do you use on the child?"

4. "Do you use oil on the child's hair?"

13. The parent of a child who has tinea capitis with a large kerion asks the nurse what a kerion is. The nurse replies it is

1. "a raised, red rash on the scalp."

2. "a moist, boggy area on the scalp."

3. "an ulcer on the scalp."

4. "a cut on the scalp."

14. A parent of a child with tinea corporis asks the nurse how it is contracted. The nurse should respond that it is contracted

1. by petting an infected kitten.

2. through a mosquito bite.

3. through a worm that has burrowed into the skin.

4. by touching a poison ivy plant.

15. The client with tinea corporis is prescribed ketoconazole (Nizoral) cream. The nurse should include which of the following in the instructions for care?

1. Apply the cream for one week

2. Use the cream for two to three days until the lesion clears

3. Continue using the cream for five to seven days after the lesion clears

4. Stop the cream as soon as the lesions clear

16. Oral ketoconazole (Nizoral) has been prescribed for a child with tinea versicolor. Which of the following instructions should the nurse give the parent and child regarding the use of the medication?

1. Take in the morning only

2. Take with a fatty meal

3. Take on an empty stomach

4. After taking the medication, exercise to work up a sweat

17. An adolescent plans to go to the beach after the appointment, and asks the nurse about the use of sunscreen. The nurse should offer which of the following instructions?

1. Apply the sunscreen after getting to the beach

2. If waterproof sunscreen is used, it does not have to be reapplied

3. Apply a thin layer of sunscreen to the body

4. Use sunscreen with a sun protection factor (SPF) of 15 or higher

18. A child taking an oral corticosteroid such as Orapred, Prelone, or Pediapred requires monthly follow-up appointments. Which of the following should be done at each visit?
Select all that apply:

[   ] 1. Monitor the weight

[   ] 2. Draw a blood sample for a CBC

[   ] 3. Assess the blood pressure

[   ] 4. Perform a physical examination

[   ] 5. Ask the client about diuresis

[   ] 6. Administer an antacid

19. The nurse is caring for a 1-month-old infant with a hemangioma on the anterior neck being treated with oral corticosteroids (Orapred, Prelone, Pediapred). Which of the following is most important to instruct the parents?

1. Administer the drug on an empty stomach

2. Avoid exposure to people who are sick

3. Do not get immunizations that contain live attenuated vaccines (MMR and varicella)

4. Go to the emergency room if stridor or difficulty breathing develops

20. The nurse should prepare a child with a port-wine stain on the face for which of the following treatments?

1. Pulsed dye laser

2. Excision

3. Injection with corticosteroids (Kenalog)

4. Oral antibiotics

21. Following laser treatment for a port-wine stain, which of the following should the nurse include in the home care instructions?

1. Keep the area moist with antibiotic ointment (Bacitracin, Polysporin)

2. The client will not experience any discomfort

3. Sun exposure will help to heal the area more quickly

4. The bruising will disappear in two days

22. A 6-month-old infant is diagnosed with impetigo. The parent asks what is necessary to prevent spreading to other family members. The nurse should tell the parent that the most effective way to prevent the spread of infection is

    1. washing bed linen after every use.
    2. good hand washing.
    3. wearing gown and gloves when holding the infant.
    4. washing the infant's skin to remove the honey crust.

23. A 6-year-old client presents with very small scaly plaques over the entire body. The diagnosis is guttate psoriasis. In taking the history, the nurse should ask if the client has recently had which of the following?

    1. Varicella
    2. Measles
    3. Strep infection
    4. Impetigo

24. A child with psoriasis asks the nurse to explain the Koebner phenomenon. The nurse replies, "The Koebner phenomenon

    1. refers to the severe itching the client experiences with psoriasis."
    2. indicates infection of the psoriatic lesions."
    3. is the clearing of scaling spontaneously."
    4. means that psoriatic lesions commonly occur at sites of trauma."

25. A 9-month-old infant brought to the clinic has bright red areas on the face, arms, and legs. The mother explains that they were at the zoo all morning. The nurse needs to instruct the parent regarding which of the following?

    1. Sun protection
    2. Eczema
    3. Psoriasis
    4. Port-wine stains

26. The registered nurse is preparing the clinical assignments for an integumentary unit. Which of the following assignments should the nurse delegate to a licensed practical nurse?

    1. Instruct a child with psoriasis to wear protective guards when participating in sports
    2. Report the characteristics of a child with a congenital nevus
    3. Assess the serum electrolyte levels in a child taking oral steroids
    4. Administer an analgesic to a child who sustained a burn

ANSWERS AND RATIONALES

1. **2.** With pediculosis capitis, nits are firmly attached to the hair shaft with a cement-like substance. The scalp must be treated with a pediculosis product. After rinsing, the hair must be combed with a fine-toothed comb to remove the nits. Scabies are itchy primarily at night.
   NP = An
   CN = He/3
   CL = An
   SA = 4

2. **2.** The best way to prevent other family members from getting lice is to wash all clothing and linens in hot water and dry them in a hot dryer to kill the lice. Items that cannot be washed can be sealed in a plastic bag for two weeks or dry cleaned.
   NP = An
   CN = He/3
   CL = An
   SA = 4

3. **1.** All family members and close contacts of a child with scabies should be treated with permethrin 5% (Elimite) even if asymptomatic. Apply the cream from the neck down in a thin layer. Leave on for 8 to 14 hours followed by showering or bathing.
   NP = Pl
   CN = He/3
   CL = Ap
   SA = 4

4. **1.** Congenital nevi are tan or brown macules or plaques that may have hair growth. There is a slightly increased risk of melanoma in a child with a small to medium congenital nevus. Following surgery for a congenital nevus, it is necessary to avoid physical activity for two to four weeks. This is to promote optimal healing and avoid dehiscence of the wound. Increased tension at the site can result in spreading of the scar.
   NP = Im
   CN = He/3
   CL = Ap
   SA = 4

5. **3.** A 16-year-old adolescent who presents with inflammatory papules and pustules is experiencing acne. Antibiotics have many adverse reactions including stomach upset, dizziness, and photosensitivity. The priority information to communicate to a potentially sexually active client is that

antibiotics may decrease the effectiveness of oral contraceptives. Untreated, acne can cause scarring.
NP = Im
CN = He/3
CL = An
SA = 4

6. **4.** There are many myths involving acne. Diet does not affect acne; however, eating sensibly is always advised. Washing the face with vigorous scrubbing and harsh soaps only irritates and inflames the skin. Cosmetics should be water-based and oil-free. Look for labels that say "noncomedogenic," which do not cause acne.
NP = Pl
CN = He/3
CL = Ap
SA = 4

7. **2.** Isotretinoin (Accutane) is a retinoid used in the treatment of severe recalcitrant acne unresponsive to standard therapy. The client should be monitored for depression, her liver, lipid, and CBC levels should be monitored, and she should be informed that there are no dietary restrictions. However, the priority intervention is to instruct the client that Accutane causes severe teratogenic effects, and two forms of birth control must be used while taking Accutane and for one month after treatment is completed.
NP = Pl
CN = Sa/1
CL = An
SA = 8

8. **1.** Atopic dermatitis is a chronic relapsing inflammation of the dermis and epidermis. In older children it is seen as dry, red, itchy patches on the flexural areas, including the antecubital spaces, the popliteal fossae, wrists, ankles, and neck. Dome-shaped, flesh-colored papules are found in molluscum contagiosum. An irregularly shaped reddish-purple macular vascular lesion is a port-wine stain. Scaly demarcated plaques over the entire body are consistent with psoriasis.
NP = Ev
CN = He/3
CL = An
SA = 4

9. **2.** Steroid ointments used to treat atopic dermatitis cannot penetrate an emollient and must be applied first. Bathing the child for a maximum of 10 minutes, applying emollients frequently during the day, and wearing cotton underwear are all appropriate interventions.

NP = Ev
CN = He/3
CL = An
SA = 4

10. **2.** Clinical manifestation of papules and vesicles on the wrists, waistline, and interdigital spaces are consistent with the diagnosis of scabies. The rash is intensely pruritic at night. A mineral oil prep is a microscopic examination that will show ova, feces, or a live mite. KOH is a potassium hydroxide test that examines hair, scales, and nails for superficial fungal infection. Wood's lamp examination of the skin with long-wave ultraviolet light causes specific substances to fluoresce.
NP = Im
CN = Ph/7
CL = An
SA = 4

11. **4.** Permethrin 5% cream (Elimite) is used in the treatment of scabies. It should be applied in a thin layer from the neck down, treating the entire body. Taking a warm shower or bath prior to application is not recommended because it may increase absorption and the possibility of toxicity.
NP = Pl
CN = He/3
CL = Ap
SA = 4

12. **1.** Tinea capitis is characterized by scaly patches, papules, and pustules and can be accompanied by hair loss.
NP = As
CN = He/3
CL = Ap
SA = 4

13. **2.** A kerion is a moist, boggy area on the scalp. It is a hypersensitivity reaction to the untreated fungus in tinea capitis.
NP = An
CN = He/3
CL = Ap
SA = 4

14. **1.** Tinea corporis is a superficial fungal infection of the skin that is spread by direct contact with an infected person, animal, or soil.
NP = An
CN = He/3
CL = Ap
SA = 4

15. **3.** Tinea corporis is a superficial fungal infection of the skin characterized by an annular, well-circumscribed scaly patch that may have a central clearing and a scaly vesicular, papular, or pustular border. Rapid improvement is often seen after application of ketoconazole (Nizoral). The cream should be continued five to seven days after the lesion clears to completely treat the tinea and to prevent recurrence.
NP = Pl
CN = Ph/6
CL = Ap
SA = 5

16. **4.** A child who has tinea versicolor should take the oral ketoconazole (Nizoral) and then exercise to work up a sweat and sleep in the sweat. Showering should be avoided until the morning. This allows the medication to work.
NP = Pl
CN = Ph/6
CL = Ap
SA = 5

17. **4.** Use sunscreen with a sun protection factor (SPF) of 15 or higher. Apply 30 minutes before sun exposure and use liberally. One ounce usually covers the average body. Reapply at least every two hours and more frequently if swimming.
NP = Pl
CN = He/3
CL = Ap
SA = 4

18. **1, 2, 3, 4.** The weight and blood pressure should be assessed at monthly follow-up appointments for a child taking an oral corticosteroid. A physical exam will be done at each visit to monitor the effectiveness and the development of adverse reactions related to treatment. Although steroids cause gastrointestinal adverse reactions, they should not be given with an antacid, because the antacid decreases the effectiveness of the steroid. Edema, not diuresis, occurs. Serum glucose and electrolytes should be assessed.
NP = Pl
CN = Ph/6
CL = Ap
SA = 5

19. **4.** The most rapid growth phase of a hemangioma is between 1 and 4 months. A hemangioma on the anterior neck may grow large enough to occlude the airway and cause respiratory distress. This is a medical emergency and should be treated in the emergency room. Oral

corticosteroids (Orapred, Prelone, Pediapred) are given to prevent growth and avoid the occluded airway and respiratory distress.

NP = Pl

CN = Ph/6

CL = Ap

SA = 5

20. **1.** Port-wine stains are capillary malformations that are present at birth. Pulsed dye laser is the treatment of choice for port-wine stains. They should be treated to prevent thickening and darkening of the stain and the development of angiomas.

NP = Im

CN = Ph/7

CL = An

SA = 4

21. **1.** Pulsed dye laser is the treatment of choice for a child with a port-wine stain. It prevents thickening and darkening of the stain and the development of angiomas. The area should be kept moist to promote healing. Sun exposure should be avoided because the area will be very sensitive to sun. Discomfort should be treated with analgesics. Bruising will take about two weeks to disappear.

NP = Pl

CN = Ph/7

CL = Ap

SA = 4

22. **2.** Impetigo is a highly contagious superficial skin infection. Good hand washing is the most effective way to prevent the spread of impetigo.

NP = Pl

CN = Ph/7

CL = An

SA = 4

23. **3.** Guttate psoriasis usually follows a strep infection and is characterized by very small scaly plaques over the entire body.

NP = As

CN = He/3

CL = An

SA = 4

24. **4.** The Koebner phenomenon refers to the fact that psoriatic lesions commonly occur at sites of repeated trauma. The most common sites are the knees, elbows, scalp, and fingernails.

NP = An

CN = He/3

CL = Ap
SA = 4

25. **1.** Since skin cancer accounts for half of all cancers diagnosed in the United States each year, sun protection is essential in skin cancer prevention.
NP = Im
CN = He/3
CL = Ap
SA = 4

26. **4.** Instructing a child, reporting disease characteristics, and assessing the serum laboratory data are tasks that should be performed by the registered nurse. A licensed practical nurse may administer a prescribed analgesic.
NP = Pl
CN = Sa/1
CL = An
SA = 8

MUSCULOSKELETAL DISORDERS - COMPREHENSIVE EXAM

1. A 9-year-old child was seen in the outpatient clinic after a fall from a tree. Radiographs ruled out a fracture of the tibia. Before sending the child home, the nurse instructs the child to do which of the following in the next 24 hours?

1. Apply a heating pad to the sore spot to increase blood flow

2. Elevate the affected extremity on a pillow while watching a video

3. Dangle the foot to increase circulation

4. Perform range-of-motion exercises and ambulate as much as possible to decrease stiffness

2. A school nurse is conducting a musculoskeletal assessment of the students in a fifth grade class. The nurse should be concerned with which of the following observations?

1. Almost 90% of the girls are taller than the boys

2. There is no significant difference in muscle strength in girls and boys

3. Boys are more interested in gross motor activity

4. Two of the girls have asymmetry of the scapula

3. A nurse is caring for a child after a bone scan. Which of the following orders should the nurse question?

1. Monitor the IV site for redness, swelling, or hematoma

2. Administer a pain medication as necessary

3. Encourage an increase in fluid intake for 24 to 48 hours

4. Elevate the extremity and limit range of motion for 24 hours

4. A nurse is caring for a child who is going to have a computerized tomography (CT) with contrast. Which action by the nurse would be the priority?

1. Ask the child and family if there are any questions about the procedure

2. Assess the child's attention span and activity level

3. Label the child's chart with an allergy to shellfish

4. Administer preprocedural sedation as ordered

5. A nurse witnessed a small boy being hit by a moving vehicle at the baseball park. The child is dazed, crying, and trying to get up and find the parents. The right leg appears fractured. Which of the following actions should the nurse take?

1. Stay with and calm the child and send someone to call for help

2. Assist the child to get up and walk to a safer place

3. Leave the child with a responsible friend and find the parents

4. Try to immobilize the extremity while manually palpating the suspected fracture site

6. Which of the following should the nurse include in the discharge teaching plan for the parents of an 8-month-old with a plaster cast?

1. Importance of cast changes at follow-up visits

2. Use a dull pencil to scratch around the top of the cast

3. Keep the cast clean by washing it and drying with a blow dryer

4. Maintain the cast in a dependent position

7. During an earlier visit, a clinic nurse gave discharge instructions about caring for a fiberglass cast to a school-age child and the parents. Which of the following statements during a follow-up visit would indicate that the child and parents need further instruction?

1. "I wouldn't let my child come into the kitchen while I was mopping the floor."

2. "We have been using a damp cloth to wipe the dirt off the cast."

3. "I had to dry the cast with a hair dryer set on cool once after taking a shower."

4. "My child loves to play hide and seek with matchbox cars and the top portion of the cast."

8. The nurse should include which of the following in the plan of care for a child in Buck's traction?

    1. Assess the skeletal traction setup

    2. Place the child in a supine position with both legs flexed slightly less than 90 degrees

    3. Perform pin site care every shift

    4. Maintain the immobilization of the extremity

9. A nurse is caring for a school-aged child in Buck's traction to the right leg. The nurse should perform which of the following interventions to prevent complications of the traction?

    1. Provide video movies and games

    2. Release the weights on the right leg once per shift

    3. Massage the skin of the extremities with antibacterial lotion morning and evening

    4. Inspect and provide pin site care once a shift

10. Which of the following assessments of the skeletal traction pin sites of a child in skeletal traction is a priority to report?

    1. Inflammation

    2. Pain at the pin site

    3. Serous drainage

    4. Pallor and coolness of toes

11. Which of the following assessment findings would the nurse discover in a 2-week-old infant with congenital clubfoot?
    Select all that apply:

    [   ] 1. Flexible range of motion of feet and ankles

    [   ] 2. Plantar flexion

    [   ] 3. Heel inversion

    [   ] 4. Bilateral pedal pulses with a positive Babinski

    [   ] 5. Adducted left forefoot

    [   ] 6. Notable pes varus of right foot

12. The nurse is providing follow-up teaching to a mother of a male newborn diagnosed with clubfoot. Which of the following statements by the mother indicates the mother does not understand the teaching and more instruction is needed?

    1. "I realize my baby will start treatment as soon as possible."

    2. "These casts are only needed until my baby outgrows this problem."

3. "I've told the people at work that I will have to bring the baby to the clinic every week."

4. "Hopefully, my baby will not require surgery but we will have to watch his feet until he is grown."

13. The nurse assesses a 4-week-old infant suspected of having congenital hip dysplasia. Which of the following clinical manifestations would be most supportive of this diagnosis?
Select all that apply:

[　] 1. Bilateral symmetry of lower femur, tibia, and fibula

[　] 2. Flexible range of motion of all extremities

[　] 3. Abduction of affected hip when the infant is supine with knees and hips flexed

[　] 4. Symmetry of the gluteal folds when prone or suspended in upright position

[　] 5. Toe walking

[　] 6. Unequal level of the pelvis

14. The nurse observes the physician assessing the infant with hip dysplasia using Ortolani's maneuver. The nurse informs the parent that this test is performed for which of the following reasons?

1. Push the femoral head out of the acetabulum

2. Evaluate range of motion of both extremities

3. Assess for length, strength, and symmetry of extremities

4. Determine the extent of dislocation by manipulating the femoral head back into the acetabulum

15. The nurse should include which of the following interventions in the post-op care for a child following surgery for hip dysplasia?

1. Assess neurovascular status with a hip spica cast

2. Teach the parents how to apply a Pavlik harness

3. Keep the child sedated for the first 24 hours after surgery

4. Prepare the child and family for traction care in the home setting

16. The nurse assessing a toddler suspects osteogenesis imperfecta (OI). Which of the following assessment findings caused the nurse to suspect this condition?

1. Normal height and weight for age

2. Blue discoloration of sclera

3. Congenital cleft lip and palate previously diagnosed

4. Stiffness of all joints of upper and lower body

17. The nurse is planning a teaching plan for the parents of a child with osteogenesis imperfecta (OI). Which of the following statements by the mother indicates a lack of knowledge related to this condition?

1. ''I use extreme care moving the joints when bathing, dressing, and diapering my child.''

2. ''We make sure that our child performs dental care each day and gets a check-up once a year.''

3. ''It was so sad and hard to take care of our child at birth because of a skull fracture.''

4. ''If I hadn't smoked and hadn't drunk alcohol while I was pregnant, we wouldn't have to deal with this.''

18. The nurse is assessing a 16-year-old high-school baseball pitcher who is complaining of ''arm pain.'' The physician determines a sprain of the elbow and shoulder with microtrauma. Which of the following home care instructions would be most appropriate?

1. Elevate the affected extremity over the head for 30 minutes three times a day

2. Apply ice to the affected joint for 20 to 30 minutes, as needed, during the first 6 to 12 hours

3. Use heat and compression to soothe the stiffness of the muscle and joint

4. Perform range-of-motion exercises twice a day for the first 24 to 48 hours to maintain looseness of the joint

19. A 10-year-old male is seen by the school nurse with a chief complaint of ''pain in right hip and top of thigh.'' Which of the following additional clinical manifestations caused the nurse to suspect Legg-Calvé-Perthes disease?

1. Equal bilateral muscle strength with flexible range of motion after rest period

2. History of strep throat 21 days ago

3. Observed limping to class after physical education class

4. Report of discomfort that is increased after periods of rest

20. During an admission, the nurse caring for a child with slipped femoral capital epiphysis (SFCE) would expect to find which of the following upon initial assessment?

1. No visible physiologic findings

2. Presence of a limp and delayed strength in range of motion

3. Observation of gait shows an external rotation of the hip

4. An absence of pain

21. The school nurse assesses children of all ages for spinal deformities. Which of the following indicates that the nurse has an appropriate understanding of spinal assessment of children?

   1. Scoliosis is a lateral curvature of the spine that becomes prominent before and during the growth spurt of juvenility

   2. An increased anterior/posterior curvature of the lumbar spine is never normal at any age

   3. Spinal deformities are generally diagnosed before the child is 4 years old

   4. All spinal deformities will require pre- and postoperative teaching plans

22. Which of the following is a priority for the nurse to include in a teaching plan for a teenage girl diagnosed with scoliosis?

   1. Carefully select physical activities to minimize the progressive curvature of the spinal defect

   2. Promote age-appropriate activities of daily living before, during, and after medical treatment

   3. Prepare the teenager for impending surgery that will occur in late adolescence after immobility management with braces

   4. Stress the importance of pursuing low-impact exercises during the adult years following treatment of scoliosis

ANSWERS AND RATIONALES

1. **2.** Therapeutic management following a fall from a tree in which a fracture was ruled out would include RICE (rest, ice, compression, and elevation). Watching a video is an age-appropriate developmental activity.
   NP = Pl
   CN = He/3
   CL = Ap
   SA = 4

2. **4.** Since girls begin a growth spurt in late school age, asymmetry of scapula or hip may be indicative of scoliosis.
   NP = An
   CN = He/3
   CL = An
   SA = 4

3. **4.** There is no activity restriction necessary after a bone scan. Monitoring the child's condition including the IV site after the procedure,

administering p.r.n. meds for discomfort, and increasing fluids are acceptable interventions.

NP = An
CN = Ph/7
CL = Ap
SA = 4

4. **3.** Contrast material for a computerized tomography (CT) scan often includes iodine or shellfish derivatives. All clients should be assessed for allergy to these prior to start of the procedure.

NP = Im
CN = Ph/7
CL = Ap
SA = 4

5. **1.** The nurse should remain with the child following a fracture of the leg to assess the child's condition. The nurse should send other observers to call for emergency help and find the parents. Before the child is moved, the leg should be immobilized.

NP = Im
CN = Ph/7
CL = An
SA = 4

6. **1.** Cast changes during clinic appointments are very important because children grow rapidly during the infant years. Scratching should never be allowed with a pencil or any other object, because this may cause injury to the skin. A hair dryer set on a cool setting may be used to reduce itching. The cast should be prevented from getting wet. Plastic wrapping or a bag may be used during bathing to prevent the cast from becoming wet. The cast should be elevated above the level of the heart to prevent swelling and improve circulation.

NP = Pl
CN = He/3
CL = Ap
SA = 4

7. **4.** Nothing should ever be put inside a cast, including objects used to scratch under the cast.

NP = Ev
CN = He/3
CL = An
SA = 4

8. **4.** Buck's traction is used for short-term immobilization to decrease muscle spasm. A boot is applied to the skin and traction applied to the boot.

Countertraction is then applied to the body. It is not a skeletal traction setup and does not lengthen bone. A child placed in Bryant's traction is in a supine position with both legs flexed slightly less than 90 degrees.

NP = Pl

CN = He/3

CL = An

SA = 4

9. **1.** Age-appropriate diversional activities are the priority for children restricted by immobility devices. Buck's traction is skin traction not a skeletal traction. Lotions and removal of weights are contraindicated unless ordered by a physician.

NP = Im

CN = He/3

CL = Ap

SA = 4

10. **4.** Although inflammation, pain at the pin site, and serous drainage may be found at the pin site, pallor and coolness of extremity may be early signs of neurovascular complications, and the priority is to report this finding.

NP = As

CN = Sa/1

CL = An

SA = 8

11. **2, 3, 5.** Plantar flexion, heel inversion, and an adducted left forefoot are the classic clinical manifestations of unilateral left clubfoot. Joints of the feet and ankles are rigid. Pes varus on toeing in may be present, but is not indicative of clubfoot. Pulses and reflexes (Babinski) are normal for an infant.

NP = As

CN = He/3

CL = Ap

SA = 4

12. **2.** Serial casting is a major part of the treatment of clubfoot. It consists of a series of casts being applied, generally over a three-month period. The casts are changed every one to two weeks until complete correction has occurred. If the condition is not corrected by casting, surgery is required. After surgery, casting is also required. After the casting, braces are required.

NP = Ev

CN = He/3

CL = An

SA = 4

13. 3, 5, 6. Classic manifestations of developmental dysplasia of the hip include abduction of the affected hip and, as the child grows, toe walking and an unequal level of the pelvis. Generally, asymmetry of thigh gluteal folds and apparent shortening of the femur are also noted. The clinical manifestations get worse the longer the condition goes undiagnosed.
NP = As
CN = He/3
CL = Ap
SA = 4

14. 4. Ortolani's maneuver for the hip allows for reduction of the head of the femur into the acetabulum and includes palpation for a click upon reduction.
NP = Im
CN = He/3
CL = An
SA = 4

15. 1. Surgery for hip dysplasia is performed to reduce the dislocated hip. Following surgery, a hip spica cast is applied. Performing a neurovascular assessment would be an appropriate intervention. A Pavlik harness is worn preoperatively. Routine pain medication, not sedation, is given as necessary. Traction is not indicated in the home pre- or postoperatively.
NP = Pl
CN = He/3
CL = Ap
SA = 4

16. 2. Osteogenesis imperfecta, also known as the brittle bone disease, is a connective tissue disorder characterized by a disturbed formation of the periosteal bone. Common clinical manifestations include scleral discoloration, hyperlaxity of ligaments, short stature, and multiple fractures.
NP = As
CN = He/3
CL = Ap
SA = 4

17. 4. Osteogenesis imperfecta, known as the brittle bone disease, is genetically transmitted. It may occur at birth or as the child grows. It is not associated with the mother smoking or drinking during pregnancy. Dental caries is an associated problem as well as multiple fractures.
NP = Ev
CN = He/3
CL = An
SA = 4

18. **2.** Medical management for a sprain is ice, compression, elevation, and support (ICES) during the first 6 to 12 hours after injury.
NP = Pl
CN = He/3
CL = Ap
SA = 4

19. **3.** Legg-Calvé-Perthes disease is an avascular necrosis of the femoral head with collapse followed by regeneration. Limited range of motion, stiffness in mornings or after rest, a limp that is aggravated by increased activity, shortened affected limb, and positive Trendelenburg sign are all clinical manifestations. Definitive diagnosis is made by x-ray and bone scan.
NP = As
CN = He/3
CL = Ap
SA = 4

20. **3.** Slipped femoral capital epiphysis is a condition in which the upper femoral epiphysis gradually slips from its functional position. Pain in extremity hip-to-thigh-to-knee is reported along with decreased range of motion and internal rotation of the hip. Gait indicates external rotation of the hip to relieve stress and pain at the joint.
NP = As
CN = He/3
CL = An
SA = 4

21. **1.** Scoliosis is a lateral curvature of the spine occurring most often during the adolescent growth spurt, which generally occurs between 11 and 14 years for girls and 13 and 16 years for boys. Lordosis is an increased anterior curvature of the lumbar spine; it is normal in toddlers and pregnant females. Conservative treatment includes bracing and exercises prior to any surgical treatment.
NP = An
CN = He/3
CL = An
SA = 4

22. **2.** The promotion of age-appropriate developmental activity is a priority of any approach to therapeutic management, and the treatment of scoliosis is no exception.
NP = Pl
CN = He/3
CL = An
SA = 4

Practice Test 3

1. The nurse caring for the child with osteomyelitis is preparing the child and parents for home management. Which of the following statements by the parent is an indication that additional teaching is needed?

    1. "At the first sign of a fever, I am going to call the pediatrician's office."

    2. "I'm glad the medicine was given in the hospital and won't have to be taken at home."

    3. "I know rest is important but I will need to get plenty of games and videos."

    4. "I'm glad we caught this early and avoided complications."

2. A 4-year-old boy has just been diagnosed with Duchenne's muscular dystrophy. The parents ask the nurse if their infant daughter will also show symptoms of the disease. The nurse's best response would be

    1. "Each of your children has a 25% chance of having the disease and a 50% chance of being a carrier."

    2. "Each of your sons has a 25% chance of having the disease, and your daughters will not be affected."

    3. "Each of your sons has a 50% chance of having the disease, and each of your daughters has a 50% chance of being a carrier."

    4. "Every child in your family has a 50% chance of having the disease."

3. A 9-year-old child has recently been diagnosed with rheumatoid arthritis. The nurse has developed a teaching plan for the child and family. Which of the following would be the priority to include in the teaching plan?

1. Develop an exercise plan for home and school

2. Organize the day with prolonged periods of rest

3. Assist the child and family in development of a diet plan high in protein, vitamin C, and other herbal supplements

4. Suggest to the child's counselor that the child be moved to a special class schedule for special education students

4. The registered nurse is delegating nursing tasks for a musculoskeletal unit. Which of the following activities should the nurse delegate to unlicensed assistive personnel?

1. Place a child with dysplasia of the hip in a Pavlik harness

2. Perform a scoliosis screening

3. Bathe a child with a hip spica cast

4. Place a child in Buck's traction

ANSWERS AND RATIONALES

1. **2.** Osteomyelitis is an infection of the bone caused by a microorganism. The child will be discharged, but will need additional oral antibiotic therapy for as long as two weeks.
NP = Ev
CN = He/3
CL = An
SA = 4

2. **3.** Duchenne's muscular dystrophy is an X-linked recessive disorder. The defective gene is transmitted through carrier females to affected sons 50% of the time, depending on which X is transmitted. Daughters have a 50% chance of becoming carriers of this disease. With autosomal recessive disorders, both parents are carriers of a trait, and each male child has a 25% chance of having the disease but the female children are unaffected.
NP = An
CN = He/3
CL = An
SA = 4

3. **1.** A child with rheumatoid arthritis should be encouraged to participate in normal activities of daily living that include exercise to promote joint mobility, muscle tone, and strength.
NP = Pl
CN = Sa/1
CL = An
SA = 4

4. 3. It is appropriate for unlicensed assistive personnel to bathe a child in a hip spica cast. Performing a scoliosis screening, placing a child in a Pavlik harness, and placing a child in Buck's traction are all tasks that require the skills of a nurse.
NP = Pl
CN = Sa/1
CL = An
SA = 8

GENITOURINARY DISORDERS - COMPREHENSIVE EXAM

1. The nurse informs the parents of a child that the primary indicator of vesicoureteral reflux is _____ .

2. The nurse is caring for a child who had a urethral stent placed during hypospadias surgery. Which of the following drugs should the nurse administer when the child experiences bladder spasms?

   1. Acetaminophen (Tylenol)

   2. Oxybutynin chloride (Ditropan)

   3. Desmopressin acetate (DDAVP)

   4. Furosemide (Lasix)

3. The nurse is caring for a 2-month-old child with an inguinal hernia. Which of the following would indicate to the nurse that the infant's hernia has strangulated?
Select all that apply:

   [ ] 1. Reddened scrotum

   [ ] 2. Bradycardia

   [ ] 3. Inconsolable crying

   [ ] 4. Abdominal distention

   [ ] 5. Pain

   [ ] 6. Lethargy

4. The parents of a child with secondary nephrotic syndrome ask the nurse what the usual treatment is. The nurse explains, ''The priority treatment for nephrotic syndrome is to promote a remission by

   1. administering corticosteroid therapy.''

   2. restricting the salt intake.''

   3. administering diuretics.''

   4. maintaining a strict intake and output.''

5. Two hours after giving birth, a mother expresses concern to the nurse that her infant has not voided. The appropriate response by the nurse is which of the following?

    1. "You need not worry unless your infant has not voided for 12 hours."

    2. "I will notify your physician of your concern."

    3. "Voiding in newborns generally occurs within 48 hours after being born."

    4. "I will offer your infant more fluids to promote voiding."

6. Which of the following should the nurse include in the education provided to the parents of a child born with cryptorchidism?
Select all that apply:

    [   ] **1.** High-birth-weight infant boys have a higher incidence

    [   ] **2.** An orchiopexy should be performed within the first three months of life to prevent infertility later in life

    [   ] **3.** There is an increased incidence of cancer of the testis as an adult

    [   ] **4.** Human chorionic gonadotropin (HCG) may be used to induce the descent of the testis

    [   ] **5.** Unilateral cryptorchidism is most common and particularly affects the right testis

    [   ] **6.** Decreased spermatogenesis is not an issue after successful treatment

7. The parents of a 3-year-old bring the child to a clinic because the child has been experiencing nocturnal enuresis. Which of the following statements by the nurse is most appropriate for these parents?

    1. "I will talk to your physician about medication to stop the enuresis."

    2. "The enuresis should be evaluated for a possible structural cause."

    3. "Voluntary control of urine may not be achieved until 5 years of age."

    4. "You need not be concerned since it is only nocturnal enuresis."

8. A male child receiving topical testosterone cream has developed engorgement of the genitalia, localized acne, and pubic hair. In determining what action to take next, which of the following factors should the nurse consider?

    1. The strength of the testosterone cream will need to be reduced

    2. These adverse reactions will resolve when the testosterone is discontinued

    3. The testosterone cream should be applied less frequently

    4. These adverse reactions will not occur if the testosterone is taken orally

9. Desmopressin acetate (DDAVP) has been prescribed for a child with cystic fibrosis and enuresis. Which of the following is the priority nursing action?

   1. Place the child on a strict intake and output

   2. Monitor the child for headaches, nausea, nasal congestion, and epistaxis

   3. Call the physician and question the order

   4. Instruct the parents to avoid over-the-counter products containing epinephrine

10. The nurse is caring for a child with acute glomerulonephritis. Which of the following measures would be essential to include in the child's plan of care?

    1. Monitor the child for dribbling after voiding

    2. Encourage small, frequent high-protein meals

    3. Weigh the child at the same time of day with similar clothes

    4. Establish a regular voiding schedule

11. Which of the following questions should the nurse ask the parents of a child with enuresis?

    1. "Did any of your other children experience enuresis?"

    2. "Have you noticed your child drinking more?"

    3. "Are you able to successfully discipline your child?"

    4. "Is your child also experiencing constipation?"

12. The nurse working on a pediatric unit is evaluating 24-hour urine outputs of four children. Which of the following 24-hour outputs should the nurse report?
    Select all that apply:

    [ ] 1. A 10-day-old infant who voided 336 ml

    [ ] 2. A 6-month-old child who voided 280 ml

    [ ] 3. A 2-year-old child who voided 450 ml

    [ ] 4. A 4-year-old child who voided 640 ml

    [ ] 5. A 7-year-old who voided 1000 ml

    [ ] 6. A 13-year-old who voided 720 ml

13. Which of the following should the nurse include when collecting a midstream urine specimen from an 8-month-old infant?

    1. Wash hands, remove diaper, and cleanse the genital area with three soapy cotton balls

    2. Moving downward with gloved hands, cleanse the penis of a male infant with soapy cotton balls

3. Moving from back to front with gloved hands, cleanse the genital area of a female infant with warm, soapy cotton balls

4. After drying the skin around the genital area, remove the adhesive from the collection bag and apply it securely

14. After applying a urine collection bag to a 3-month-old infant for a midstream urine specimen, the nurse should monitor the bag for a minimum of how many ml of urine to ensure that the laboratory has an adequate sample for a culture and sensitivity test?_____

15. Which of the following should the nurse include in a class for the parents of children recently diagnosed with renal failure?
    1. Renal failure is generally transient, caused by dehydration, and responds to the administration of fluids
    2. Bradypnea, anxiousness, and muscle irritability are common manifestations in acute renal failure
    3. A diet with foods high in potassium and protein should be served in an attractive manner
    4. Hypotension, excessive energy, and menorrhagia are common clinical manifestations of chronic renal failure

16. The nurse should monitor a child receiving imipramine hydrochloride (Tofranil) for which of the following adverse reactions?
    Select all that apply:
    [ ] 1. Dry mouth
    [ ] 2. Changes in personality
    [ ] 3. Listlessness
    [ ] 4. Diarrhea
    [ ] 5. Polyuria
    [ ] 6. Insomnia

17. The nurse is admitting a child with bladder exstrophy. Which of the following assessments would be essential to make this diagnosis?
    1. Difficulty walking and a waddling gait
    2. Visible deformity
    3. Undescended testes
    4. Absence of a vagina

18. When working with a child who has hypospadias, the nurse should include which of the following considerations in planning the goals of of care?

1. Surgery is the treatment of choice generally performed before the child reaches the age of 18 months

2. Circumcision should be done within the first two days of life

3. Desmopressin acetate (DDAVP) should routinely be administered in the care of the child

4. Human chorionic gonadotropin (HCG) may be given for a short period of time after the diagnosis is made

19. Which of the following should the nurse include in the plan of care of a 7-year-old child with a urinary tract infection?

    1. Increase fluids to 50 ml/kg or 25 ml/lb of body weight

    2. Instruct the parents to have the child wear nylon underwear

    3. Monitor the child for urinary hesitancy and retention

    4. Instruct the parents to avoid giving the child bubble baths

20. The nurse is evaluating the laboratory results of four pediatric clients. Which of the following results should the nurse report?

    1. A creatinine level of 0.9 mg/dl in a 16-year-old adolescent

    2. A blood urea nitrogen (BUN) of 20 mg/dl in a newborn

    3. A potassium level of 3.8 mEq/L in a 6-year-old child

    4. A sodium level of 142 mEq/L in a 1-year-old infant

21. When preparing a 1-year-old child with chronic renal failure for an intravenous pyelography (IVP), it would be essential for the nurse to plan to explain which of the following aspects of the procedure?

    1. NPO after midnight the day before the procedure

    2. A Fleet enema will be administered the evening before the procedure

    3. The procedure will be performed early in the morning

    4. Withhold solid food but not fluids for eight hours before the procedure

22. The nurse is observing a staff member preparing a 6-year-old male child for the insertion of a Foley catheter. Which of the following would indicate the staff member is performing the task correctly?

    1. Lift the penis to a 45 degree angle to the body

    2. Hold the penile shaft on top of the glans

    3. Apply a lubricant to the end of the urethra prior to the insertion of the catheter

    4. Insert a size 8 Foley catheter

23. The nurse is collecting a nursing history on a child suspected of having acute glomerulonephritis. Which of the following questions would elicit the most accurate information?

1. "Does your child have a diet high in protein?"

2. "Has your child recently had a streptococcal infection?"

3. "Did your child recently sustain an injury to the flank area?"

4. "Does you child drink a sufficient amount of fluids daily?"

24. The nurse should assist a child with acute glomerulonephritis make which of the following menu selections?

    1. Baked ham, baked potato, broccoli, orange, and whole milk

    2. Peanut butter sandwich, potato chips, pickle, and skim milk

    3. Grilled pork chop, mashed potato, green beans, banana, and tea

    4. Turkey sandwich, carrot and celery sticks, apple, and tea

25. The mother of a child suspected of having nephrotic syndrome asks the nurse why her 4-year-old seems to continually be gaining weight and "puffy." Which of the following should the nurse consider before responding to the mother?

    1. Abdominal swelling and lower extremity edema is common during the day

    2. Rapid weight gain is common at this age

    3. Children of this age have high-fat, high-calorie diets

    4. A slow development of generalized edema may initially be confused with normal growth

26. Which of the following should the nurse include in the plan of care for a child with chronic renal failure?
    Select all that apply:

    [ ] 1. Encourage vitamin A, E, and K supplements

    [ ] 2. Administer prescribed aluminum hydroxyl gel

    [ ] 3. Administer prescribed oxybutynin chloride (Ditropan)

    [ ] 4. Assess for dental complications

    [ ] 5. Monitor the blood pressure

    [ ] 6. Offer a high-protein diet

27. The registered nurse is preparing to delegate the nursing tasks on a genitourinary unit. Which of the following tasks should the nurse delegate to a licensed practical nurse?

    1. Insert a Foley catheter into a child

    2. Assess a child for complications of renal failure

    3. Monitor the laboratory data on a client in hemolytic uremic syndrome

    4. Instruct the parents of a child with acute glomerulonephritis on the dietary management

ANSWERS AND RATIONALES

1. **recurrent urinary tract infections.** Recurrent urinary tract infections are the primary indicators of vesicoureteral reflux. Less common clinical manifestations include urinary incontinence, flank pain, and abdominal pain. These are vague indicators that often are associated with other disorders.
   NP = Im
   CN = He/3
   CL = An
   SA = 4

2. **2.** Following hypospadias surgery, a urethral stent may be inserted to ensure urinary drainage and facilitate patency. Oxybutynin chloride (Ditropan) is the drug of choice to alleviate bladder spasms associated with the stent and surgery. Acetaminophen (Tylenol) is a nonopioid analgesic generally used to treat mild to moderate pain. Desmopressin acetate (DDAVP) is a synthetic analog of vasopressin used in the treatment of nocturnal enuresis that acts by increasing water retention and urine concentration. Furosemide (Lasix) is a potent diuretic used to increase urinary output.
   NP = Pl
   CN = Ph/6
   CL = An
   SA = 4

3. **1, 3, 4, 5.** A hernia becomes strangulated when the herniated intestines become trapped, edematous, and twisted, which results in the blood supply being cut off. Ischemia and obstruction of the bowel may lead to necrosis and perforation. Clinical manifestations of a strangulated hernia include a scrotum that has become red, a distended abdomen, extreme irritability, and a child that cannot be consoled. Other, more vague, clinical manifestations include vomiting and tachycardia.
   NP = An
   CN = Ph/7
   CL = An
   SA = 4

4. **1.** The priority treatment for nephrotic syndrome is to administer corticosteroids, particularly prednisolone (Prelone) to promote a remission. Corticosteroids decrease the inflammation and the loss of protein, and restore oncotic pressure while promoting diuresis. Restricting the salt intake and maintaining a strict intake and output are

important interventions, but are not the priorities. Diuretics are not administered unless severe edema is present.

NP = An
CN = Sa/1
CL = An
SA = 4

5. **3.** Renal blood flow significantly increases after birth, with the kidney taking over the role of the placenta. Voiding generally occurs within 48 hours after birth.

NP = An
CN = He/3
CL = An
SA = 4

6. **3, 4, 5.** Cryptorchidism, or undescended testis, is the failure of one or both testes to descend into the scrotum. Normally, the testes descend into the scrotum during the third trimester. Typically, cryptorchidism occurs in premature infants and is unilateral, affecting the right testis. There is an increased incidence of both infertility and cancer of the testis later in life. Treatment generally includes waiting to see if the testis descends within the first year of life. Human chorionic gonadotropin (HCG) may also be given to increase the production of testosterone to assist in the descent of the testis.

NP = Pl
CN = He/3
CL = An
SA = 4

7. **3.** Voluntary control of urine should not be considered abnormal until after the age of 5 years.

NP = An
CN = He/3
CL = An
SA = 4

8. **2.** Common adverse reactions that occur with testosterone cream include enlargement and growth of the genitalia, localized acne, and growth of pubic hair. All of these adverse reactions will resolve when the cream is discontinued.

NP = An
CN = Ph/6
CL = An
SA = 5

9. 3. The priority nursing intervention is for the nurse to question an order for desmopressin acetate (DDAVP) for a child with cystic fibrosis. DDAVP is contraindicated for a child with cystic fibrosis or renal disease because fluid and electrolyte imbalances are potential adverse reactions. DDAVP is a pituitary hormone that works to increase water retention and urine concentration. Placing the child on a strict intake and output and monitoring the child for adverse reactions, such as headaches, nausea, nasal congestion, and epistaxis, are important interventions but are not the priorities. Avoiding over-the-counter products containing epinephrine is also an important intervention, because products containing epinephrine decrease the effectiveness of the DDAVP.
NP = Im
CN = Sa/1
CL = Ap
SA = 4

10. 3. Weighing the child at the same time of day with similar clothes is important in the plan of care for a child with glomerulonephritis. An increase in weight reflects fluid retention and a decrease in weight reflects a return of normal renal function or an intake that is not sufficient to meet the demands of the body. The appropriate diet should be low in both sodium and protein. Dribbling after voiding and establishing a voiding schedule are interventions that are useful in the treatment of enuresis.
NP = Pl
CN = He/3
CL = Ap
SA = 4

11. 4. It is essential to assess if a child experiencing enuresis is also experiencing constipation. Enuresis and constipation should be treated simultaneously to obtain a resolution of both. To treat only one problem may result in a failure to show improvement.
NP = As
CN = He/3
CL = An
SA = 4

12. 2, 3, 6. A 10-day to 2-month-old newborn should normally void between 250 ml and 400 ml in a 24-hour period. A 2-month- to 1-year-old infant should void 400 ml to 500 ml. A child who is 1 to 3 years of age should void between 500 ml and 600 ml. A child who is 3 to 5 years of age should void 600 ml to 700 ml. A child who is 5 to 8 years of age should void between 700 ml and 1000 ml. A child who is 8 years of age should void 800

ml to 1400 ml. Any deviations from these norms should be reported as abnormal, necessitating further evaluation.

NP = An
CN = Ph/7
CL = An
SA = 4

13. **4.** Before obtaining a urine specimen by a midstream catch, gloves should be donned and the existing diaper removed. The nurse should then wash the hands and don fresh gloves to cleanse the genital area. The nurse should cleanse toward the penis in a male infant and from front to back in a female infant with one warm soapy cotton ball at a time. After drying the skin around the genital area, the adhesive should be removed and the collection bag should be securely applied.

NP = Pl
CN = Ph/7
CL = Ap
SA = 4

14. **20.** A minimum of 20 ml should be collected when performing a midstream urine specimen for a culture and sensitivity test.

NP = As
CN = Ph/7
CL = An
SA = 4

15. **1.** Renal failure is an uncommon disorder that is generally transient and most frequently caused by dehydration. It responds to the administration of fluids. Common clinical manifestations of acute renal failure include tachypnea, listlessness, and hypocalcemia (muscle twitching is an indication of hypercalcemia). A diet with foods low in potassium and protein should be offered in an attractive manner. Hypertension, loss of energy, and amenorrhea are clinical manifestations of chronic renal failure.

NP = Pl
CN = He/3
CL = An
SA = 4

16. **1, 2, 6.** Imipramine hydrochloride (Tofranil) is a tricyclic antidepressant used in the treatment of enuresis to decrease the depth of sleep in the latter part of the night. Decreasing the depth of sleep in the latter part of the night would permit the child to awaken more easily and get to the bathroom to prevent enuresis. Common adverse reactions to imipramine hydrochloride (Tofranil) include dry mouth, changes in personality, nervousness, constipation, urinary retention, and insomnia.

NP = As
CN = Ph/6
CL = Ap
SA = 5

17. **2.** Bladder exstrophy is a rare and severe congenital anomaly characterized by an exposed urinary urethra and bladder, pelvic bone separation, and genital and anal abnormalities. Although a difficulty walking, waddling gait, undescended testes, and the absence of a vagina are clinical manifestations, the diagnosis is made on the visible defect.
NP = As
CN = Sa/1
CL = An
SA = 4

18. **1.** Hypospadias is a common congenital defect in which the urethral meatus appears on the ventral surface of the penis. Surgery is the treatment of choice before the child reaches the age of 18 months. Circumcision is avoided in these infants. Desmopressin acetate (DDAVP) is a synthetic analog vasopressin used in the treatment of enuresis that acts by promoting the retention of water and urine concentration. Human chorionic gonadotropin (HCG) is administered in the care of cryptorchidism, the failure of one or both testes to normally descend into the scrotum, to induce the descent of the testes.
NP = Pl
CN = He/3
CL = An
SA = 4

19. **4.** Fluids should be increased to 100 ml/kg or 50 ml/lb of body weight in a child with a urinary tract infection. Children should wear cotton underwear, and bubble baths are to be avoided. Urinary frequency would be a common clinical manifestation.
NP = Pl
CN = He/3
CL = Ap
SA = 4

20. **2.** A blood urea nitrogen (BUN) level of 20 mEq/L is extremely elevated in a newborn and should be promptly reported. A normal level in a newborn is 3 mg/dl to 12 mg/dl. A BUN level reflects the nitrogen in the blood which is an end product of protein metabolism. An elevated level indicates renal disease, dehydration, increased catabolism of protein, hemorrhage, or corticosteroid therapy. A normal creatinine level, a byproduct of protein metabolism, is 0.5 mg/dl to 1.0 mg/dl in an adolescent. A normal

potassium level in a child is 3.4 mEq/L to 4.7 mEq/L. A normal sodium level in a newborn is 139 mEq/L to 146 mEq/L.
NP = An
CN = Ph/7
CL = An
SA = 4

21. 3. The preparation of an infant under the age of 2 years for an intravenous pyelography (IVP) includes performing the test early in the day after withholding the morning bottle and solid food to prevent fluid restriction. Withholding food and fluids for two to eight hours is appropriate in a child over the age of 2 years. A cathartic may be administered the evening before the procedure but a Fleet enema is contraindicated in a child with chronic renal failure because of hyperphosphatemia.
NP = Pl
CN = Ph/7
CL = An
SA = 4

22. 4. A size 8 Foley catheter should be used for a child aged 4 to 8 years. The penis should be lifted to a 90 degree angle to the body, and the penile shaft should be held under the glans to prevent contaminating the area with the foreskin. A lidocaine applicator is inserted 1 cm to 2 cm into the urethra, 5 ml to 10 ml of lubricant is applied, and the end of the penis is held closed for two to three minutes.
NP = Ev
CN = Ph/7
CL = Ap
SA = 4

23. 2. Glomerulonephritis is a postinfectious inflammation of the glomeruli within the kidney caused by a streptococcal, pneumococcal, or viral infection.
NP = As
CN = He/3
CL = An
SA = 4

24. 4. The appropriate diet for a child with acute glomerulonephritis is low in salt, protein, and potassium. A turkey sandwich, carrot and celery sticks, apple, and tea are lower in salt, protein, and potassium than a diet including ham, pork chop, peanut butter sandwich, potatoes, green leafy vegetables, oranges, bananas, and milk.
NP = Im
CN = Ph/5
CL = An
SA = 4

25. 4. Nephrotic syndrome results from a glomerular injury and primarily occurs in children between the ages of 2 and 6 years. Although weight gain, edema (generally periorbital), abdominal swelling, and lower extremity edema are clinical manifestations of nephrotic syndrome, a slow, generalized edema may initially be confused with normal growth.
NP = An
CN = He/3
CL = An
SA = 4

26. 2, 4, 5. Nursing interventions for chronic renal failure include administering aluminum hydroxyl gel to bind with phosphorus, encourage frequent dental care and assess for complications, and monitor the blood pressure. Fat-soluble vitamins (A, E, and K) are to be avoided because they may accumulate. Oxybutynin chloride (Ditropan) is an anticholinergic used for children who have a small bladder capacity. The diet should be low in protein.
NP = Pl
CN = He/3
CL = Ap
SA = 4

27. 1. A registered nurse should perform all tasks that involve assessment, monitoring, and instructing. A licensed practical nurse may insert a Foley catheter into a child.
NP = Pl
CN = Sa/1
CL = An
SA = 8

ONCOLOGY DISORDERS - COMPREHENSIVE EXAM

1. A child needs human leukocyte antigen (HLA) typing, and the child's parents ask what this means. When responding, the nurse should explain, "HLA refers to the

   1. type of stem cell transplant the child will receive."
   2. antigens that help the body identify foreign cells."
   3. antibodies that the body develops during stem cell transplantation."
   4. changes that occur after exposure to foreign cells."

2. The nurse is caring for a child with astrocytoma who has developed diabetes insipidus. Which of the following is the priority treatment goal?

   1. Maintain fluid and electrolyte balances

   2. Maintain normal body weight

   3. Restrict sodium intake

   4. Restrict oral fluid intake

3. The nurse is assessing a child with posterior fossa syndrome. The nurse should assess the child for which of the following?
   Select all that apply:

   [ ] 1. Abdominal distention

   [ ] 2. Speech alterations

   [ ] 3. Constipation

   [ ] 4. Circulation, motion, sensitivity (CMS) checks distal to operative site

   [ ] 5. Postoperative intensive care unit psychosis

   [ ] 6. Emotional lability 24 to 48 hours postoperatively

4. When preparing an adolescent for a bone marrow aspiration, the nurse should

   1. instruct the adolescent not to eat or drink after midnight the day of the procedure.

   2. instruct the adolescent to lie flat for one hour after the procedure.

   3. administer prophylactic antibiotics one hour prior to the procedure.

   4. position the adolescent prone with a folded blanket under the adolescent's pelvis.

5. The parent of a school-aged child with mild mucositis is having difficulty with menu selection. The nurse helps the parent choose which of the following lunch selections?
   Select all that apply:

   [ ] 1. Cheeseburger

   [ ] 2. Potato chips

   [ ] 3. Cream of chicken soup

   [ ] 4. Beef broth

   [ ] 5. Jell-O

   [ ] 6. Vanilla pudding

6. The nurse is collecting a nursing history from a parent of an infant admitted with retinoblastoma. The nurse should question the parent about

   1. family history.
   2. birth history.
   3. ophthalmic injury.
   4. number of siblings.

7. The nurse is caring for a child with a chest tube inserted after a thoracotomy for metastatic osteosarcoma. Which of the following would indicate to the nurse that the child's condition is deteriorating?
   1. Decreased breath sounds and oxygen saturation of 90%
   2. Shallow respirations and guarding during respiratory assessments
   3. Increased chest tube output in the last 4 hours
   4. Hemoptysis

8. An infant is diagnosed with Stage I neuroblastoma. Which of the following should the nurse tell the parents their child will require?
   1. "Monitoring only, as the tumor may regress or maturate."
   2. "Palliative care, as stage I neuroblastoma is a terminal disease."
   3. "Radiation therapy to the tumor site only, due to the child's age."
   4. "Chemotherapy to shrink the tumor."

9. The nurse is caring for an infant with a brain tumor who has a ventriculoperitoneal (VP) shunt. The child has a bulging fontanel, fever, is vomiting, irritable, and inconsolable. The nurse should report this as which of the following?
   1. A feeding intolerance
   2. VP shunt malfunction
   3. Dehydration
   4. An abdominal abscess

10. In postprocedure care for a child who has had a lumbar puncture, which of the following is the priority intervention?
   1. Monitor the bandage for cerebral spinal fluid leakage
   2. Maintain the integrity of the dressing for 24 hours after the procedure
   3. Instruct the child to lie flat for 30 minutes postprocedure
   4. Instruct the child to resume a normal diet

11. When obtaining a nursing history on a child with Wilms' tumor, the nurse should inquire about which of the following?
   1. Bone pain
   2. Changes in neurological status

3. Genital malformations

4. Previous urinary tract or kidney infections

12. The nurse is caring for a child who will be discharged with a venous port in the left subclavicular region. The discharge instructions should include which of the following statements?

    1. "The child is not allowed to go swimming in a chlorinated pool."

    2. "The child will not have full range of motion of the left upper extremity."

    3. "The venous port requires an occlusive dressing."

    4. "The venous port needs to be accessed with a special needle."

13. The nurse is admitting an adolescent who has had intermittent fevers, fatigue, weight loss, and night sweats for the past three or four months. The nurse should report this as a suspected case of

    1. Ewing's sarcoma

    2. Hodgkin's disease

    3. Wilms' tumor

    4. Osteosarcoma

14. The nurse identifies which of the following children to be a priority for needing a stem cell transplant?

    1. A child with acute myelogenous leukemia

    2. An adolescent with osteosarcoma

    3. An adolescent with Hodgkin's disease

    4. A child with Wilms' tumor

15. The nurse evaluates which of the following as indicating that a child with an external central line catheter has an infection?

    1. Blistering skin underneath the occlusive dressing

    2. Erythematous skin underneath the occlusive dressing

    3. Petechiae noted around central line exit site

    4. Tenderness when manipulating the catheter

16. An adolescent is admitted with newly diagnosed osteosarcoma. Which of the following questions should the nurse ask?

    1. "Do you have any trouble breathing?"

    2. "Do you live near electromagnetic fields?"

    3. "What kinds of calcium-rich foods to you eat or drink?"

    4. "How long have you had pain with activity?"

17. The nurse is caring for a child admitted with a brain tumor. The child's parents inquire about the incidence of brain tumors in children. Which of the following would be the nurse's best response?

    1. "Brain tumors are the leading type of cancer in children."
    2. "Brain tumors are commonly seen in children who live near nuclear plants."
    3. "Brain tumors are the most common solid tumors in children."
    4. "Brain tumors are extremely rare in children."

18. The nurse is caring for a child with acute myelogenous leukemia who is complaining of a headache. Which of the following should be included in the nursing assessment?

    1. Review the most recent complete blood count results
    2. Perform cranial nerve testing
    3. Obtain orthostatic blood pressures
    4. Auscultate quality of respirations

19. During the preoperative care of a child with Wilms' tumor, which of the following nursing goals should have priority?

    1. Promotion of nutrition
    2. Prevention of abdominal trauma
    3. Prevention of infection
    4. Maintain renal function

20. A child with newly diagnosed acute lymphocytic leukemia is experiencing tumor lysis syndrome. Which of the following is the priority treatment goal?

    1. Administer antibiotics
    2. Decrease tumor burden
    3. Increase cardiac output
    4. Prevent renal failure

21. The parents of a 3-year-old child receiving cranial radiation therapy inquire about adverse reactions that might affect their child's growth and development. The nurse's best response would be

    1. "Cranial radiation therapy will not affect the child's growth or development."
    2. "Cranial radiation therapy only affects the growth and development of infants."
    3. "Your child will be closely monitored for linear growth; however, cranial radiation should not affect cognitive development."

4. "Your child will be closely monitored for linear growth and neurocognitive development, as cranial radiation can affect both areas."

22. When educating a group of parents about pediatric malignancies, which of the following statements best describes the origin of pediatric malignancies?

   1. Embryonic in nature

   2. Epithelial in nature

   3. Associated with environmental factors

   4. Arising from inherited genetic abnormalities

23. When explaining the treatment of children diagnosed with neuroblastoma who have had stem cell transplantation, the nurse should state, "Biologic modifiers are administered to

   1. prevent rejection after the stem cell transplant."

   2. provide systemic protection from residual neuroblastoma cells."

   3. induce growth arrest and apoptosis (cell death) of residual neuroblastoma cells."

   4. assist in the healing process of traumatized tissue."

24. The child is having an autologous stem cell transplantation for recurrent Wilms' tumor. Which of the following is the priority treatment goal?

   1. Increase the effectiveness of pretransplant chemotherapy and radiation

   2. Replace the defective hematopoietic system

   3. Replenish the hematopoietic system with host cells after high-dose chemotherapy

   4. Infuse donor cells to re-create the lymphatic system

25. The nurse is caring for a child with newly diagnosed acute lymphocytic leukemia who is scheduled for a chest x-ray. When the parents ask why radiographic testing is necessary, the nurse should explain that children with leukemia

   1. "often have enlarged hearts."

   2. "may have masses in their chests that can affect their respiratory status."

   3. "may have masses in their chests that require immediate surgical resection."

   4. "may have lymph node enlargement easily identified on chest x-ray."

26. The registered nurse is delegating the nursing tasks for a pediatric oncology unit. Which of the following nursing tasks should the nurse delegate to a licensed practical nurse?

1. Crush and mix prednisone in applesauce before administering to a child with leukemia

2. Prepare a child for an autologous bone marrow transplant

3. Instruct the parents of a child receiving chemotherapy about the adverse reactions to chemotherapy

4. Instruct the parents of a child receiving radiation about the care provided during radiation

ANSWERS AND RATIONALES

1. 2. Human leukocyte antigens (HLA) are unique to each individual and assist the body in recognizing "self" from "foreign." The type of stem cell transplant would be allogeneic or autologous. Antibodies that the body develops during stem cell transplantation and changes that occur after exposure to foreign cells cannot be predicted before transplantation.
NP = An
CN = He/3
CL = An
SA = 4

2. 1. Fluid and electrolyte imbalances can lead to uncontrolled seizures and alter cardiac functioning, which can be life-threatening events for a child with astrocytoma. Maintaining normal body weight is not a priority in treating diabetes insipidus. Restricting sodium and oral fluid intake are maintenance interventions once fluid and electrolytes are properly balanced.
NP = Pl
CN = Sa/1
CL = An
SA = 8

3. 2, 6. Speech alterations and emotional lability are hallmark clinical manifestations of posterior fossa syndrome. Abdominal distention and constipation are general postoperative manifestations. Circulation, motion, and sensitivity (CMS) checks are performed when a surgical intervention has been performed on a child's extremity. ICU psychosis occurs after a prolonged hospitalization.
NP = As
CN = He/3

CL = Ap
SA = 4

4. **4.** Positioning the child prone with pelvic support allows the practitioner performing the bone marrow aspiration easy access to the posterior iliac crest. Nothing by mouth after midnight is applicable to procedures for which the client is anesthetized. Positioning the client flat is the postprocedure intervention for lumbar puncture. Prophylactic antibiotic administration is appropriate for solid organ transplant clients.
    NP = Im
    CN = Ph/7
    CL = Ap
    SA = 4

5. **3, 6.** Cream of chicken soup and vanilla pudding offer nutritional support from a soft diet for a child with epithelial injury to the oral cavity such as that which occurs in mucositis. Cheeseburger and potato chips can cause mechanical injuries, and mastication can exacerbate pain. Beef broth and Jell-O do not contain the nutritional support required for wound healing.
    NP = Im
    CN = Ph/5
    CL = Ap
    SA = 4

6. **1.** Retinoblastoma has a strong familial link. Birth history, ophthalmic injury, and number of siblings are important components to obtain in a nursing history, but are not directly linked to retinoblastoma.
    NP = As
    CN = He/3
    CL = Ap
    SA = 4

7. **1.** While caring for a child who has metastatic osteosarcoma and has had a thoracotomy with a chest tube, a change in breath sounds and a drop in saturation are signs that the oxygenation and compensatory efforts have been ineffective, and immediate intervention is required. Shallow respirations and guarding are expected behaviors from a child postoperatively. Increased chest tube output and hemoptysis are expected following thoracic surgery.
    NP = An
    CN = Ph/7
    CL = An
    SA = 4

8. **1.** Neuroblastoma is a tumor that originates from the adrenal medulla and sympathetic nervous system. A Stage I neuroblastoma is a localized tumor

confined to the area of origin and will often regress in infants. It requires only monitoring.

NP = An
CN = He/3
CL = An
SA = 4

9. 2. When a child who has a brain tumor and a ventriculoperitoneal shunt develops a bulging fontanel, fever, and is vomiting, irritable, and inconsolable, there is a blockage in the flow of cerebral spinal fluid, which leads to these clinical manifestations of hydrocephalus. Feeding intolerance and abdominal abscess will not produce a bulging fontanel. Dehydration would produce a sunken fontanel.

NP = An
CN = Ph/7
CL = An
SA = 4

10. 1. The priority intervention following a lumbar puncture is to monitor the bandage for cerebral spinal fluid leakage. Such a leakage predisposes the child to a central nervous system infection and must be corrected immediately. Although maintaining the integrity of the dressing for 24 hours, instructing the child to lie flat for 30 minutes, and instructing the child to resume a normal diet following the procedure are all correct interventions, they are not the priority.

NP = Pl
CN = Sa/1
CL = An
SA = 8

11. 3. Wilms' tumor is the most common type of childhood cancer of the kidney. A high incidence of genital malformations is associated with Wilms' tumor. Bone pain is associated with bone tumors or bony infiltrates, such as leukemia. Neurological status is associated with central nervous system malignancies. Previous urinary tract or kidney infections suggest genitourinary dysfunctions or obstructions and are not associated with a malignancy.

NP = As
CN = He/3
CL = Ap
SA = 4

12. 4. The venous port is implanted under the subcutaneous tissue and requires access with an angled needle. Instructing a child to avoid swimming in a chlorinated pool and using an occlusive dressing both

apply to an external central line. Central line placement of any kind does not limit range of motion after the initial placement.
NP = Pl
CN = He/3
CL = Ap
SA = 4

13. **2.** Ewing's sarcoma is present in older children and young adults. The usual clinical manifestation is pain and swelling at the site. Wilms' tumor is most common between the ages of 2 and 3 years and presents with abdominal distention. Osteosarcoma presents with a bony, palpable mass with associated pain. Hodgkin's disease is a lymphoma that originates in the cervical lymph node and spreads to other lymph nodes. If Hodgkin's disease goes untreated, it may spread to the organs. Characteristic manifestations include intermittent fevers, fatigue, weight loss, and night sweats generally over a period of three to four months.
NP = An
CN = He/3
CL = An
SA = 4

14. **1.** Children with acute myelogenous leukemia require stem cell transplantation if they have a matched related donor or if they are Philadelphia positive. Stem cell transplantation is not a part of the primary treatment modality for osteosarcoma, Hodgkin's disease, or Wilms' tumor.
NP = As
CN = Sa/1
CL = An
SA = 4

15. **4.** Pain is one of the first signs of an infection in an immunocompromised child and would indicate an infection in a child with a central line catheter. Blistering skin and erythematous skin underneath the occlusive dressing indicate an inflammatory response to the dressing. Petechiae indicate a low platelet count.
NP = Ev
CN = Ph/7
CL = An
SA = 4

16. **4.** Osteosarcoma is a tumor of the bone in the growth metaphysis or the end of the long bones. Pain with activity is the primary clinical manifestation that will bring a child to a health care provider and is associated with pathogenesis. Trouble breathing does not address bone pain. Electromagnetic fields have no direct correlation with malignant

processes. Calcium intake does not predispose a child to malignancies of the bone or give pertinent information regarding the child's current complaint.

NP = As
CN = He/3
CL = An
SA = 4

17. **3.** Brain tumors are the most common type of solid tumor in children. Leukemia is the leading type of cancer in children. Environmental causes have not been supported in the literature. Brain tumors are the second most common type of childhood malignancy.

NP = An
CN = He/3
CL = Ap
SA = 4

18. **1.** It is appropriate to review the blood counts in a child with acute myelogenous leukemia. It may reveal anemia, for which headache may be a manifestation. Cranial nerve testing is not indicated for neurologic manifestations. Orthostatic blood pressures are assessed when the child complains of dizziness. Auscultation of breath sounds will produce other marked clinical manifestations before a headache if the respiratory status is compromised.

NP = As
CN = He/3
CL = An
SA = 4

19. **2.** Wilms' tumor is the most common type of cancer of the kidney in children. Abdominal trauma may rupture the encapsulated tumor, spilling malignant cells into the abdominal cavity. Promotion of nutrition, prevention of infection, and maintaining renal function are all appropriate interventions, but not the priority.

NP = Pl
CN = Sa/1
CL = An
SA = 8

20. **4.** Tumor lysis syndrome can quickly lead to acute renal failure if no interventions are implemented when a child has acute lymphocytic leukemia. Administering antibiotics and increasing cardiac output are appropriate interventions for septic shock. Decreasing tumor burden is an appropriate intervention for superior vena cava syndrome or spinal cord compression.

NP = Pl
CN = Sa/1

CL = An
SA = 8

21. **4.** Cranial radiation has stunting effects, physical and cognitive, on the growing brain of a child.
NP = An
CN = He/3
CL = An
SA = 4

22. **1.** Histologically, pediatric cancers arise from embryonal tissue. Adult malignancies are epithelial in nature. That environmental factors lead to cancers is a theoretical assumption not supported in the literature. Inherited genetic abnormalities can be extrapolated from various forms of pediatric cancers, such as retinoblastoma; however, most pediatric malignancies arise from embryonal tissue.
NP = Ev
CN = He/3
CL = Ap
SA = 4

23. **3.** Biologic modifiers induce growth arrest and apoptosis (cell death) of residual neuroblastoma. Preventing rejection is the action of an immunosuppressive agent. Biologic modifiers do not provide systemic protection or promote healing.
NP = Ev
CN = Ph/6
CL = Ap
SA = 5

24. **3.** Host cells are infused after high-dose chemotherapy in order to replenish the hematopoietic system. Stem cell transplantation is not correlated with an increased effectiveness of pretransplant therapy. A defective hematopoietic system is not the area of concern. The high-dose chemotherapy is given to eradicate the tumor. Infusing cells to re-create the lymphatic system is not necessary, as it is the hematopoietic system that needs replenishing after high-dose chemotherapy.
NP = Pl
CN = Sa/1
CL = An
SA = 4

25. **2.** Children with leukemia may have mediastinal masses that impair their respiratory status. A child with an enlarged heart would require an echocardiogram. Immediate surgical resection is incorrect, because initiation of chemotherapy will shrink the chest mass. Lymph node

identification requires a computerized tomography (CT) with contrast for visualization of the lymphatic system.

NP = Ev

CN = Ph/7

CL = Ap

SA = 4

26. 1. A licensed practical nurse may crush prednisone, which has a very bitter taste, and mix it in applesauce before administering it to a child with leukemia. A registered nurse should prepare a child for an autologous bone marrow transplant and instruct a parent about chemotherapy and radiation.

NP = Pl

CN = Sa/1

CL = An

SA = 8

HEMATOLOGICAL DISORDERS - COMPREHENSIVE EXAM

1. The nurse is evaluating an adolescent with anemia. Which of the following subjective findings would the nurse recognize as significant?

    1. Diet includes a variety of fruits, vegetables, and meats

    2. Appendectomy three years ago

    3. Takes ibuprofen (Motrin) for frequent headaches

    4. Menstrual flow usually lasts three days

2. The nurse should assess a child exposed to prolonged anemia to be at risk for which of the following?

    1. Darkened skin

    2. Growth retardation

    3. Bradycardia

    4. Lymphadenopathy

3. The nurse should consider which of the following laboratory results in a client's chart when evaluating the child's response to therapy for anemia?

    1. Hemoglobin electrophoresis

    2. Platelet count

    3. Prothrombin time (PT)

    4. Reticulocyte count

4. The parent of a child with iron deficiency anemia asks the nurse about the treatment of this condition. Which of the following should the nurse describe as the primary goal of therapy?

   1. To replenish body's iron stores

   2. To prevent impairment in intellectual development

   3. To improve the child's diet

   4. To enroll all eligible children in WIC

5. Which of the following should the nurse recommend in the education given to the parents of a newborn with sickle cell anemia?

   1. A multivitamin with iron

   2. The Prevnar vaccine

   3. Daily aspirin therapy

   4. A diet high in fiber

6. The nurse assists a child with sickle cell anemia who has gallstones to make which of the following menu selections?
   Select all that apply:

   [ ] 1. Cheeseburger

   [ ] 2. Turkey sandwich

   [ ] 3. Pretzels

   [ ] 4. Custard

   [ ] 5. French fries

   [ ] 6. Chocolate shake

7. An 18-year-old female adolescent with sickle cell disease is concerned because all of her friends have started menstruating, but she has not. The nurse's best response would be

   1. "We should send you for an endocrine evaluation."

   2. "Have you been exercising a lot?"

   3. "You will achieve puberty, but later than your peers."

   4. "It is a result of a poor dietary intake."

8. The nurse is screening children suspected of having beta thalassemia major. Based on an understanding of the risk factors associated with this disease, the nurse suspects which of the following children to have beta thalassemia major?

   1. A 4-year-old child of African-American descent

   2. A 5-year-old child of Asian descent

3. A 3-year-old child of Scandinavian descent

4. A 1-year-old child of Mediterranean descent

9. Before planning the care of a child with beta thalassemia major, the nurse should consider which of the following as potential complications?
Select all that apply:

[ ] **1.** Infection

[ ] **2.** Intracranial hemorrhage

[ ] **3.** Congestive heart failure

[ ] **4.** Pathologic fractures

[ ] **5.** Iron overload

[ ] **6.** Hypovolemic shock

10. The nurse is caring for a child with von Willebrand's disease. Which of the following drugs should the nurse prepare to administer to this child?

1. Cyclosporine (Neoral, Sandimmune)

2. Deferoxamine (Desferal)

3. Meperidine (Demerol)

4. Desmopressin (DDAVP, Stimate)

11. The nurse assesses a child with aplastic anemia to have which of the following clinical manifestations?
Select all that apply:

[ ] **1.** Pallor

[ ] **2.** Frontal bossing

[ ] **3.** Amenorrhea

[ ] **4.** Increased bruising

[ ] **5.** Fever of 39.4°C, or 103°F

[ ] **6.** Priapism

12. The nurse receives an order to administer which of the following prescribed drugs to a child with aplastic anemia?

1. Baby aspirin

2. Aminocaproic acid (Amicar)

3. Antihemophilic factor (Humate-P)

4. Cyclosporine (Neoral, Sandimmune)

13. The mother of a child with hemophilia A is expecting her second child, a daughter. She wants to know what the chances are that this child will have the same condition. The nurse responds

1. "There is a 25% chance that this child will have the disorder."
2. "There is a 50% chance that this child will have the disorder."
3. "It is highly unlikely that this child will have the disorder."
4. "There is a 75% chance that this child will have the disorder."

14. The nurse is discharging a client with hemophilia A. Which of the following should the nurse include in the child's discharge instructions?

    1. Avoid all forms of physical activity
    2. Seek immediate medical attention for a fever of 38.3°C, or 101°F
    3. Avoid iron supplements
    4. Use a soft-bristled toothbrush for oral hygiene

15. A child is being admitted to the hematology unit of the hospital with suspected idiopathic thrombocytopenic purpura (ITP). The nurse recognizes that which of the following assessment findings is most commonly associated with this condition?

    1. Cheilosis
    2. Hepatomegaly
    3. Petechiae
    4. Hematuria

16. The mother of a child with von Willebrand's disease asks the nurse if any special precautions should be taken prior to visiting the dentist for a routine cleaning. The nurse's best response would be

    1. "Dental cleanings should be avoided."
    2. "Administer desmopressin (DDAVP) as prescribed by your physician before the appointment."
    3. "It is recommended that your child have a CBC checked prior to the cleaning."
    4. "You should see a hematologist first for a possible platelet transfusion prior to the appointment."

17. The nurse caring for a child with acute idiopathic thrombocytopenic purpura (ITP) should prepare the child for which of the following treatments?

    1. Bone marrow transplant
    2. Cryoprecipitate
    3. Monthly transfusion therapy
    4. Oral prednisone

18. The nurse is admitting a child with a diagnosis of abdominal pain who is also experiencing hypotension and bleeding from puncture sites, the nose,

and the mouth. The nurse suspects these assessment findings are indicators of which of the following disorders?

1. Acute disseminated intravascular coagulation (DIC)
2. Acute idiopathic thrombocytopenic purpura (ITP)
3. Chronic disseminated intravascular coagulation (DIC)
4. Chronic idiopathic thrombocytopenic purpura (ITP)

19. When preparing a client for a bone marrow aspiration, which of the following nursing measures should the nurse include?

1. Maintain sterile technique
2. Avoid restraining the child
3. Avoid using conscious sedation
4. Cleanse the site with sterile water

20. After assessing four clients on the hematology unit of the hospital, the nurse anticipates a client with which of the following conditions will require a bone marrow aspiration to confirm a diagnosis prior to beginning treatment?

1. Hemophilia A
2. Beta thalassemia major
3. Idiopathic thrombocytopenic purpura (ITP)
4. Sickle cell anemia

21. The nurse is caring for a child with sickle cell anemia. The child's parents ask the nurse why their child is anemic. The nurse should explain, "Anemia of sickle cell disease results from

1. underproduction of red blood cells."
2. destruction of red blood cells."
3. chronic bleeding resulting from capillary damage."
4. a lack of iron in the red blood cells."

22. The nurse caring for a client with aplastic anemia should evaluate what laboratory test to determine the presence of a systemic infection? _____ .

23. The nurse should include which of the following adverse reactions to the medication instructions given to the parents and child taking an oral iron supplement?
Select all that apply:

[ ] 1. Flushing
[ ] 2. Nausea
[ ] 3. Urticaria

[   ] **4.** Abdominal cramps

[   ] **5.** Headache

[   ] **6.** Constipation

24. The nurse is assessing a child with sickle cell disease who is experiencing pain. Which of the following nursing measures should receive priority in this child's care?

   1. Give a prescribed analgesic immediately

   2. Conclude that the pain is due to a vasoocclusive episode

   3. Perform a thorough examination to rule out other causes of the pain

   4. Recommend that the client is a candidate for hydroxyurea (Hydrea) therapy

25. The nurse should monitor the complete blood count of an adolescent who has been on trimethoprim and sulfamethoxazole (Bactrim) for several months in the treatment of severe acne for which of the following blood dyscrasias?

   1. Aplastic anemia

   2. Iron deficiency anemia

   3. Von Willebrand's

   4. Beta thalassemia

26. The registered nurse is preparing to make the clinical assignments for a pediatric hematology unit. Which of the following assignments should the nurse delegate to a licensed practical nurse?

   1. Provide the care for a child in a sickle cell crisis

   2. Evaluate the complete blood count in a child suspected of having a blood dyscrasia

   3. Assist a child with iron deficient anemia to mark a menu

   4. Assess a client taking prednisone for adverse reactions

ANSWERS AND RATIONALES

1. **3.** Ibuprofen (Motrin) may lead to gastrointestinal bleeding, especially if taken frequently, which could lead to anemia. A healthy, balanced diet, including a variety of meats and vegetables, would not likely lead to anemia. Although bleeding is a result of surgery, a surgery performed three years ago would not contribute to anemia. A heavy menstrual flow may lead to anemia but a history of a three-day flow does not support this as a cause for the anemia.

   NP = As

   CN = He/3

CL = Ap
SA = 4

2. **2.** Children who experience anemia for an extended period are likely to have delays in both height and weight. Darkened skin is not the result of prolonged anemia. Anemia is usually associated with tachycardia and not bradycardia. Lymphadenopathy is most commonly associated with malignant conditions, not anemia.
NP = As
CN = Ph/7
CL = An
SA = 4

3. **4.** The reticulocyte count is a measure of how quickly the body is producing new red blood cells. This is routinely used in the evaluation of the resolution of anemia. The platelet count may give clues to the cause of bleeding in a child but not to the response to therapy. Hemoglobin electrophoresis is a test used to determine the presence of hemoglobinopathies. Prothrombin time (PT) is utilized in the diagnosis of coagulation disorders.
NP = Ev
CN = Ph/7
CL = Ap
SA = 4

4. **1.** The goal of therapy in the treatment of iron deficiency anemia is to correct the cause of anemia and to replenish the body's iron stores. Preventing impairment of intellectual development and improvement of the child's diet may indirectly result from treating the anemia but are not the primary goals. WIC may be beneficial for some clients, but is not the primary goal of therapy.
NP = Pl
CN = He/3
CL = Ap
SA = 4

5. **2.** Prevnar and Pneumovax are both vaccines aimed to prevent pneumococcal infection in children with sickle cell disease. Children with sickle cell disease usually possess a higher stored iron level due to increased destruction of red blood cells, so excess iron in a multivitamin is of no added benefit. Daily aspirin therapy is not recommended for sickle cell clients. A diet high in fiber is a good idea for everyone, but is not especially important in the management of sickle cell disease.
NP = Pl
CN = He/3

CL = Ap
SA = 4

6. **2, 3, 4.** Pain with gallstones is most often precipitated by eating a meal high in fat. A meal of cheeseburger, French fries, and a chocolate shake has the highest fat content. This meal would be most likely to cause an episode of nausea or vomiting in a child with sickle cell disease who has gallstones. A turkey sandwich, pretzels, and custard would be the most appropriate food selections.
NP = Im
CN = Ph/5
CL = Ap
SA = 4

7. **3.** It is normal for adolescents with sickle cell disease to grow and develop more slowly than their peers do. This often results in the delay of sexual maturation, including the start of menstruation. Children with sickle cell disease will achieve puberty, but most often later than their peers. An endocrine evaluation is not necessary in these adolescents. Excessive exercise is often a cause of amenorrhea in athletes; however, children with sickle cell disease are not able to tolerate such strenuous activity. A poor dietary intake has no effect on the menstrual cycle.
NP = An
CN = He/3
CL = An
SA = 4

8. **4.** Beta thalassemia major is an autosomal recessive disorder that most often affects children of Mediterranean descent. It usually manifests itself during the second 6 months of life and clinical manifestations of severe anemia become apparent as the child grows older.
NP = Im
CN = He/3
CL = Ap
SA = 4

9. **3, 4, 5.** Children with beta thalassemia major are at risk of developing congestive heart failure, pathologic fractures, and iron overload due to chronic blood transfusions. Infection is not associated with beta thalassemia. Intracranial hemorrhage is most commonly associated with hemophilia. Hypovolemic shock is most commonly associated with disseminated intravascular coagulation (DIC).
NP = An
CN = Ph/7
CL = An
SA = 4

10. **2.** Von Willebrand's disease is the most common congenital disorder of homeostasis. It results from a deficient von Willebrand's factor (a protein that facilitates an adhesion between platelets and injured vessels). Desmopressin (DDAVP, Stimate) is used to manage bleeding episodes in children with this disorder. Cyclosporine (Neoral, Sandimmune) is a drug used for immunosuppression. Deferoxamine (Desferal), a chelation agent that helps the body excrete excess iron to prevent organ damage, is the drug indicated in children with beta thalassemia major who are on a chronic transfusion regimen. Meperidine (Demerol) is used for the treatment of pain.
NP = Pl
CN = Ph/6
CL = An
SA = 5

11. **1, 4, 5.** Aplastic anemia is a disorder in which there is an injury or abnormal stem cells that results in an inadequate number of erythrocytes, leukocytes, and platelets. Pallor, increased bruising, and fever of 39.4°C, or 103°F are characteristic of aplastic anemia and result from a decrease in hematocrit, WBC count, and platelet count. Frontal bossing may occur with prolonged anemia. Amenorrhea may be achieved by the use of oral contraceptives and is not a result of this condition. Priapism is a clinical manifestation associated with sickle cell anemia.
NP = As
CN = He/3
CL = Ap
SA = 4

12. **4.** Aplastic anemia is autoimmune in nature, and cyclosporine (Neoral, Sandimmune) is an immunosuppressive agent used in the treatment of this disorder. Baby aspirin is contraindicated in children with aplastic anemia because the resulting decrease in platelet count increases the risk for bleeding. Aminocaproic (Amicar) is used for prolonged bleeding of mucous membranes in patients with hemophilia. Antihemophilic factor (Humate-P) is used to treat prolonged bleeding in children with von Willebrand's disease who do not respond to DDAVP.
NP = Im
CN = Ph/6
CL = An
SA = 5

13. **3.** Hemophilia A is an X-linked recessive disorder that only affects males. Since the mother is expecting a female offspring, she can be reassured that her baby will not be affected by the condition.

NP = An
CN = He/3
CL = An
SA = 4

14. **4.** Children with hemophilia should use a soft-bristled toothbrush to prevent trauma to oral tissues. Children with hemophilia A should be encouraged to participate in physical activity to increase flexibility and strength. However, they should avoid contact sports. Fevers are not common to this condition. Iron supplementation is often recommended for clients with hemophilia to correct the iron deficiency that occurs from bleeding episodes.
NP = Pl
CN = He/3
CL = Ap
SA = 4

15. **3.** Petechiae are the result of microscopic areas of bleeding under the skin due to the rapid destruction of platelets in idiopathic thrombocytopenic purpura (ITP). Cheilosis is associated with anemia. Hepatomegaly is not common in clients with idiopathic thrombocytopenic purpura (ITP). Hematuria is possible in idiopathic thrombocytopenic purpura (ITP), but is not common.
NP = As
CN = He/3
CL = Ap
SA = 4

16. **2.** Von Willebrand is a genetic disorder in children that results in a deficiency in the circulating protein (von Willebrand's factor) that facilitates adhesions between platelets and injured vessels. Children should receive the desmopressin (DDAVP) prior to dental procedures to decrease the likelihood of bleeding from dental trauma. Dental cleanings are permitted in children with von Willebrand's disease as long as the appropriate precautions are followed. Reviewing the results of a CBC prior to a dental evaluation is not necessary because it will not influence actions to be taken prior to the dental appointment. Platelet transfusions are not used to treat clients with this disorder.
NP = An
CN = He/3
CL = An
SA = 4

17. **4.** A short course of oral corticosteroids, such as prednisone, is the treatment of choice for children with acute idiopathic thrombocytopenic purpura (ITP). Bone marrow transplant is not indicated for clients with

ITP, since it is usually a brief, self-limited disorder. Cryoprecipitate is traditionally used in the treatment of clients experiencing acute bleeding episodes as a result of hemophilia or von Willebrand's disease. Monthly transfusion therapy with IVIG may be used in clients with chronic, not acute, ITP.

NP = Im
CN = He/3
CL = An
SA = 4

18. **1.** Acute disseminated intravascular coagulation (DIC) is manifested by oozing from puncture sites; bleeding from the nose, mouth, and eyes; purpura and petechiae; GI bleeding; hypotension; and organ dysfunction. Chronic disseminated intravascular coagulation (DIC) is manifested by jaundice, hypoxia, oliguria, and changes in mental status. Acute and chronic idiopathic thrombocytopenic purpura (ITP) are both less severe than acute disseminated intravascular coagulation. The clinical manifestations are similar for both conditions, which are often associated with petechiae and purpura.

NP = As
CN = He/3
CL = An
SA = 4

19. **1.** Sterile technique must be maintained during a bone marrow aspiration to avoid the possibility of infection at the insertion site. The nurse is often needed during the procedure to help restrain the child. Sedation is often necessary in children and is commonly achieved with the use of Versed. The site should be cleansed thoroughly with alcohol and Betadine prior to beginning the procedure.

NP = Pl
CN = Ph/7
CL = Ap
SA = 4

20. **3.** A diagnosis of idiopathic thrombocytopenic purpura (ITP) must be confirmed with bone marrow aspiration prior to beginning steroid therapy, because the anti-inflammatory properties of prednisone can mask a developing malignancy. Hemophilia is a bleeding disorder diagnosed via family history and coagulation testing. Beta thalassemia major and sickle cell anemia are both hemoglobinopathies diagnosed with hemoglobin electrophoresis.

NP = An
CN = Ph/7
CL = An
SA = 4

21. **2.** With sickle cell anemia, the red blood cells are not healthy and are destroyed rather quickly. The lifespan of a normal, healthy red blood cell is 120 days. In children with sickle cell anemia, the lifespan of the red blood cell is approximately 20 to 30 days. Children with sickle cell disease often have elevated reticulocyte counts and produce large numbers of red blood cells. Children with sickle cell disease do sustain capillary damage from sickled cells, but bleeding does not occur. Red blood cells produced by children with sickle cell disease contain adequate amounts of iron, due to the increase in iron stores in these children.
NP = An
CN = He/3
CL = An
SA = 4

22. **WBC with differential.** A white blood cell count with a differential is the best method of determining the presence or absence of infection, since it gives the number of circulating white cells in addition to a breakdown of the different types that are present.
NP = Ev
CN = Ph/7
CL = Ap
SA = 4

23. **2, 4, 6.** Flushing, urticaria, and headache are adverse reactions commonly associated with parenteral, not oral iron administration. The adverse reactions commonly associated with oral iron supplementation include nausea, epigastric discomfort, abdominal cramps, constipation, diarrhea, and black, tarry stools. Giving the medication after a meal can minimize these adverse reactions.
NP = Pl
CN = Ph/6
CL = Ap
SA = 5

24. **3.** A complete, thorough history and physical examination should be completed prior to identifying the source of pain. The source should be treated accordingly. It would be a mistake to administer an analgesic immediately, because the analgesic would mask the pain and make identifying the source of the pain impossible. Not every ache and pain experienced by children with sickle cell disease is due to a vasoocclusive crisis. Children with sickle cell disease can experience all normal childhood illnesses and injuries. Hydroxyurea (Hydrea) is a drug reserved for those children who are frequently hospitalized for pain and do not respond to usual treatment.
NP = Pl
CN = Sa/1

CL = An
SA = 8

25. **1.** Aplastic anemia can be either hereditary or acquired. There are many pharmacologic agents that can cause a client to develop aplastic anemia. Sulfonamides, such as trimethoprim and sulfamethoxazole (Bactrim), are some of these agents. Iron deficiency anemia is not caused by antibiotic therapy. Beta thalassemia and von Willebrand's are genetic disorders.
NP = As
CN = Ph/6
CL = An
SA = 4

26. **3.** Providing care to a child in a sickle cell crisis, evaluating a complete blood count, and assessing a client taking prednisone for adverse reactions require the skills of a registered nurse. A licensed practical nurse may assist a child in marking a menu.
NP = Pl
CN = Sa/1
CL = An
SA = 8

INFECTIOUS AND COMMUNICABLE DISORDERS - COMPREHENSIVE EXAM

1. The nurse is admitting a child suspected of having a skin wound contaminated with animal feces. Which of the following are the two early clinical manifestations indicating the child is experiencing tetanus? _____

2. The nurse is assessing four children. Which of the following children does the nurse evaluate to have *Giardia*?

   1. A 3-year-old child in a day care center

   2. A 17-year-old adolescent who engages in unprotected sexual intercourse

   3. An infant exposed to the disease through the birth process

   4. A 16-year-old adolescent who is a drug addict

3. The nurse is caring for a child with a multiple-resistant organism with methicillin-resistant *Staphylococcus aureus* (MRSA). Which of the following is a priority for the nurse to include in this child's plan of care? Select all that apply:

   [   ] **1.** Meticulous hand washing

   [   ] **2.** Private room

[   ] **3.** High-protein diet

[   ] **4.** Increased fluids

[   ] **5.** Disposable equipment

[   ] **6.** Continuous isolation precautions

4. The nurse assesses which of the following clinical manifestations to be present in a client suspected of having severe acute respiratory syndrome (SARS)?
Select all that apply:

[   ] **1.** Malaise

[   ] **2.** Cough

[   ] **3.** Dyspnea

[   ] **4.** Watery diarrhea

[   ] **5.** Coughing up blood

[   ] **6.** Temperature of 38.3°C, or 101°F

5. The mother of an adolescent with tuberculosis does not want her child to go through the treatment for tuberculosis. Which of the following should be the priority response by the nurse?

1. "Your child will not be contagious in the latent stage."

2. "Your child may be asymptomatic in the latent stage."

3. "Active disease may develop later in life if treatment was never received."

4. "Blood in the sputum is an indication of a complication."

6. Which of the following dosing schedules for acetaminophen (Tylenol) indicates the nurse understands how the Tylenol should be administered to a child?

1. Administer every three hours on a routine schedule

2. Administer 10 to 15 mg/kg/dose every four hours

3. Administer 20 to 30 mg/kg/dose every four hours but not over five times a day

4. Administer at the request of the child

7. Which of the following is a priority question to ask the adolescent female client receiving a measles, mumps, and rubella (MMR) vaccine?

1. "Are you pregnant?"

2. "Did you miss your last scheduled immunization?"

3. "How did you react to your last immunization?"

4. "How old were you at your last scheduled immunization?"

8. The mother of a child asks the nurse why her child must receive the polio vaccine because she thought polio has been eradicated. Which of the following is the most appropriate response by the nurse?

   1. "Receiving the polio vaccine is now optional."

   2. "Although the polio vaccine is optional, it is recommended."

   3. "It is still given because polio is still active in other parts of the world."

   4. "The polio vaccine is given in one dose and will last for a lifetime."

9. Which of the following interventions should the nurse include in the plan of care for a child with chickenpox?

   1. Perform cool baths with baking soda

   2. Administer acetylsalicylic acid (aspirin) as an analgesic

   3. Dress the child in warm clothing

   4. Maintain a warm environment

10. The nurse is delegating clinical assignments on a pediatric infectious and communicable disease unit. Which of the following assignments should the nurse delegate to a licensed practical nurse?

   1. Outline the immunization schedule with the mother of a newborn

   2. Instruct the mother of a child with *Giardia* on future preventive measures

   3. Assess a child suspected of having severe acute respiratory syndrome

   4. Administer acetaminophen (Tylenol) to a child with chickenpox

11. The nurse should monitor a child with rubella (German measles) for which of the following complications?

   1. Transient polyarthralgia

   2. Seizures

   3. Red maculopapular discrete rash

   4. Obstructive laryngotracheitis

12. The nurse is caring for four children on an infectious and communicable disease unit. For which of the following children should the nurse inform the parent that a carrier state is possible?

   1. Rotavirus

   2. Hepatitis B

   3. *Giardia*

   4. *Enterobius* (pinworm)

13. The nurse should assess a child suspected of erythema infectiosum (Fifth's disease) for which of the following?

    1. Cervical lymphadenopathy

    2. Red facial rash

    3. Koplik's spots

    4. Obstructive laryngotracheitis

14. The nurse should implement which of the following precautions when admitting a child with mumps?

    1. Respiratory

    2. Enteric

    3. Protective

    4. Contact

15. A client who is pregnant asks the nurse when childhood immunizations should begin. Which of the following is the appropriate response by the nurse? "Childhood immunizations begin at

    1. birth."

    2. 3 months."

    3. 6 months."

    4. 9 months."

16. A mother asks the nurse how the polio vaccine is administered, because she heard the way it is administered has changed. Which of the following would be the most appropriate response by the nurse?

    1. "The polio vaccine is not recommended as it once was, because poliomyelitis is essentially nonexistent."

    2. "The oral polio vaccine is the only available vaccine, is proven to be safe, and is universally used."

    3. "There are several different types of polio vaccines that can be given and the type selected is determined by client preference."

    4. "Inactivated polio virus vaccine has primarily replaced the oral vaccine, because it eliminates the risk of vaccine-associated polio paralysis."

17. The nurse informs a mother that her child who has vertically transmitted HIV infection contracted the condition in which of the following ways?

    1. Through sexual intercourse

    2. Through contaminated needles

    3. A weakened immune system

    4. Intrauterine from maternal infection

18. The nurse is teaching a class to new mothers on childhood immunizations. Which of the following should the nurse include in the class?

    1. After completing the infant immunizations, lifetime immunity to diphtheria is present and no further injections are necessary.

    2. Measles vaccine is first given at 2 months followed by another vaccine at 6 months.

    3. Four doses of the polio vaccine are recommended before the child enters school.

    4. Pertussis vaccine cannot be given until the child reaches 7 years of age.

19. Which of the following should the nurse include in the instructions given to a group of student nurses about methicillin-resistant *Staphylococcus aureus* (MRSA) and vancomycin-resistant *Enterococcus* (VRE)?

    1. MRSA and VRE are infections that occur in clients with weakened immune systems

    2. There is no known antibiotic treatment for MRSA and VRE

    3. MRSA and VRE mutate very rapidly

    4. MRSA and VRE are transmitted by contaminated hands and gloves from health care workers

20. The nurse identifies which of the following considerations as the priority before administering a vaccine to an infant?

    1. Store all vaccines in the refrigerator

    2. Deep penetration of the muscle for deposition of the drug intramuscularly

    3. Inform the parents of the reactions possible from the vaccines

    4. Protect all vaccine vials from light by storing them in the boxes they came in

21. When teaching a human sexuality class, the nurse should instruct an adolescent client that the most common sexually transmitted disease among adolescents in America today is

    1. syphilis.

    2. gonorrhea.

    3. human papillomavirus.

    4. chlamydia.

22. Which of the following should the nurse inform a newly pregnant woman about a potential cytomegalovirus (CMV) infection?

    1. There is a high risk when exposed to the urine and saliva of a CMV infected child

    2. The incubation period for CMV is 7 to 10 days after exposure

3. If an infection develops, treatment is successful with antibiotics

4. CMV poses no threat to the developing fetus

23. A client questions the nurse about diphtheria. The nurse responds appropriately by stating, "Diphtheria

1. is spread by intimate contact with bodily discharges."

2. does not require treatment."

3. no longer exists since worldwide immunization began."

4. is treated with a tetanus injection."

24. The nurse should instruct a mother to monitor her infant for which of the following reactions to the diphtheria, pertussis, and tetanus (DPT) immunization?
Select all that apply:

[ ] 1. Anorexia

[ ] 2. Low-grade fever

[ ] 3. Arthralgia

[ ] 4. Behavioral changes

[ ] 5. Tenderness at the injection site

[ ] 6. Erythema and swelling

25. The nurse should inform an adolescent client suspected of having infectious mononucleosis that it is contracted by which of the following routes?

1. Contact with another's oral secretions

2. Changing the diapers of an infected child

3. Wiping tears

4. Casual contact with an infected individual

26. When an infant client is admitted to the hospital in respiratory distress, with a high-pitched inspiration and coughing paroxysms, which of the following are the most appropriate nursing interventions the nurse should initiate?
Select all that apply:

[ ] 1. Initiate strict isolation

[ ] 2. Provide respiratory therapy

[ ] 3. Don a mask

[ ] 4. Provide diphtheria, pertussis, and tetanus (DPT) immunization

[ ] 5. Initiate droplet/airborne isolation

[ ] 6. Have emergency respiratory equipment available

27. The nurse should inform the parents of a child admitted with a suspected diagnosis of respiratory syncytial virus that this disorder is

    1. common and never dangerous.

    2. of concern only in infants under 6 months of age.

    3. the most common cause of bronchiolitis and pneumonia among infants.

    4. no longer contagious after symptoms appear.

28. The nurse is admitting a 1-year-old client with a fever, runny nose, and cough. The nurse should initially suspect and report which of the following disorders?

    1. Diphtheria

    2. Measles

    3. Tetanus

    4. Respiratory syncytial virus

29. Which of the following should the nurse monitor in a child admitted with suspected *Enterobius* (pinworms)?
    Select all that apply:

    [ ] **1.** Nocturnal anal itching

    [ ] **2.** Abdominal pain

    [ ] **3.** Sleeplessness

    [ ] **4.** Nausea

    [ ] **5.** Diarrhea

    [ ] **6.** Dehydration

30. A client asks the nurse about the normal infectious period for tuberculosis. Which of the following is the appropriate response by the nurse?

    1. A client with confirmed pulmonary tuberculosis will always be contagious

    2. A client with tuberculosis is contagious for seven days after the onset of clinical manifestations

    3. A client with tuberculosis is contagious until appropriate antibiotic therapy is completed

    4. Tuberculosis is not contagious

31. Which of the following should the nurse include in the plan of care for a child with respiratory syncytial virus (RSV) being managed at home?

    1. IV rehydration

    2. Oxygen therapy

3. Symptomatic treatment
4. Ribavirin therapy

ANSWERS AND RATIONALES

1. **Headache and restlessness.** Tetanus is caused by a spore-forming bacillus that produces a neurotoxin that is transmitted through a wound in the skin from contact with soil contaminated by animal feces. Early clinical manifestations are headache and restlessness followed by spasms of chewing muscles, difficulty in opening the mouth (trismus), dysphagia, and opisthotonos (severe spasm of the back muscles, causing the back to arch and the head to bend back on the neck).
NP = As
CN = Sa/2
CL = Ap
SA = 4

2. **1.** *Giardia* is more common in children than adults through hand-to-mouth transfer of cysts from feces from an infected individual. It is associated with day care centers and residential institutions. Clinical manifestations include chronic or relapsing diarrhea. Gonorrhea is a sexually transmitted disease that may be spread through unprotected sexual intercourse. Syphilis may be transmitted congenitally during pregnancy or at the time of delivery. Human immune deficiency virus is spread through contact with infected blood or body fluids, sexual contact, dirty needles, and perinatal transmission.
NP = Ev
CN = Sa/2
CL = An
SA = 4

3. **1, 2, 5, 6.** It is a priority to use meticulous hand washing when caring for a client with methicillin-resistant *Staphylococcus aureus*. A private room, disposable equipment or equipment that is adequately cleaned between clients, and continuous isolation are also a part of the care in multiple-resistant organisms.
NP = Pl
CN = Sa/1
CL = An
SA = 8

4. **1, 3, 6.** Severe acute respiratory syndrome is a communicable disease in which one or more clinical findings or respiratory illness is present and a temperature greater than 38°C, or 100.4°F. Clinical manifestations of West

Nile virus include malaise, anorexia, nausea, and vomiting. Clinical manifestations of rotavirus are vomiting, watery diarrhea, and abdominal pain. Coughing up blood or sputum, weakness, and weight loss are clinical manifestations found in tuberculosis.
NP = As
CN = Sa/2
CL = Ap
SA = 4

5. 3. Active tuberculosis may develop later in life if the infected adolescent does not receive treatment for the tuberculosis at the time of the infection. The client may be asymptomatic and will not be contagious in the latent stage. Coughing up blood in the sputum is a clinical manifestation in the active stage of tuberculosis.
NP = An
CN = Sa/1
CL = An
SA = 8

6. 2. The recommended dose of acetaminophen (Tylenol) for infants and children is 10 to 15 mg/kg/dose every four hours but not over five times a day. Liver toxicity results from overdose. Careful attention must be paid to over-the-counter products, because many of them have Tylenol in them.
NP = Ev
CN = Ph/6
CL = Ap
SA = 5

7. 1. It is a priority that the nurse asks a female adolescent client before giving the measles, mumps, and rubella (MMR) vaccine if she is pregnant. This vaccine is teratogen-interfering with normal prenatal development. After administering the vaccine, the nurse should caution the client to avoid pregnancy for three months.
NP = As
CN = Sa/1
CL = An
SA = 8

8. 3. Although polio has been eradicated in the United States, it is still present in other parts of the world. If the disease were accidentally introduced into the United States and individuals were not vaccinated, there could be an epidemic.
NP = As
CN = He/3
CL = An
SA = 4

9. **1.** Cool baths with baking soda or oatmeal are performed for children with chickenpox to promote skin care comfort. Salicylates are contraindicated because of their link to Reye's syndrome. The environment should be kept cool and the child should be dressed in cool, light clothing to promote comfort.
NP = Pl
CN = Sa/2
CL = Ap
SA = 4

10. **4.** Outlining an immunization schedule and tasks of instructing and assessing require skills of the registered nurse. A licensed practical nurse may administer acetaminophen (Tylenol) to a child.
NP = Pl
CN = Sa/1
CL = An
SA = 8

11. **1.** Transient polyarthralgia is a complication of rubella (German measles). Seizures are a complication of roseola (human herpes virus 6). A red maculopapular discrete rash is an anticipated finding with German measles. Obstructive laryngotracheitis is a clinical manifestation found in diphtheria.
NP = As
CN = Sa/2
CL = An
SA = 4

12. **2.** Hepatitis B is a carrier state disease. Rotavirus is the most common cause of severe diarrhea in children. *Giardia* is a protozoan infection spread by hand-to-mouth transfer of cysts from feces from infected persons. *Enterobius* (pinworm) is the most common helminth infection in the United States.
NP = Im
CN = Sa/2
CL = An
SA = 4

13. **2.** Cervical lymphadenopathy is present in infectious mononucleosis. A red facial rash typically appearing as a "slapped check" is present in erythema infectiosum (Fifth's disease). Koplik's spots are a clinical manifestation in measles. Obstructive laryngotracheitis occurs in diphtheria.
NP = As
CN = Sa/2

CL = Ap
SA = 4

14. 1. Mumps are spread by droplets or direct contact with respiratory secretions, so respiratory precautions should be implemented.
NP = Im
CN = Sa/2
CL = Ap
SA = 4

15. 1. Childhood immunizations should begin at birth with a hepatitis B vaccine.
NP = An
CN = Sa/2
CL = Ap
SA = 4

16. 4. An inactivated polio vaccine has been developed and is the method of administration. It does eliminate the risk of vaccine-associated polio paralysis.
NP = An
CN = Sa/2
CL = An
SA = 4

17. 4. HIV infection in adults is transmitted through sexual intercourse, contaminated needles, or a weakened immune system. Vertical transmission refers to the transmission of an infection through the placental barrier or through the birth process from mother to infant.
NP = Im
CN = Sa/2
CL = An
SA = 4

18. 3. Four doses of the polio vaccine are recommended before the child enters school. Lifetime immunity to diphtheria is not possible. The first measles vaccine is not given until after 12 months of age. The second vaccine is routinely given between ages 4 and 6 years. The first pertussis vaccine is given at 2 months.
NP = Pl
CN = Sa/2
CL = An
SA = 4

19. 4. Many individuals carry methicillin-resistant *Staphylococcus aureus* (MRSA) and vancomycin-resistant *Enterococcus* (VRE) in the normal flora without having signs of clinical illness. There are effective antibiotic

treatments available, but the course is prolonged, and the bacteria could develop resistance against the strongest antibiotics. It is not known how rapidly the bacteria mutate. Methicillin-resistant *Staphylococcus aureus* (MRSA) and vancomycin-resistant *Enterococcus* (VRE) are multiple-resistant organisms (MROs) and are transmitted from person to person in health care situations, frequently causing clinical illness among those in chronic or weakened physical states while producing no clinical manifestations in healthier individuals.
NP = Pl
CN = Sa/2
CL = An
SA = 4

20. **2.** Children have smaller muscle masses for injectable drugs than adults. Deep penetration of the muscle for deposition of the drug intramuscularly is the preferred way of administrating a vaccine to an infant. Administering the vaccine this way also decreases the pain and adverse reactions to the vaccines.
NP = An
CN = Sa/2
CL = An
SA = 4

21. **4.** Chlamydia occurs in 236 out of 100,000 individuals and, according to the CDC, it is the most common sexually transmitted disease in persons under 25 years of age. Syphilis is least common, occurring in 2.6 out of 100,000 individuals. Gonorrhea is second most common, next to chlamydia, and occurs in 132 out of 100,000 individuals. Human papillomavirus occurs in 50 out of 100,000 individuals.
NP = Im
CN = Sa/2
CL = Ap
SA = 4

22. **1.** Pregnant women who have never had a cytomegalovirus (CMV) infection are most at risk. The virus is shed through the urine and oral secretions of infected children. The incubation period for CMV is unknown. Antibiotics are ineffective in the treatment of the viruses. While most infants with congenital CMV are asymptomatic, 5% have significant manifestations of fetal damage, including psychomotor retardation, microcephaly, and learning disabilities.
NP = Im
CN = Sa/2
CL = An
SA = 4

23. **1.** Diphtheria is spread through intimate contact with infected secretions. Diphtheria can be treated with antibiotics erythromycin or penicillin benzathine. Although greatly reduced, diphtheria continues to exist, especially in nonimmunized or inadequately immunized individuals. The tetanus vaccination is given in combination with the diphtheria vaccination in the injection DT (diphtheria-tetanus). The vaccination is preventive and not a method of treatment.
NP = An
CN = Sa/2
CL = An
SA = 4

24. **2, 4, 5, 6.** Reactions to the diphtheria, pertussis, and tetanus (DPT) immunization (an inactivated antigen) occur within the first few hours or days of administration. These reactions include low-grade fever, local tenderness, erythema, swelling at the injection site, and behavioral changes.
NP = Im
CN = Sa/2
CL = Ap
SA = 4

25. **1.** Mononucleosis is caused by the Epstein-Barr virus (EBV) and is transmitted through contact with oral secretions. Changing the diapers of an infected child, wiping away tears, and casual contact with an infected individual are not modes of transmission for mononucleosis.
NP = Im
CN = Sa/2
CL = Ap
SA = 4

26. **3, 5, 6.** When an infant client is admitted to the hospital in respiratory distress, with a high-pitched inspiration and coughing paroxysms, a mask should be donned, droplet/airborne isolation should be initiated, and having emergency respiratory equipment available are the appropriate interventions. Strict isolation is not required. The diphtheria, pertussis, and tetanus (DPT) immunization is preventive and not appropriate if the child is presenting with an active infection.
NP = Pl
CN = Sa/2
CL = Ap
SA = 4

27. **3.** Respiratory syncytial virus (RSV) is frequently serious, especially in infants. It is the most common cause of bronchiolitis and pneumonia among infants. It can infect people of all ages, but produces the most

severe clinical manifestations in children under 2 years of age. By the age of 2 years, most children have been exposed to RSV and the subsequent illness becomes less severe. RSV is highly contagious through contact with respiratory secretions.

NP = Im
CN = Sa/2
CL = An
SA = 4

28. **4.** Respiratory syncytial virus (RSV) is the most common respiratory infection for small children. Because diphtheria is relatively uncommon, it would not be the first condition to rule out. Measles is also relatively uncommon and would not be expected if the infant has no history of exposure. Tetanus is not consistent with the presentation of upper respiratory clinical manifestations.

NP = An
CN = Sa/2
CL = An
SA = 4

29. **1, 3.** The classic features of *Enterobius* (pinworms) are nocturnal anal itching and sleeplessness. Nausea and vomiting are not common clinical manifestations of intestinal parasites. Abdominal pain, flatulence, and diarrhea are common clinical manifestations of *Giardia*. Dehydration may occur if diarrhea is severe.

NP = As
CN = Sa/2
CL = Ap
SA = 4

30. **3.** Tuberculosis is an infectious disease caused by *Mycobacterium tuberculosis* and generally involves the lungs. A client is placed in respiratory isolation and considered infectious until effective drug therapy has been initiated. The five drugs primarily used are isoniazid (INH), rifampin (Rifamate), pyrazinamide, streptomycin, and ethambutol (Myambutol).

NP = An
CN = Sa/2
CL = An
SA = 4

31. **3.** Respiratory syncytial virus (RSV) is a respiratory disorder managed at home with symptomatic treatment. Children with RSV typically do not require intravenous hydration. They are able to take fluid orally, unless their respiratory rates are increased to a rate requiring support. Respiratory support is not consistent with mild disease. Ribavirin is administered in a

hospital setting and is usually reserved for very young infants or children with cardiac conditions.

NP = Pl

CN = Sa/2

CL = Ap

SA = 4